ANATOMY OF ACUPUNCTURE
AN ILLUSTRATED POINT LOCATION WORKBOOK

WRITTEN BY:

MATTHEW ENRIGHT, AP, DOM (FL)
LANDON AGOADO, AP, DOM (FL)
ANDREW AGOADO, AP, DOM (FL)

MEDICAL ILLUSTRATIONS BY:

MATTHEW ENRIGHT, AP, DOM (FL)

EDITED BY:

LUPITA GARRAMBONE, AP, DOM (FL)

I

This book is not meant for the purpose of self-diagnosis or self-treatment. Patients should not use this book without direct supervision of a trained medical professional.

This book was created and designed by Acupuncturists, for Acupuncturists (both students and practitioners).

Printed in the United States of America

DEDICATION

This book was merley an idea in 2002. With the support of my mother and father, my family, colleagues, patients and friends, it has come to fruition. I would like to dedicate this book to all of those who have helped, guided, listened and supported me throughout my life and career. To my mother, thank you for encouraging me to go get my first acupuncture treatment, this along with your guidance and support thoroughout my life have molded me into the person I am today. To my wife Kelly, my daughters Kaitlin and Kendall; you are the reason I wake up every morning with the drive, determination and motivation to make a difference. I hope and pray I have the same impact on your lives as you do mine and anyone I am blessed to come in contact with.

Matthew Enright

This book is dedicated to my professors who taught me the power and the art of Traditional Chinese medicine. To my mentor and brother Dr. Fu Di who believed in me from the very beginning, who gave me wings to fly and soar in a profession that was met with skepticism 15 years ago, yet has now persevered into main stream. To my family for showing unconditional support and sacrifice. To my wife for always being my rock, for encouraging and pushing me to make my dreams a reality. Lastly, to my children, my heart walking outside of my body, for humbling me and inspiring me everyday.

Landon Agoado

I would like to take this opportunity to dedicate this book to my family, my friends, and the colleagues who have gone on this journey with me. Specifically, to my parents: You have sacrificed more for your children then most parents would. Not a day goes by that we are not grateful for everything you've done, and continue to do so.
To my brother: You have always found the time to tutor, mentor, and share in all of life's ups and down's with me.
To my dearest Benita: You are my quintessential wife and have brightened my life in so many ways. Your love is stimulating; your support is inspiring; and the best is yet to come.

Andrew Agoado

TABLE OF CONTENTS

LU 1
ZHONGFU

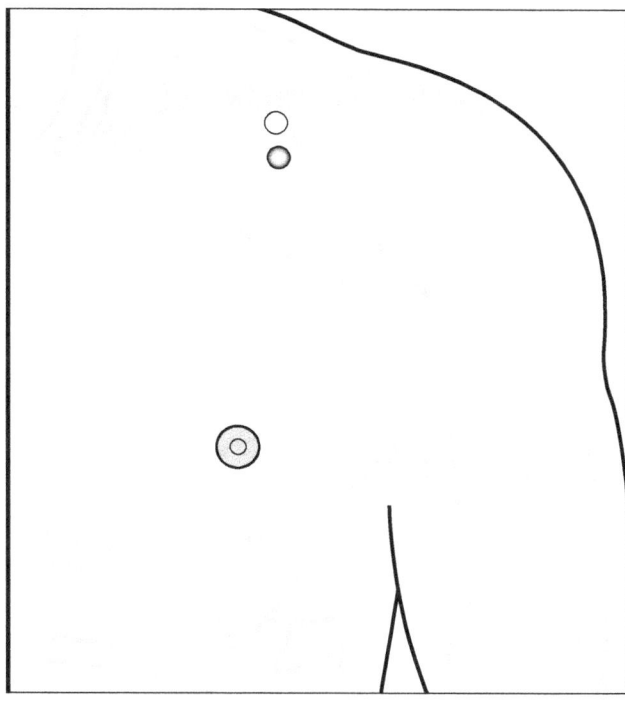

Location: On the upper lateral chest, below the acromial extremity of the clavicle, 1 cun below LU 2, level in the first intercostal space, 6 cun lateral to the midline of the chest (Ren Channel).

Functions: Tonifies and regulates the Lungs (Qi and yin), regulates upper jiao and tonifies ancestral Qi, stops cough and wheezing, disperses and descends Lung Qi, transforms phlegm and clears heat.

Indications: Asthma, cough, wheezing, neck, shoulder, back and chest pain, fullness of chest.

Attributes: Front Mu and Entry Point of the Lung.

Notes
_____
_____
_____
_____
_____
_____
_____
_____

Point Combinations
_____
_____
_____
_____
_____
_____

LU 2
YUNMEN

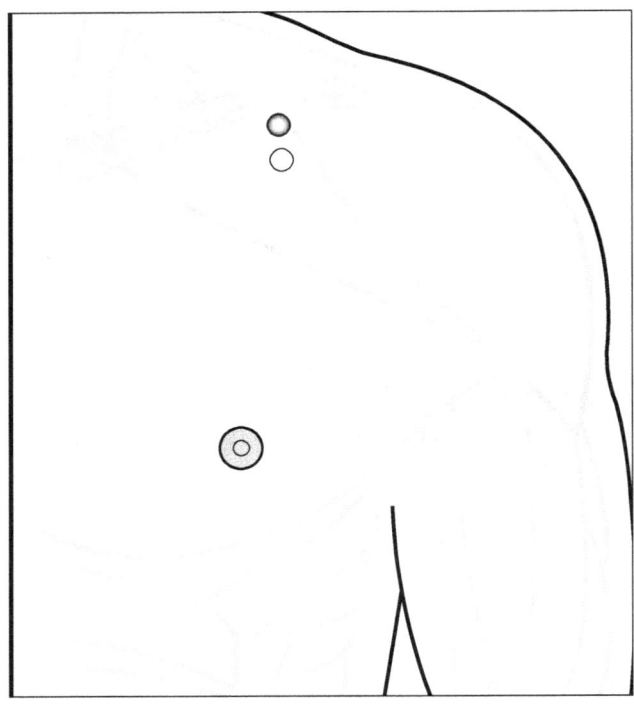

Location: On the upper lateral chest, below the acromial extremity of the clavicle, in the depression below the acromial extremity of the clavicle, 6 cun from the midline of the chest (Ren Channel).

Functions: Clears Lung heat, disperses and descends Lung heat, drains heat from limbs and opens joints and disperses fullness of the chest.

Indications: Asthma, cough, wheezing, shoulder, back and chest pain, fullness of the chest.

Notes
_____
_____
_____
_____
_____
_____
_____
_____
_____

Point Combinations
_____
_____
_____
_____
_____
_____
_____

LU 3
TIANFU

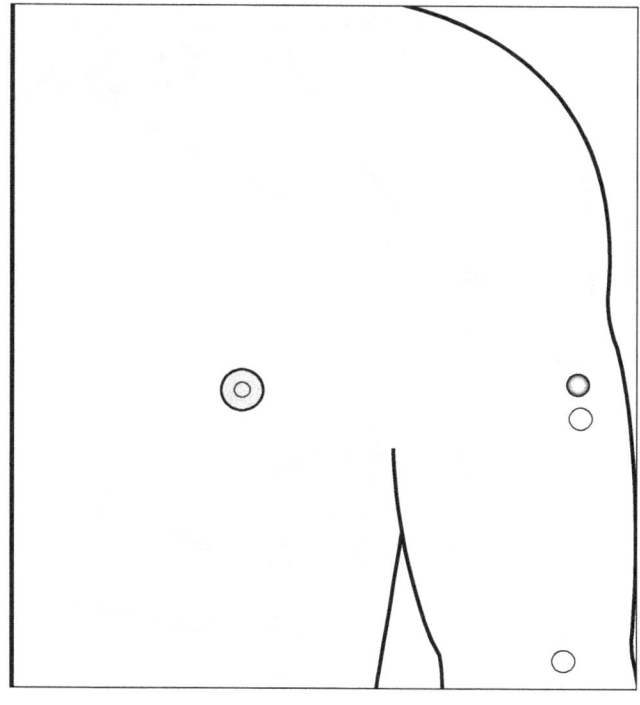

Location: On the medial upper arm, on the radial side of the biceps brachii muscle, 3 cun below the axillary fossa.

Functions: Clears Lung heat (excess or deficient type) regulates Lung Qi, cools blood and stops bleeding.

Indications: Asthma, Epistaxis, Hemoptysis, Pain in the medial aspect of upper arm, LU related spirit issues "sorrow, excessive sadness or grief".

Attributes: Window of the Sky point.

Notes

_____
_____
_____
_____
_____
_____
_____
_____
_____

Point Combinations

_____
_____
_____
_____
_____
_____

LU 4
XIABAI

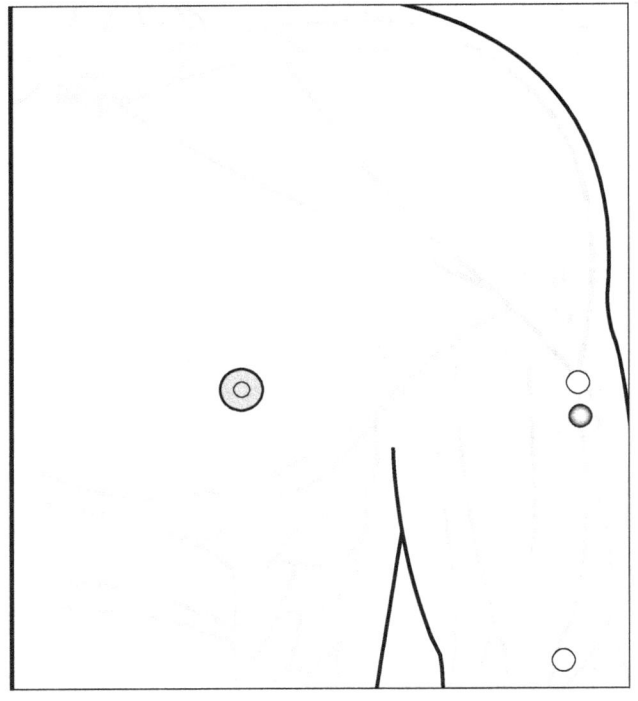

Location: On the medial upper arm, on the radial side of the biceps brachii muscle, 4 cun below the axillary fossa (1 cun directly below LU-3 Tianfu or 5 cun directly above the cubital crease).

Functions: Regulates Lung Qi, relieves pain, regulates blood and Qi.

Indications: Cough, congestion, fullness of chest, shortness of breath, pain in the medial upper arm.

Notes
_____
_____
_____
_____
_____
_____
_____
_____

Point Combinations
_____
_____
_____
_____
_____
_____
_____

LU 5
CHIZE

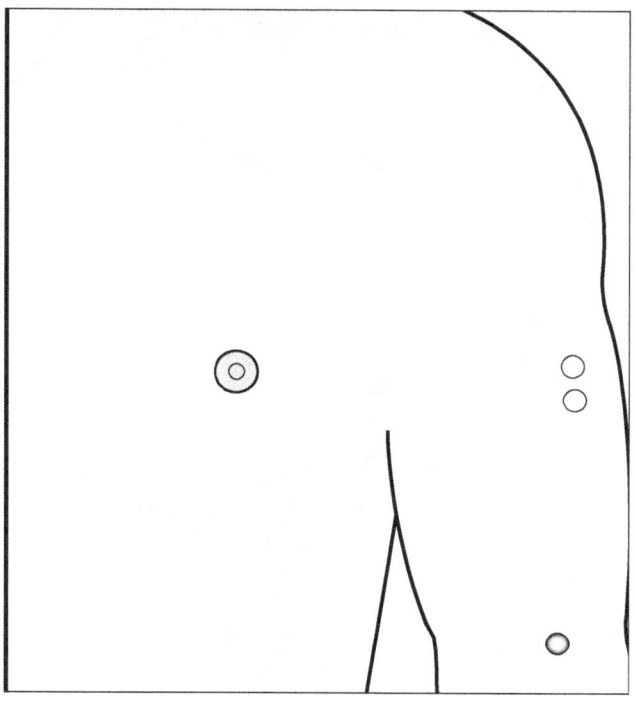

Location: On the cubital crease of the elbow, on the radial side of the biceps brachii tendon.

Functions: Descends and disperses Lung Qi and counter flow Qi, expels phlegm from the Lungs, relaxes the sinews and relieves pain, clears Lung heat/fire.

Indications: Spasmodic pain of elbow (tennis elbow) and arm, infantile convulsions, cough, afternoon fever, asthma, sore throat, hemoptysis, mastitis, fullness in chest, Qi counterflow, upper Jiao edema.

Attributes: Water point, He-Sea point.

Notes

_____

_____

_____

_____

_____

_____

_____

_____

Point Combinations

_____

_____

_____

_____

_____

_____

_____

LU 6
KONGZUI

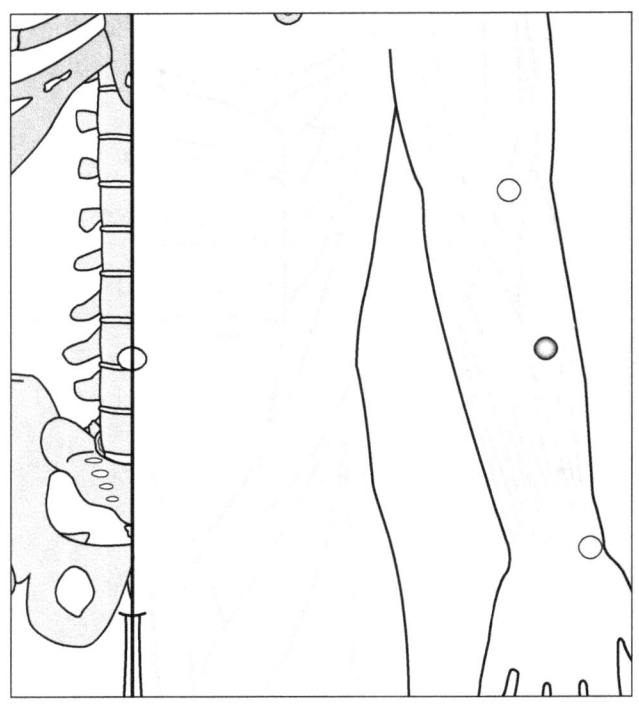

Location: On the radial side of the forearm, 7 cun above LU-9 Taiyuan, on the line joining LU-5 Chize and LU-9 Taiyuan.

Functions: Descends and disperses Lung Qi and counter flow Qi, moistens the Lungs and stops bleeding, clears Lung heat and resolves the exterior.

Indications: Acute cough (dry hacking, nighttime), pain in the chest, asthma, hemoptysis, sore throat, spasmodic pain of arm and elbow.

Attributes: Xi-Cleft point.

Notes
_____

_____

_____

_____

_____

_____

_____

_____

Point Combinations
_____

_____

_____

_____

_____

_____

LU 7
LIEQUE

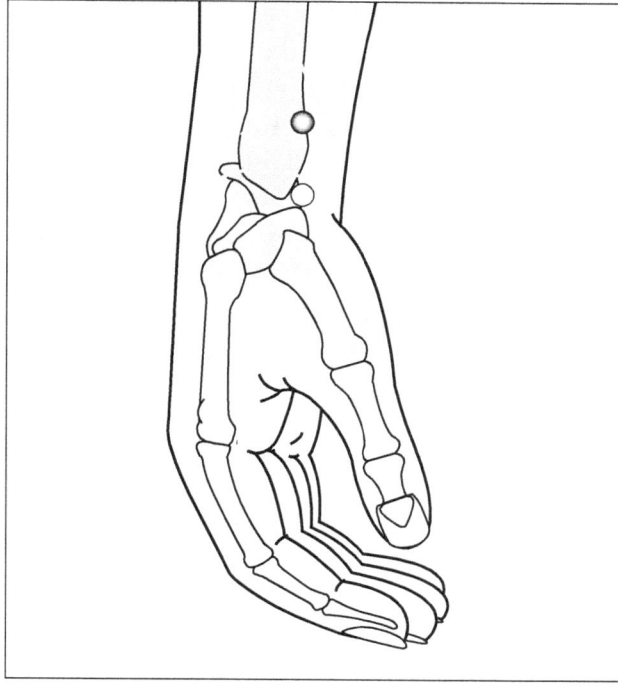

Location: On the radial side of the forearm, proximal to the styloid process of the radius, 1.5 cun above the crease of the wrist, between the brachioradial muscle and the tendon of the long abductor muscle of the thumb.

Functions: Descends and disperses Lung Qi, opens Lungs, expels wind cold, strengthens Wei Qi, releases the exterior, opens and regulates the Ren channel, courses channel to free connecting channel, opens water passages.

Indications: Headache, migraines, neck stiffness, cough, asthma, sore throat (deficient type), facial paralysis (Bell's palsy), toothache, pain and weakness of the wrist, internal and external wind.

Attributes: Luo-Connecting point, Master point of the Ren channel, Exit point, Command point of the Head and back of Neck regions.

Notes

_____
_____
_____
_____
_____
_____
_____
_____

Point Combinations

_____
_____
_____
_____
_____
_____
_____

LU 8
JINGQU

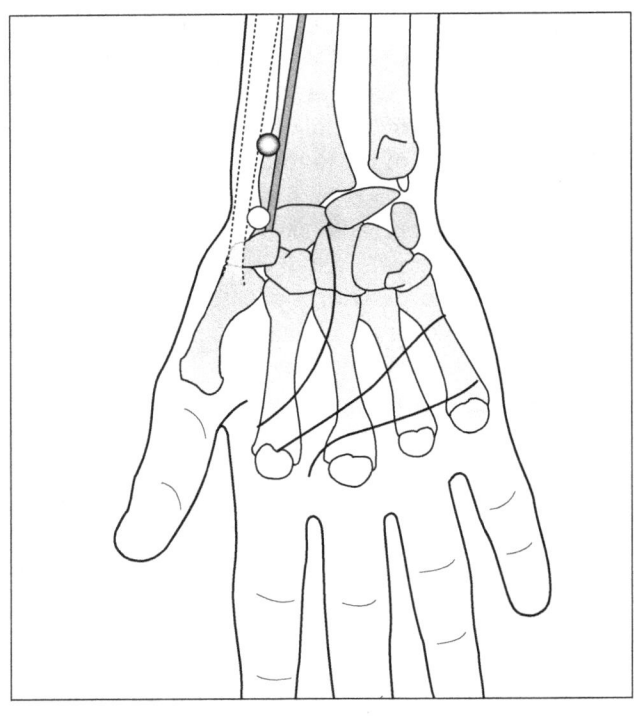

Location: On the radial side of the forearm, 1 cun above the crease of the wrist.

Functions: Descends Lung Qi, opens the Lungs, courses wind and releases the exterior.

Indications: Cough, asthma, fever, distention and pain in the chest, sore throat, wrist pain, carpal tunnel syndrome.

Attributes: Metal point, Jing River point.

Notes
_____

_____

_____

_____

_____

_____

_____

_____

Point Combinations
_____

_____

_____

_____

_____

_____

LU 9
TAIYUAN

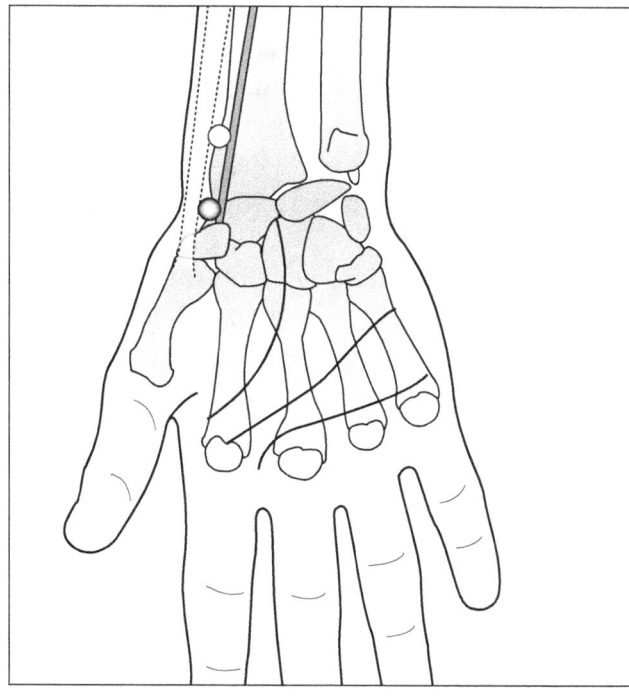

Location: On the radial side of the crease of the wrist, on the radial side of the radial artery.

Functions: Dispels wind and transforms phlegm, regulates the Lung Qi, stops cough, tonify Lung Qi and Lung yin.

Indications: Cough, asthma, hemoptysis, sore throat, shortness of breath, wheezing, palpitation, pain in the chest, wrist and arm, circulatory issues.

Attributes: Shu Stream Point, Yuan-Source Point, Influential Point of the pulse and vessels.

Notes
_____
_____
_____
_____
_____
_____
_____
_____
_____

Point Combinations
_____
_____
_____
_____
_____
_____
_____

LU 10
YUJI

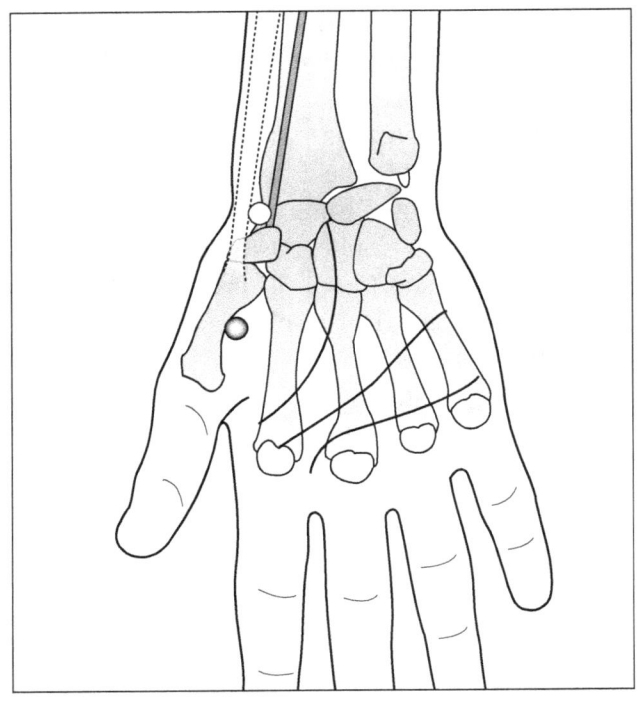

Location: On the radial side of the thumb, at the midpoint of the 1st metacarpal bone and the junction of the red and white skin.

Functions: Clears heat in the Lungs (excess or deficient), clears heat in the throat, clears blood heat.

Indications: Cough, hemoptysis, sore throat, loss of voice, fever, feverish sensation in the palms.

Attributes: Fire point, Ying Spring point.

Notes

Point Combinations

LU 11
SHAOSHANG

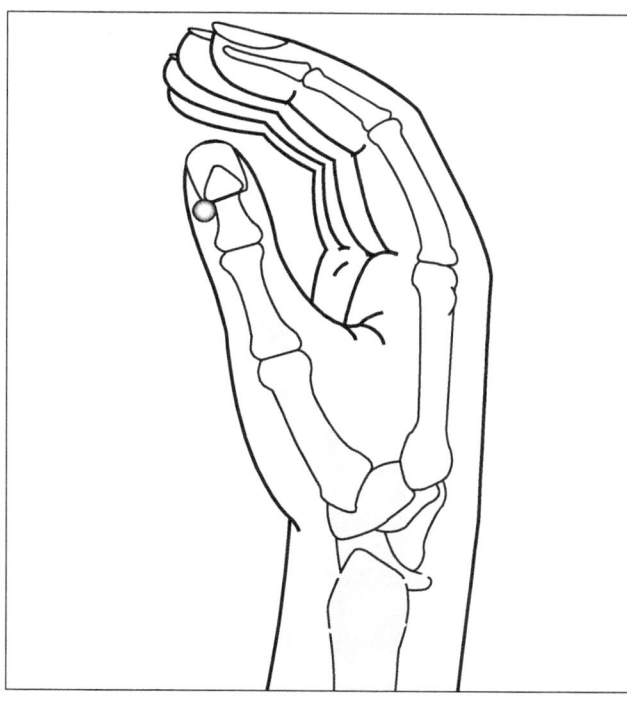

Location: On the radial side of the distal segment of the thumb, 0.1 cun from the corner of the fingernail.

Functions: Promotes resuscitation (revives fainting), opens the throat, clears heat in the Lungs.

Indications: Sore throat, cough, asthma, epistaxis, fever, loss of consciousness, mania, spasmodic pain of the thumb.

Attributes: Wood point, Jing Well point, Ghost point.

Notes
_____
_____
_____
_____
_____
_____
_____
_____

Point Combinations
_____
_____
_____
_____
_____
_____

LI 1
SHANGYANG

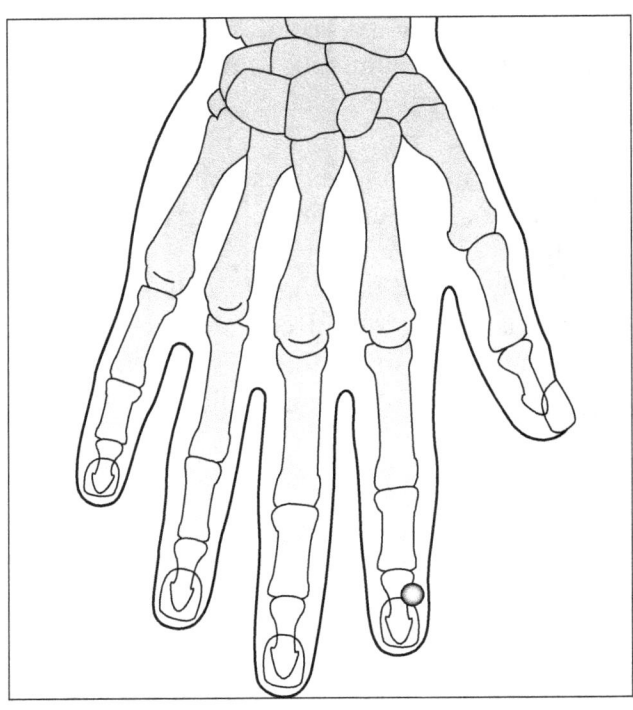

Location: On the radial side of the distal segment of the index finger, 0.1 cun from the corner of the nail.

Functions: Clears interior and exterior heat, removes blockages, reduces swelling and pain, expels wind and cold from the channel, moistens the throat.

Indications: Sore throat, loss of consciousness due to wind stroke, restores collapsed yang, pain in the finger (heat and numbness).

Attributes: Wood point, Jing Well point.

Notes

Point Combinations

LI 2
ERJIAN

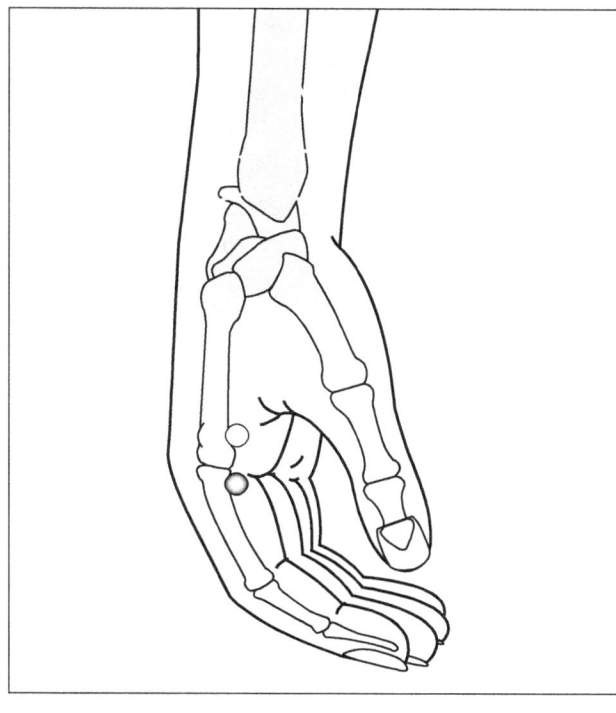

Location: On the radial side of the index finger, in the depression distal to the metacarpophalangeal joint (at the junction of the red and white skin).

Functions: Clears heat, expels wind and reduces pain and swelling.
Indications: Toothache, sore throat, febrile disease, pain and stiffness of shoulders and back, Trigeminal Neuralgia.
Attributes: Fire point, Ying Spring point, Sedating point

Notes
_____
_____
_____
_____
_____
_____
_____
_____

Point Combinations
_____
_____
_____
_____
_____
_____
_____

LI 3
SANJIAN

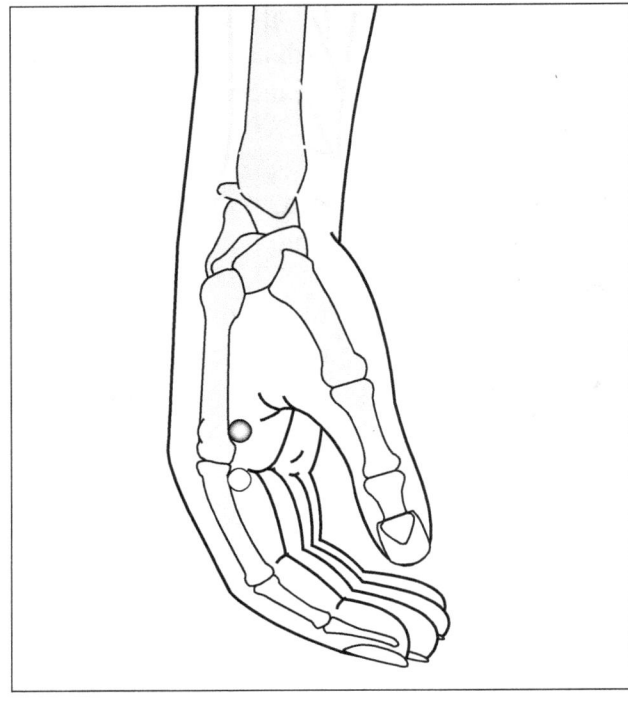

Location: On the radial side of the index finger, in the depression proximal to the metacarpophalangeal joint.

Functions: Expels wind and heat.

Indications: Acute stiff neck, swelling and/or redness of the fingers or dorsum of the hand, benefits the throat and teeth, and treats diarrhea.

Attributes: Wood point, Shu Stream point.

Notes
_____
_____
_____
_____
_____
_____
_____
_____
_____

Point Combinations
_____
_____
_____
_____
_____
_____

LI 4
HEGU

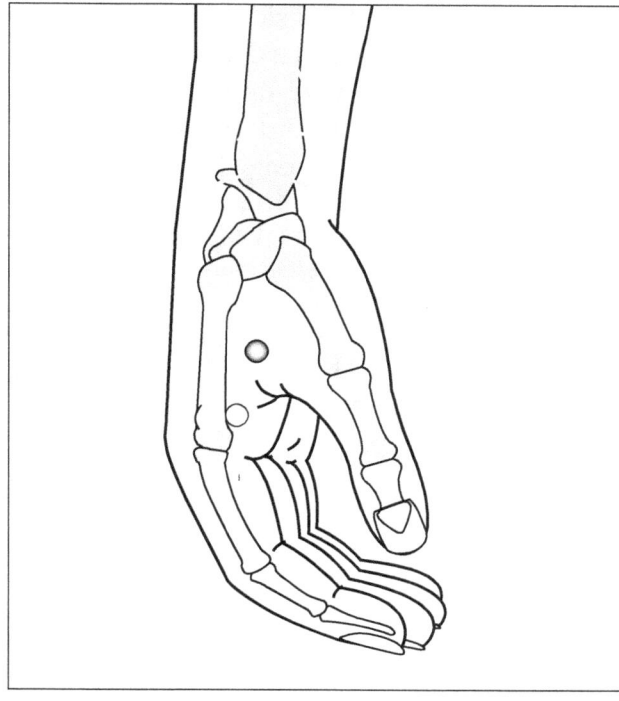

Location: On the dorsum of the hand, between the 1st and 2nd metacarpal bones, and on the radial side of the midpoint of the 2nd metacarpal bone.

Functions: Removes blockages in the channel, expels wind and releases the exterior, regulates ascending of yang and descending of yin, tonifies Qi.

Indications: Headache, hypertension, exterior wind-cold or wind-heat, febrile disease without sweating, pain anywhere, hemiplegia, amenorrhea, throat or tooth pain of the lower jaw.

Attributes: Yuan Source Point, Entry Point, Command Point of the face and mouth.

*Contraindicated in any stage pregnancy until delivery, induces labor.

Notes

_____

_____

_____

_____

_____

_____

_____

_____

Point Combinations

_____

_____

_____

_____

_____

_____

LI 5
YANGXI

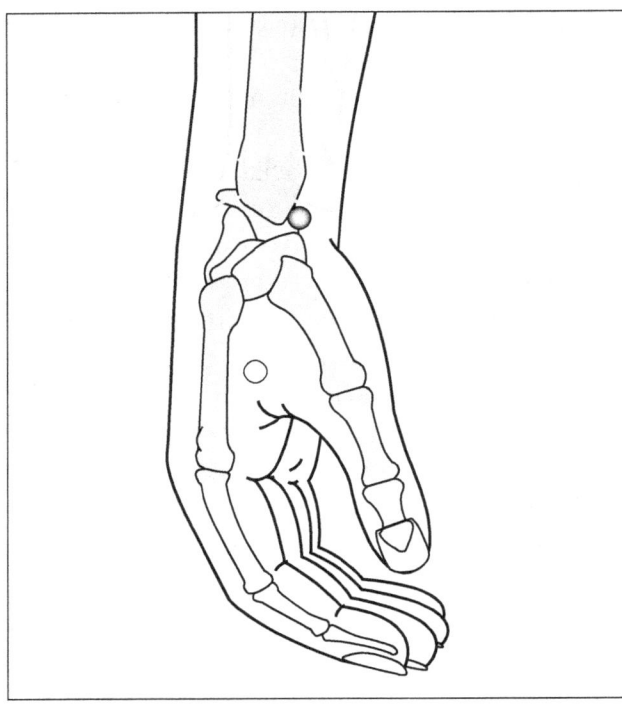

Location: On the radial side of the wrist in the depression between the tendons of the extensor pollicis longus and brevis muscles, found when the thumb is tilted upward (classic location is in the center of the anatomical snuffbox).

Functions: Calms the spirit, benefits the wrist and reduces pain, clears heat and yangming fire, expels wind and releases the exterior.

Indications: Wrist pain, sore throat, nosebleed, pain and swelling of the eye, tinnitus or deafness, depression or fear, cough, febrile disease without sweating.

Attributes: Fire point, Jing River point.

Notes
_____
_____
_____
_____
_____
_____
_____
_____

Point Combinations
_____
_____
_____
_____
_____
_____

LI 6
PIANLI

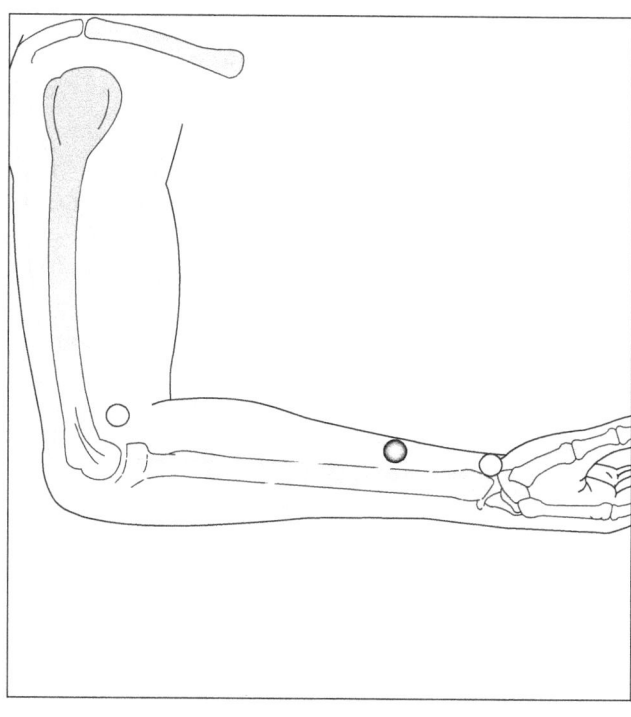

Location: On the radial side of the forearm, 3 cun above the wrist crease, on the line joining LI-5 Yangxi and LI-11 Quchi.

Functions: Opens and harmonizes water passages, expels wind and heat.

Indications: Edema of the hands and face, pain of the wrist and elbow, tinnitus or deafness, difficult urination, borborygmus with edema, ascites, malaria.

Attributes: Luo-Connecting Point.
*Especially used for mania and manic depression.

Notes

Point Combinations

LI 7
WENLIU

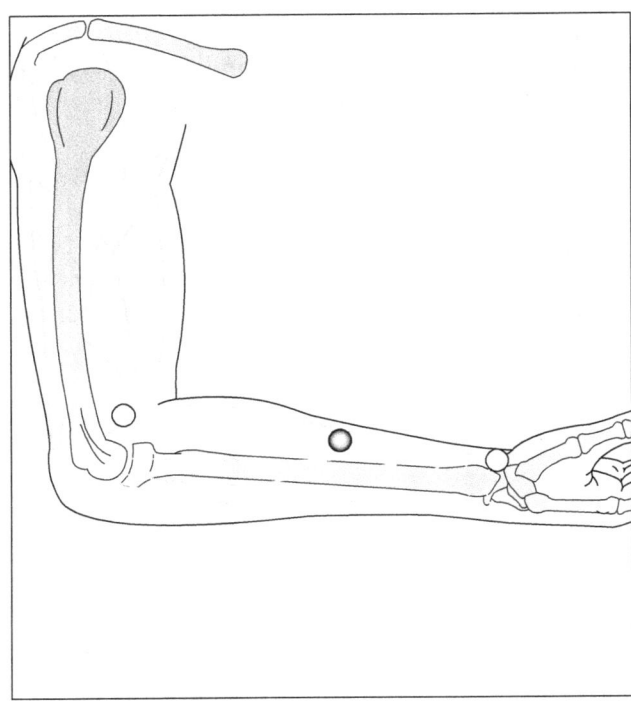

Location: On the radial side of the forearm, 5 cun above the wrist crease, on the line joining LI-5 Yangxi and LI-11 Quchi.

Functions: Clears heat and yangming fire, calms the spirit, harmonizes intestines and stomach, reduces pain and removes blockages from the channel.

Indications: Pain in the arm or shoulder, headache, sore throat, swollen tonsils, deviation, pain, or swelling of face or mouth, loss of voice, borborygmus with abdominal pain, abdominal distention, frequent laughter, "seeing ghosts".

Attribute: Xi-Cleft Point.

Notes

Point Combinations

LI 8
XIALIAN

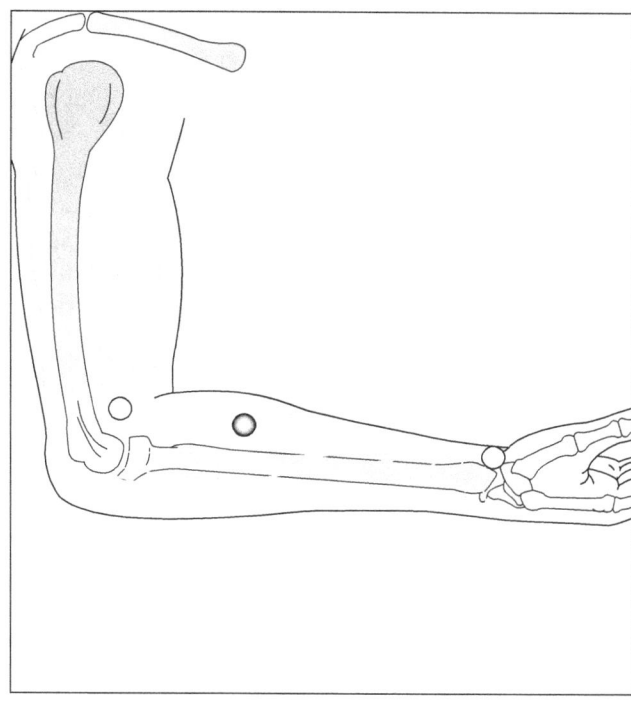

Location: On the radial side of the forearm, 4 cun below the cubital crease (LI-11 Quchi), on the line joining LI-5 Yangxi and LI-11 Quchi.

Functions: Clears heat and yangming fire, calms the spirit, harmonizes Small Intestine.

Indications: Headache, dizziness, pain in arm, elbow, or lower abdomen, borborygmus, difficult urination, diarrhea with undigested food or blood in the stool.

Attributes: Only point on Large Intestine channel used to treat breast abscess.

Notes

_____

_____

_____

_____

_____

_____

_____

_____

_____

Point Combinations

_____

_____

_____

_____

_____

_____

_____

LI 9
SHANGLIAN

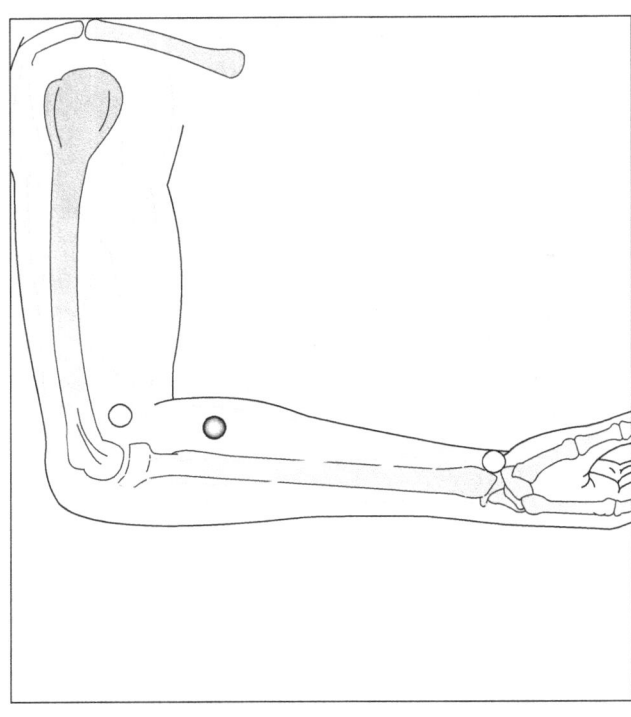

Location: On the radial side of the forearm, 3 cun below the cubital crease (LI-11 Quchi), on the line joining LI-5 Yangxi and LI-11 Quchi.

Functions: Removes blockages from the channel, reduces pain, harmonizes the Large Intestine.

Indications: Pain or numbness of the shoulder, arm, or elbow, abdominal pain, difficult urination, hemiplegia, dizziness.

Attributes: Pair with LI-8 Xianlian to treat difficult urination.

Notes
_____
_____
_____
_____
_____
_____
_____
_____

Point Combinations
_____
_____
_____
_____
_____
_____

LI 10
SHOUSANLI

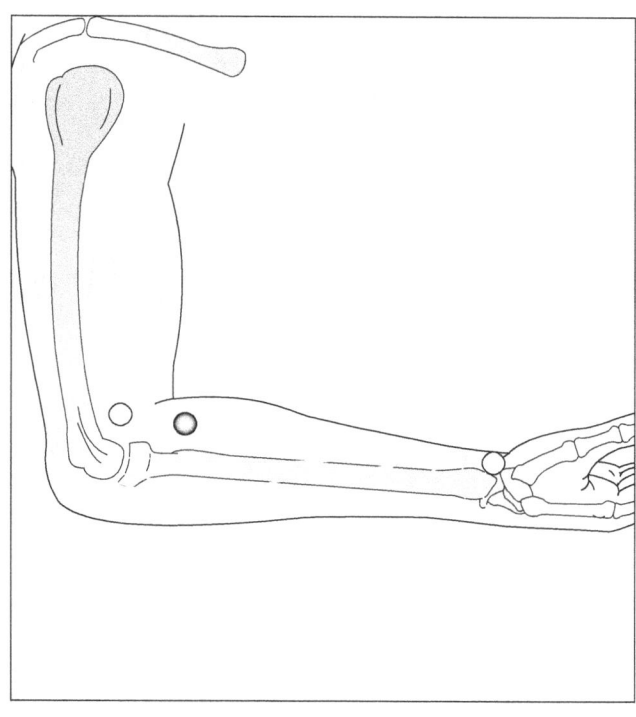

Location: On the radial side of the forearm, 2 cun below the cubital crease (LI-11 Quchi), on the line joining LI-5 Yangxi and LI-11 Quchi.

Functions: Removes blockages from the channel, reduces pain, harmonizes intestines and Stomach, manages Qi and blood.

Indications: Pain, numbness, or paralysis of arm, pain in the neck, loss of voice, abdominal pain, diarrhea, vomiting.

Attributes: Main point to treat all muscular issues affecting hands and forearms.

Notes

_____
_____
_____
_____
_____
_____
_____
_____
_____

Point Combinations

_____
_____
_____
_____
_____
_____

LI 11
QUCHI

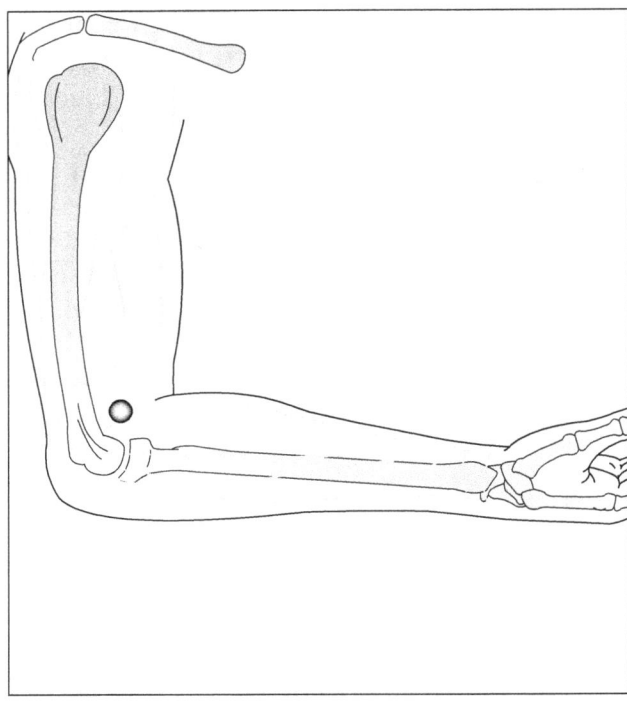

Location: With the elbow flexed, at the lateral end of the cubital crease, at the midpoint of the line connecting LU-5 Chize and the external humeral epicondyle.

Functions: Drains heat, damp and cools blood, expels wind, manages Qi and blood, benefits tendons and joints, stops itching.

Indications: Any febrile disease, hypertension, paralysis, pain in arm, sore throat, dry, itchy skin, goiter, malaria, measles.

Attributes: Earth point, He-Sea point, Tonifying point.

*Main point for any issues of the upper extremity and diseases affecting the skin.

Notes

Point Combinations

LI 12
ZHOULIAO

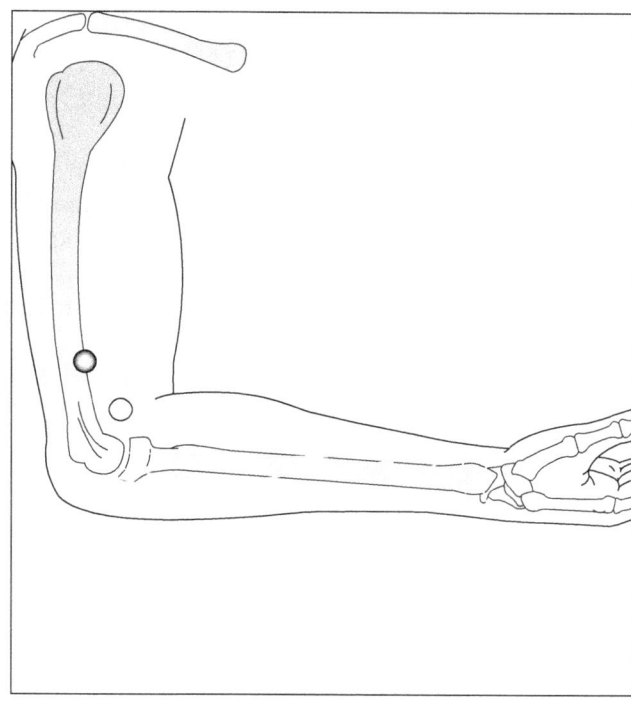

Location: With the elbow flexed, on the lateral side of the arm, on the border of the humerus, 1 cun above LI-11 Quchi.

Functions: Removes blockages from the channel, reduces pain, benefits the elbow.
Indications: Pain, numbness, spasm of the arm or elbow, immobility of the arm.
Attributes: Major point for tennis elbow.

Notes

_____

_____

_____

_____

_____

_____

_____

_____

Point Combinations

_____

_____

_____

_____

_____

_____

LI 13
SHOUWULI

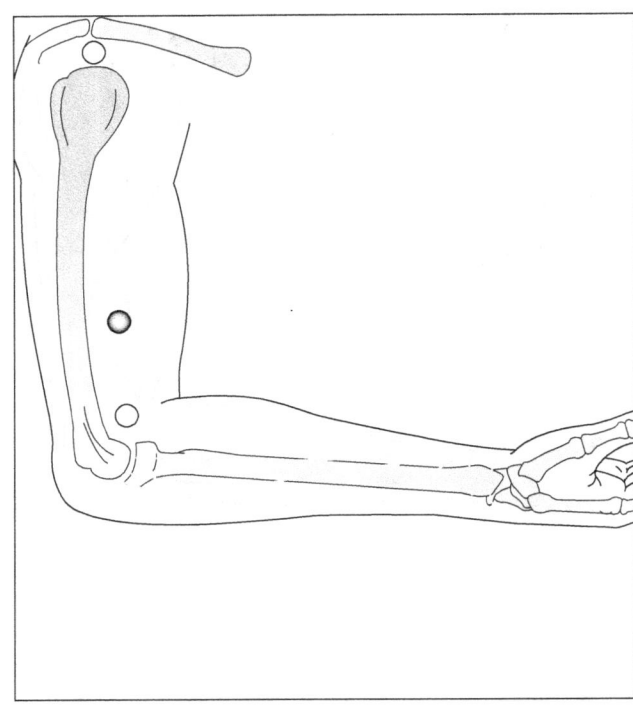

Location: On the lateral side of the arm, 3 cun above the cubital crease (LI-11 Quchi), on the line joining LI-11 Quchi and LI-15 Jianyu.

Functions: Removes blockages from the channel, reduces pain, reduces cough, manages Qi, drains damp, transforms phlegm, benefits the elbow.

Indications: Hemoptysis, pain of the arm and elbow, scrofula.

Notes

_____

_____

_____

_____

_____

_____

_____

_____

Point Combinations

_____

_____

_____

_____

_____

_____

LI 14
BINAO

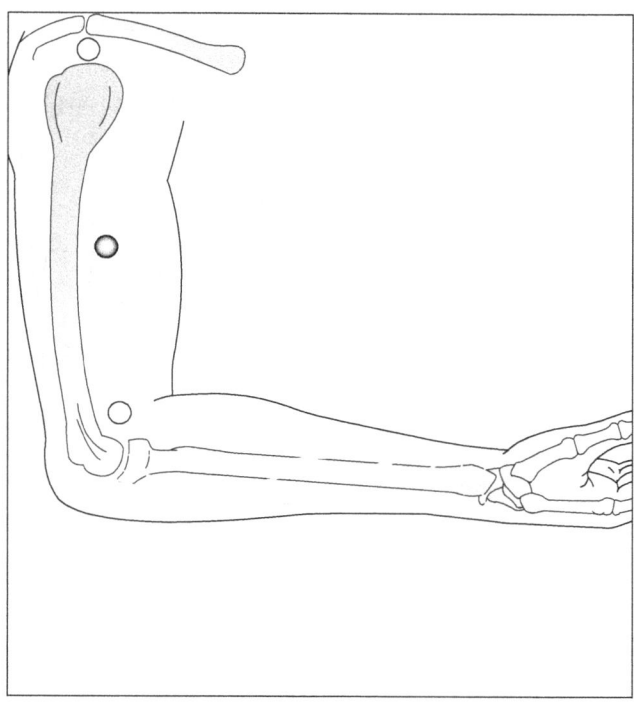

Location: On the lateral side of the arm, 7 cun above the cubital crease (LI-11 Quchi) at the insertion point of the deltoid muscle, on the line joining LI-11 Quchi and LI-15 Jianyu.

Functions: Removes blockages from the channel, benefits vision, transforms phlegm.
Indications: Neck stiffness, pain in the shoulder and arm, redness and swelling of the eyes, scrofula, goiter.

Notes

Point Combinations

LI 15
JIANYU

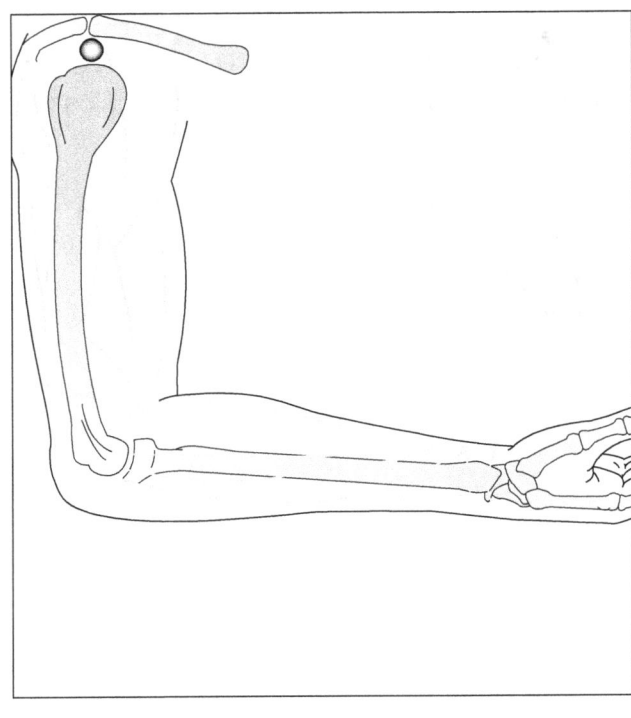

Location: On the shoulder, superior to the deltoid muscle, in the depression anterior and inferior to the acromion when the arm is abducted or raised to the level of the shoulder.

Functions: Expels wind and wind-damp, courses Qi, manages Qi and blood, transforms phlegm, reduces pain and benefits the muscles, tendons and joint of the shoulder.

Indications: Any issues of the shoulder, scrofula, goiter, hypertension.

Notes _____
_____
_____
_____
_____
_____
_____
_____

Point Combinations _____
_____
_____
_____
_____
_____
_____

LI 16
JUGU

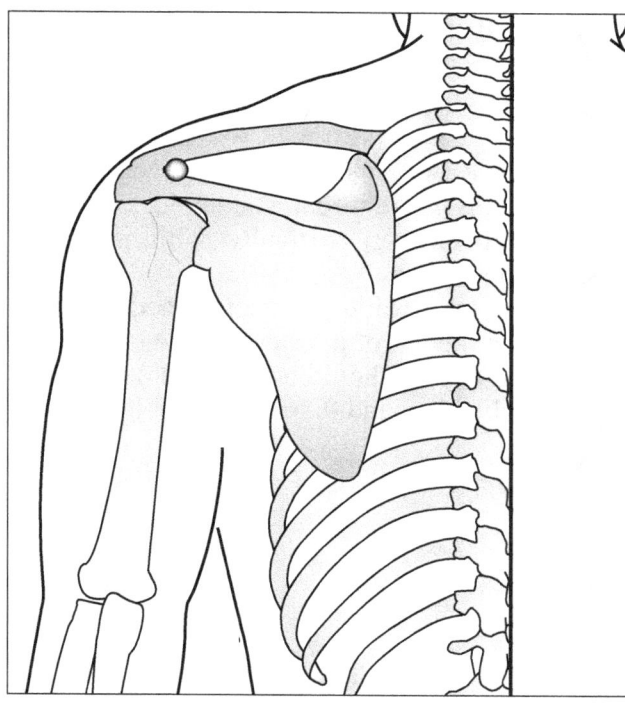

Location: On the shoulder, in the depression between the lateral acromial extremity of the clavicle and the spine of the scapula.

Functions: Removes blockages from the channel, reduces pain and benefits the muscles, tendons, and joint of the shoulder, descends lung Qi, manages Qi and blood, transforms phlegm.

Indications: Any issues of the shoulder, epilepsy, shortness of breath, cough, asthma, scrofula, goiter, vomiting blood.

Attributes: Meeting point of Large Intestine channel and Yang Qiao channels.

Notes

Point Combinations

LI 17
TIANDING

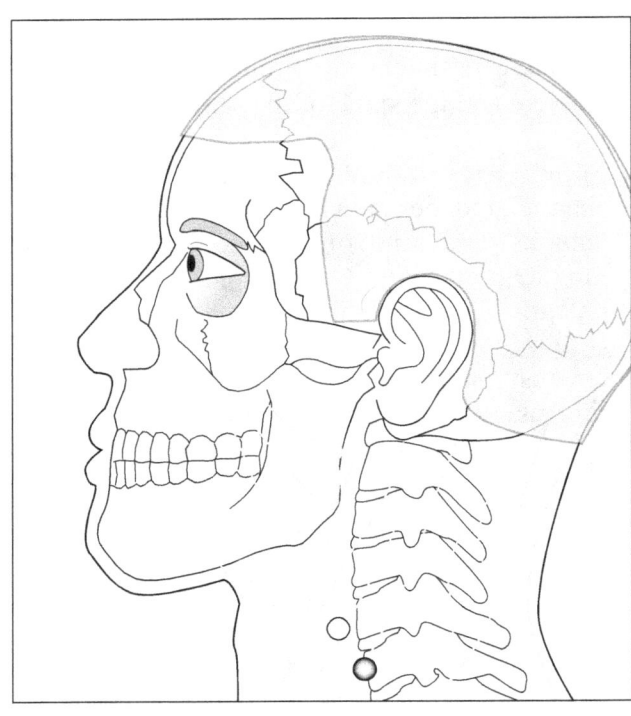

Location: On the lateral side of the neck, on the posterior border of the sternocleidomastoid muscle, 1 cun below LI-18 Futu.

Functions: Benefits throat and voice.

Indications: Sore throat, sudden loss of voice, labored breathing, difficulty with ingestion, goiter, scrofula.

Attributes: *Caution deep needling can puncture the carotid artery or jugular vein. Insertion depths should not exceed 0.3-0.5 cun (perpendicular), and 0.5-0.8 cun (oblique).

Notes

_____
_____
_____
_____
_____
_____
_____
_____

Point Combinations

_____
_____
_____
_____
_____
_____

LI 18
FUTU

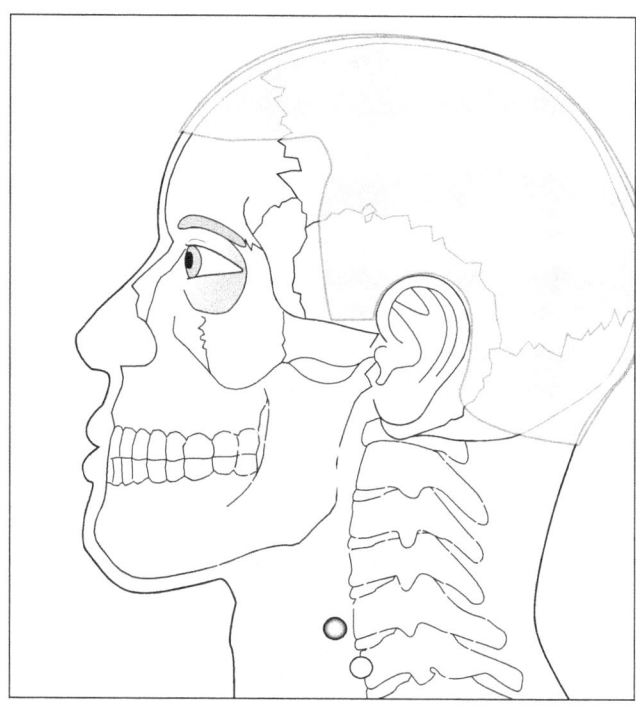

Location: On the lateral side of the neck, beside the tip of the laryngeal protuberance, between the anterior and posterior borders of the sternocleidomastoid muscle.

Functions: Benefits throat and voice.
Indications: Coughing, wheezing, asthma, hoarse voice, goiter, laryngitis, aphasia.
Attributes: Window of the Sky point.
*Caution- deep needling can puncture the carotid artery or jugular vein. Insertion depths should not exceed 0.3-0.5 cun (perpendicular), and 0.5-0.8 cun (oblique).

Notes

_____
_____
_____
_____
_____
_____
_____
_____
_____

Point Combinations

_____
_____
_____
_____
_____
_____
_____

LI 19
KOUHELIAO

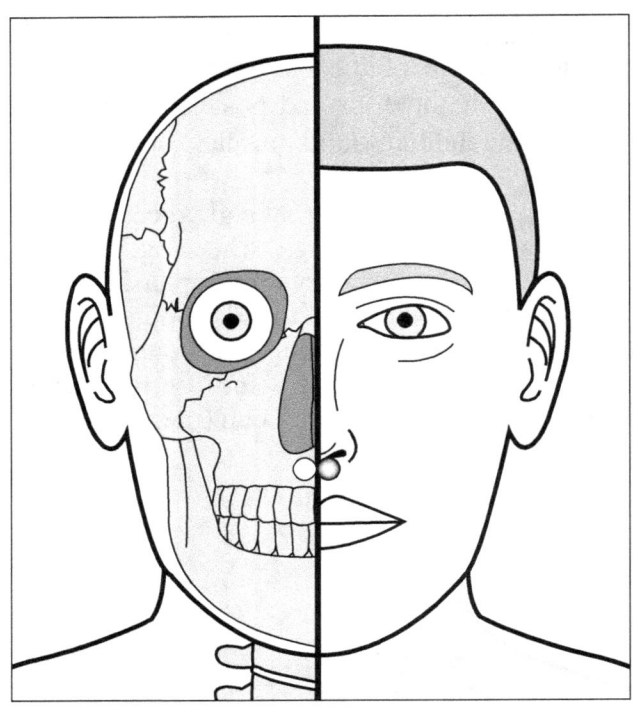

Location: On the face, directly below the lateral margin of the nostril, level with DU-26 Shuigou.

Functions: Expels wind, opens nose and nasal passages, moves Qi stasis and clears heat from the lung, lifts spirit.

Indications: Epistaxis, nasal obstruction, deviation of the mouth.

Attributes: *Moxa is contraindicated.

Notes
_____
_____
_____
_____
_____
_____
_____
_____

Point Combinations
_____
_____
_____
_____
_____
_____

LI 20
YINGXIANG

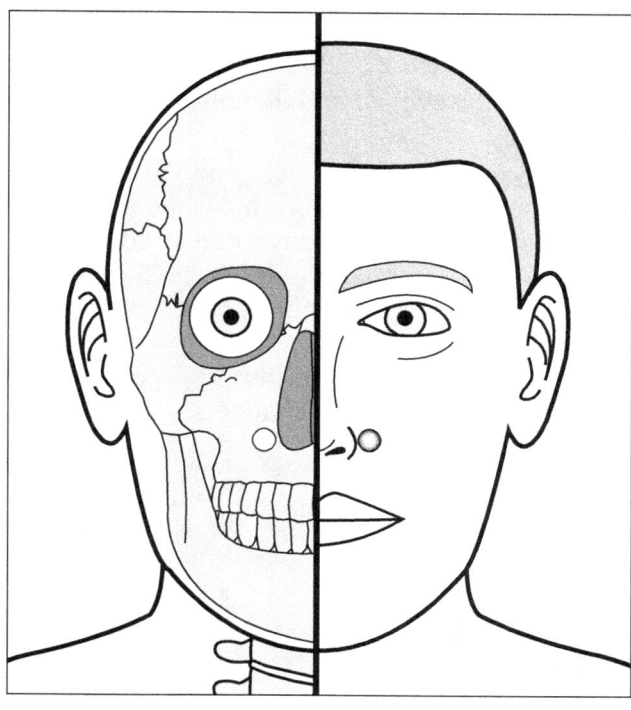

Location: On the face, in the nasolabial groove, beside the midpoint of the lateral border of the nasal ala.

Functions: Expels wind and heat, opens nose and nasal passages,

Indications: For instant clearing of sinuses, trigeminal neuralgia, tics, nasal obstruction, sneezing, runny nose, nasal polyps, allergic rhinitis, stuffy nose, sinusitis, rhinitis, rhinorrhea, itching and swelling of the face, loss of smell, epistaxis.

Attributes: Exit Point

*Moxa is contraindicated.

Notes

Point Combinations

ST 1
CHENGQI

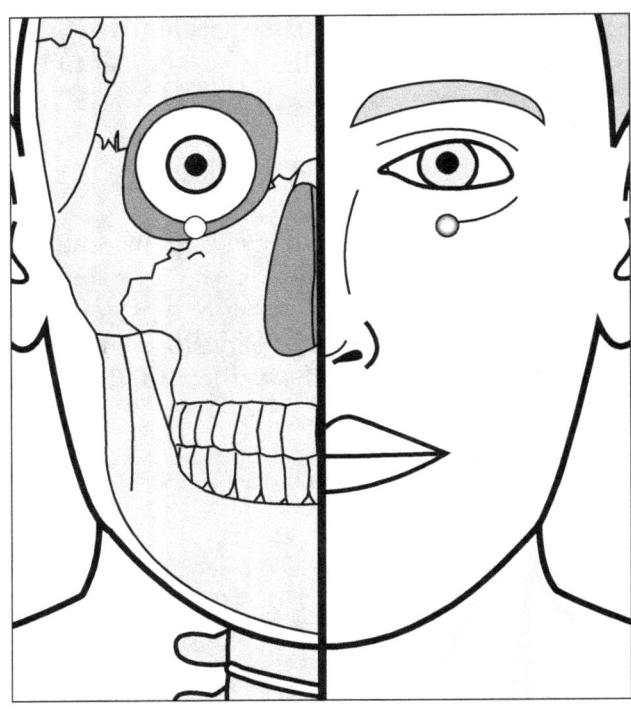

Location: On the face, directly below the pupil when the eyes are looking directly forward, between the eyeball and the infraorbital ridge.

Functions: Clears fire/heat and dispels wind, courses pathogens and brightens the eyes.

Indications: Treats any eye issue, stops excessive lacrimation, dryness, redness, itchiness, twitching, night blindness, visual disturbances, swelling.

Attributes: Entry point, meeting point of the ST, CV and Yang Qiao channels.

Notes

Point Combinations

ST 2
SIBAI

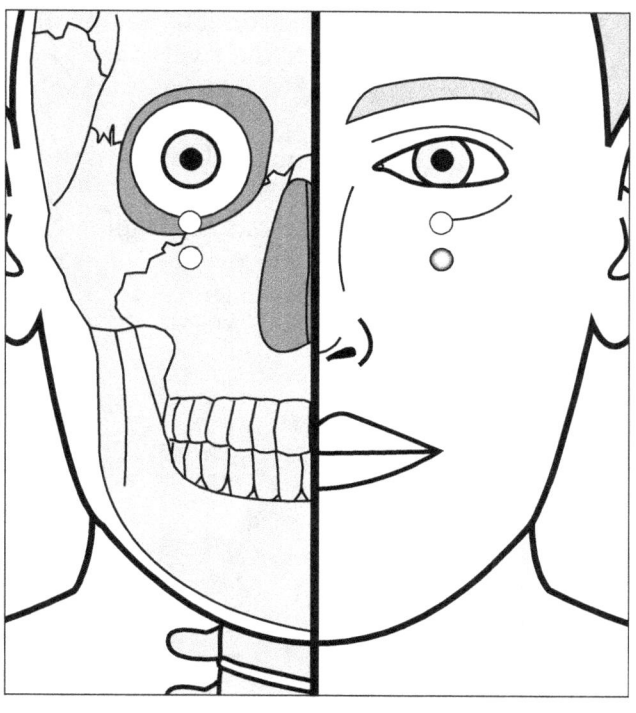

Location: On the face, 1 cun below the pupil, in the depression at the infrorbital foramen.

Functions: Dissipates fire, clears heat and expels wind, courses pathogens and brightens the eyes.

Indications: Treats any eye issue, myopia, corneal opacity, stops excessive lacrimation, dryness, redness, itchiness, twitching, night blindness, visual disturbances, swelling, facial paralysis, facial pain.

Attributes: Empirical point for biliary asceris-parasites.

Notes

_____
_____
_____
_____
_____
_____
_____
_____

Point Combinations

_____
_____
_____
_____
_____
_____

ST 3
JULIAO

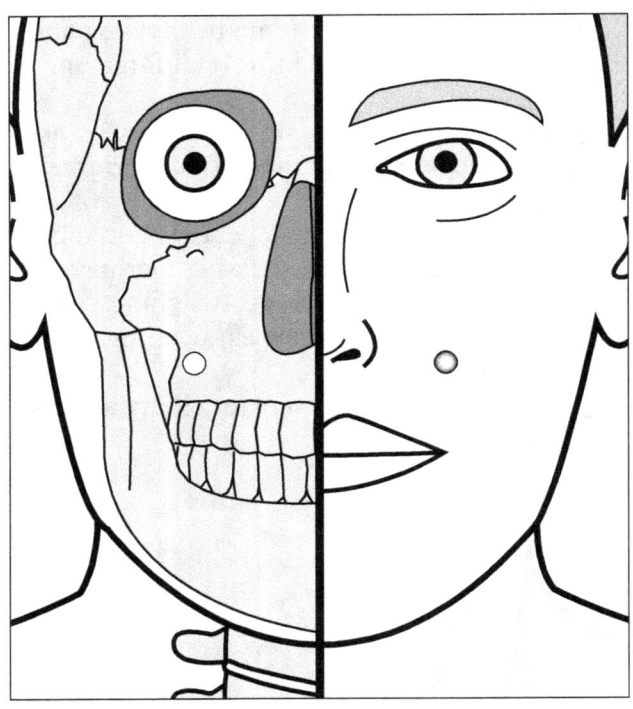

Location: On the face, directly below the pupil, in the depression at the level of the lower border of the ala nasi.

Functions: Dispels wind, relieves swelling, relieves pain.

Indications: facial paralysis, deviation from stroke, twitching of the eyelids, epistaxis, toothache, swelling of the knee.

Attributes: Meeting point of the ST, LI and Yang Qiao channels.

Notes

_____
_____
_____
_____
_____
_____
_____
_____

Point Combinations

_____
_____
_____
_____
_____
_____
_____

ST 4
DICANG

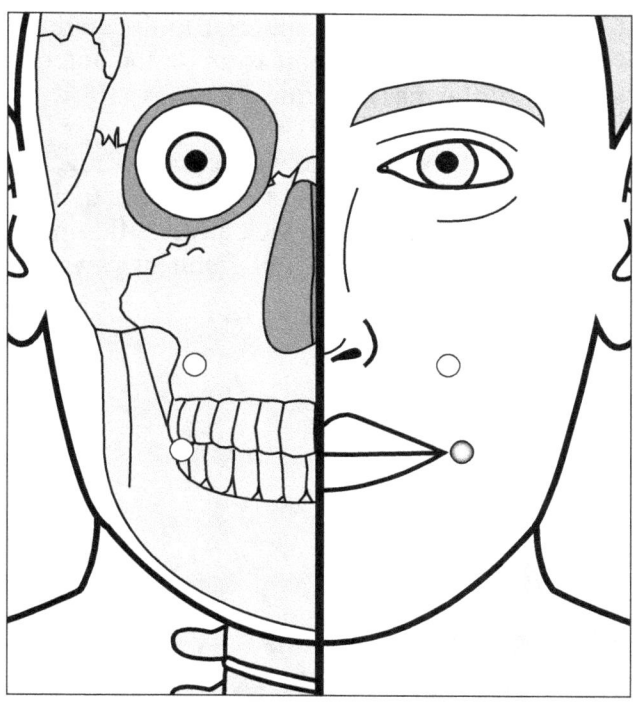

Location: On the face, directly below the pupil, beside the mouth angle (lateral to the corner of the mouth).

Functions: Dispels wind, relieves pain, activates the channel.

Indications: Wry mouth, salivation, twitching of the eyelids, twitching of the corner of the mouth, facial paralysis, toothache, inability to close the eye, itching, night blindness, inability to eat, helpful to treat atrophy and/or issues with the movement of the legs, knees.

Attributes: Meeting point of the ST, LI and Yang Qiao channels.

Notes

_____

_____

_____

_____

_____

_____

_____

_____

Point Combinations

_____

_____

_____

_____

_____

_____

ST 5
DAYING

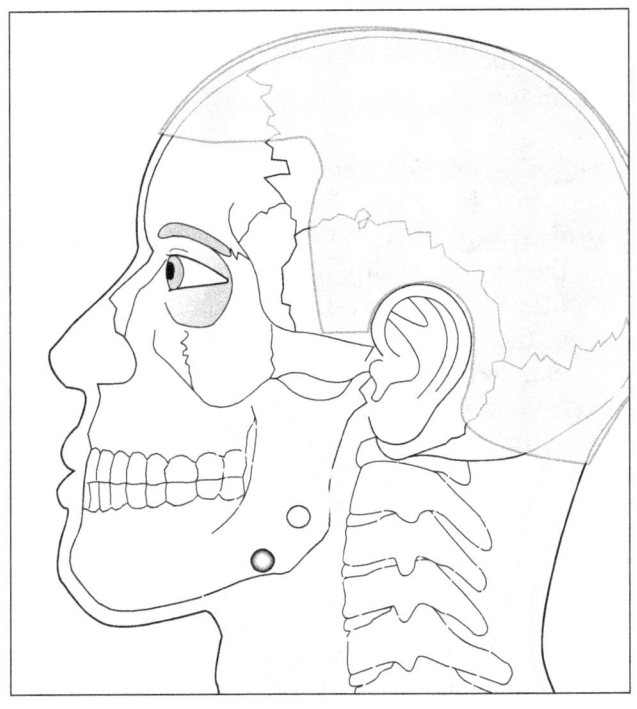

Location: On the face, anterior to the angle of the mandible, in the depression on the anterior border of the masseter muscle.

Functions: Expels wind, reduces swelling.
Indications: Toothache, wry mouth, trismus (lock jaw), neck pain, lock jaw, stiff tongue leading to speech problems, frequent yawning, difficulty closing eye.

Notes

_____
_____
_____
_____
_____
_____
_____
_____

Point Combinations

_____
_____
_____
_____
_____
_____
_____

ST 6
JIACHE

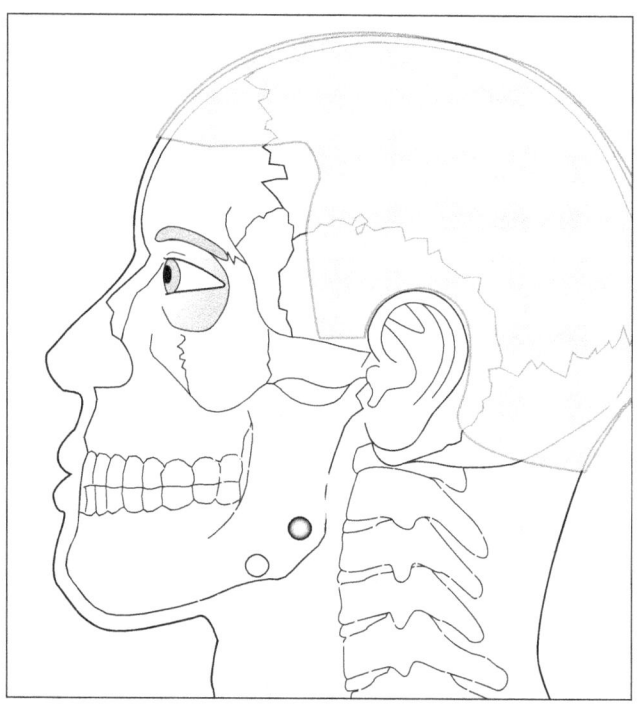

Location: On the face, one finger breadth anterior and superior to the angle of the mandible at the depression on the belly of the masseter muscle with the teeth clenched.

Functions: Expels wind, clears obstruction in the channel, opens channel, relieves pain.

Indications: Benefits the jaw and teeth, swelling of the cheek, wry mouth, toothache in the lower jaw, trismus (lock jaw), TMJ, difficulty in opening the mouth, facial paralysis, loss of voice, mumps.

Notes

_____

_____

_____

_____

_____

_____

_____

_____

Point Combinations

_____

_____

_____

_____

_____

_____

ST 7
XIAGUAN

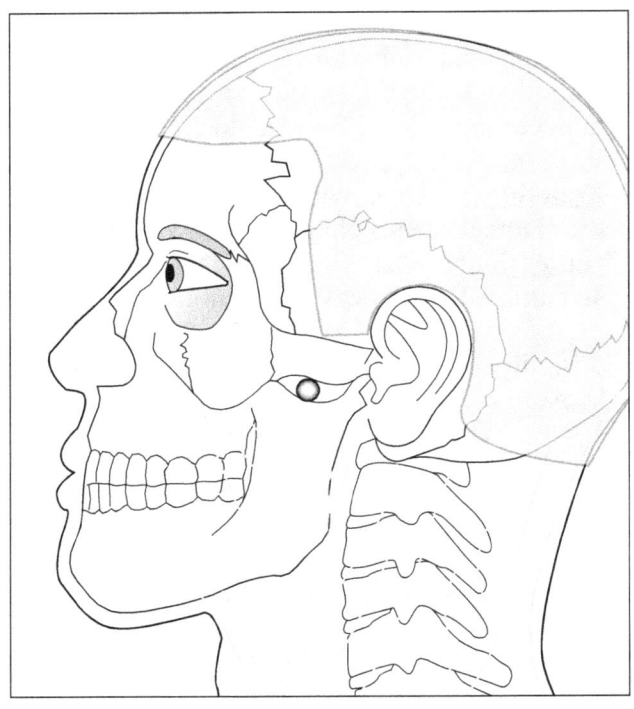

Location: On the face, anterior to the ear, in the depression between the zygomatic arch and mandibular notch.

Functions: Clears obstruction in the channel.
Indications: Benefits the ears, jaw and teeth, deafness, tinnitus, toothache, nasal congestion, wry face, difficulty opening mouth, pain in the face, TMJ, trigeminal neuralgia, ear infections.

Notes

_____
_____
_____
_____
_____
_____
_____
_____

Point Combinations

_____
_____
_____
_____
_____
_____
_____

ST 8
TOUWEI

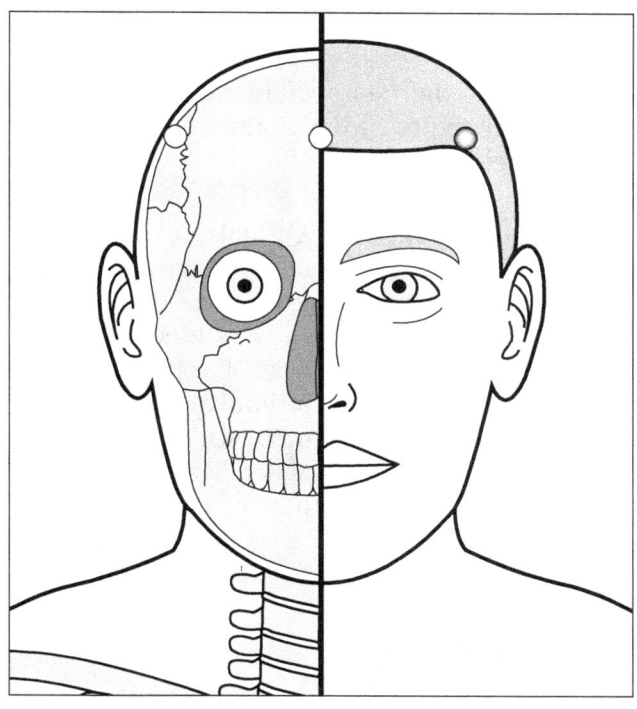

Location: On the forehead, .5 cun above the anterior hairline at the corner of the forehead, 4.5 cun lateral to the anterior midline of the head.

Functions: Expels wind, clears the head and brightens the eyes.

Indications: Headaches, migraines, poor vision, twitching eyelids, eye pain, excessive tearing, dizziness, hair loss.

Attributes: Meeting point of the ST and GB channels.

Notes
_____
_____
_____
_____
_____
_____
_____
_____

Point Combinations
_____
_____
_____
_____
_____
_____

ST 9
RENYING

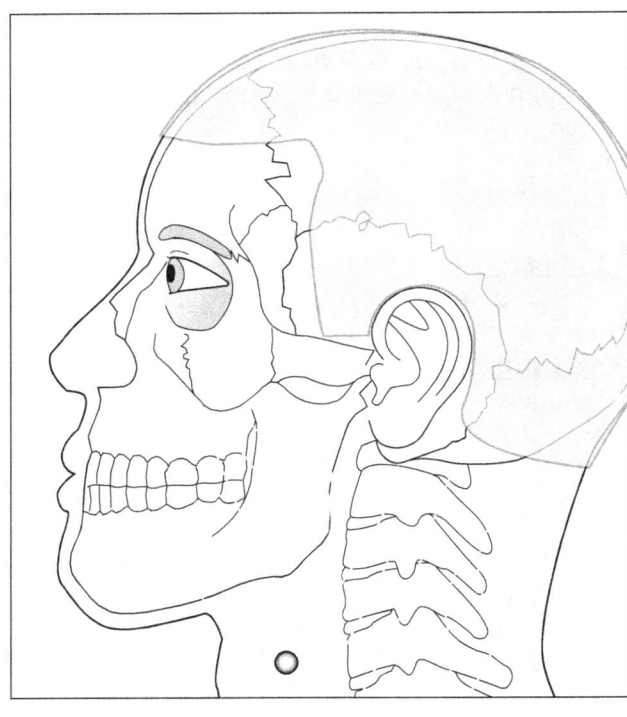

Location: On the neck, lateral to the laryngeal prominence (Adam's apple), on the anterior border of the sternocleidomastoid muscle, (where the pulse of the common carotid artery can be felt).

Functions: Regulates Qi and blood, subdues rebellious Qi, benefits the throat and neck, dissipates goiter.

Indications: Regulates/lowers blood pressure, headaches, dizziness, sore throat, vomiting, coughing, hiccups, acute lumbar sprain, lower back pain, chest tightness, asthma, scrofula, goiter, hemiplegia, apoplexy, hemoptysis.

Attributes: Meeting point of the ST and GB channels, Window of the Sky point, Sea of Qi point.

Notes

Point Combinations

ST 10
SHUITU

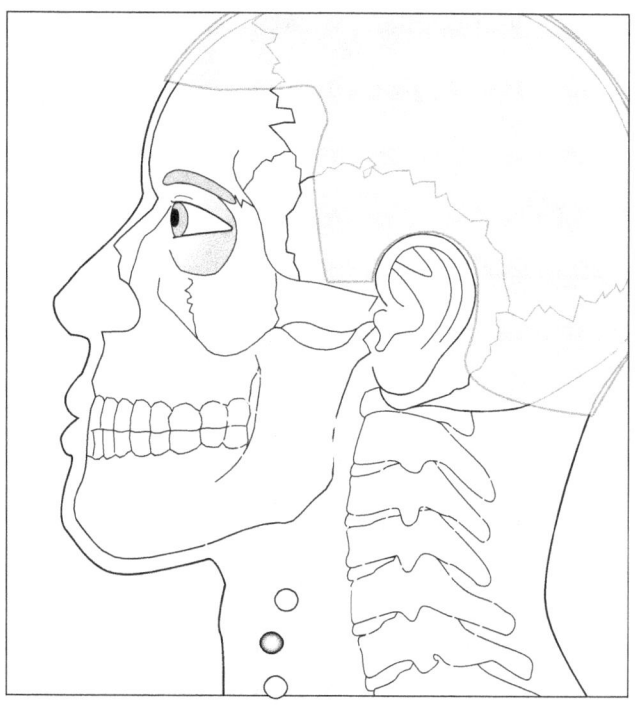

Location: On the neck, on the anterior border of the sternocleidomastoid muscle, at the midpoint of the line joining ST-9 Renying and ST-11 Qishe.

Functions: Decends Lung Qi, benefits the throat and neck.

Indications: Swollen/sore throat, cough, asthma, shortness of breath, goiter, scrofula.

Notes

_____

_____

_____

_____

_____

_____

_____

_____

_____

Point Combinations

_____

_____

_____

_____

_____

_____

_____

ST 11
QISHE

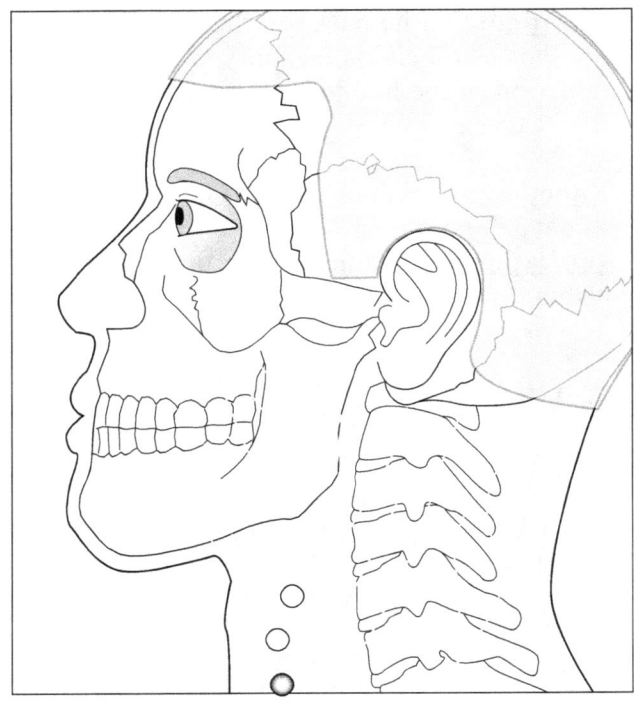

Location: On the neck, on the superior border of the clavicle, between the sternal head and clavicular head of the sternocleidomastoid muscle.

Functions: Descends Qi, benefits the throat and neck, relieves cough, Qi counterflow.

Indications: Chest congestion, cough, asthma, goiter, scrofula, pain and rigidity of the neck, dyspnea, hiccups, reflux.

Notes

Point Combinations

ST 12
QUEPEN

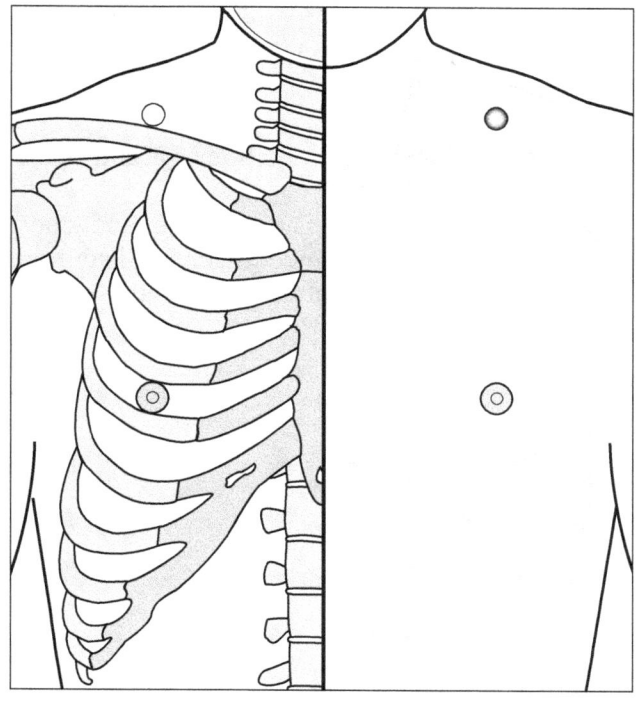

Location: On the chest, at the midpoint of the supraclavicular fossa, 4 cun lateral to the anterior midline.

Functions: Descends Lung Qi, activates the channels and relieves pain.

Indications: Cough, asthma, swollen/sore throat, scrofula, pain in the supraclavicular fossa, hiccups, mumps.

Notes

Point Combinations

ST 13
QIHU

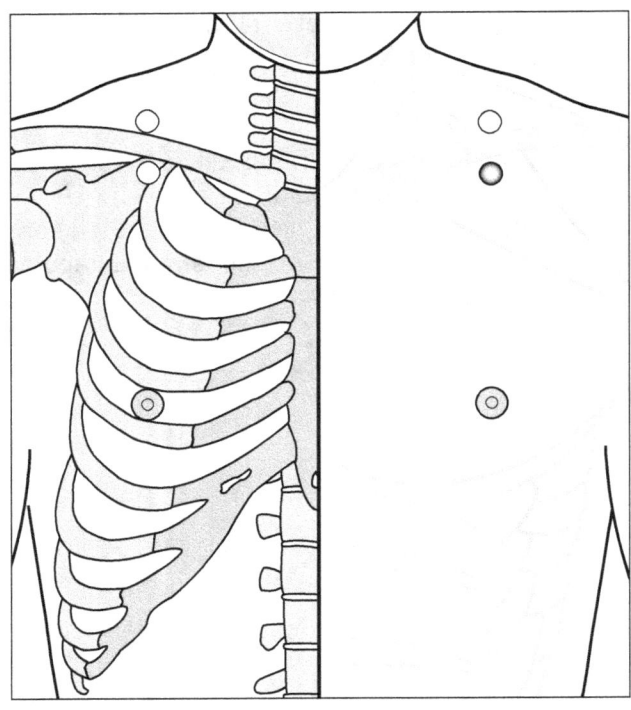

Location: On the chest, at the midpoint of the lower border of the clavicle, 4 cun lateral to the anterior midline.

Functions: Descends rebellious Qi and opens the chest.

Indications: Cough, asthma, pain and chest congestion, wheezing, hiccups, chest distention, rib pain, neck pain, inability to turn the head.

Notes

_____

_____

_____

_____

_____

_____

_____

Point Combinations

_____

_____

_____

_____

_____

_____

ST 14
KUFANG

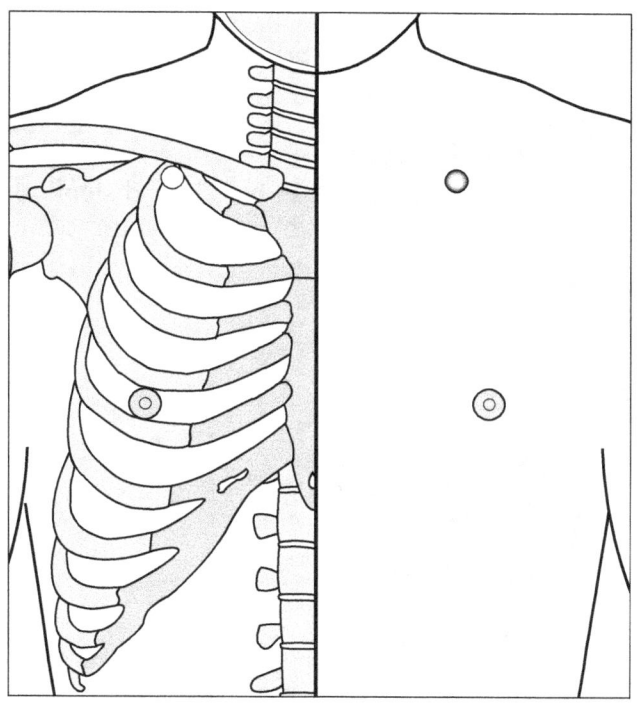

Location: On the chest, in the 1st intercostal space, 4 cun lateral to the anterior midline.

Functions: Descends rebellious Qi, opens the chest.

Indications: Cough, asthma, chest distention, pain in the chest and hypochondrium.

Notes

_____

_____

_____

_____

_____

_____

_____

_____

_____

Point Combinations

_____

_____

_____

_____

_____

_____

_____

ST 15
WUYI

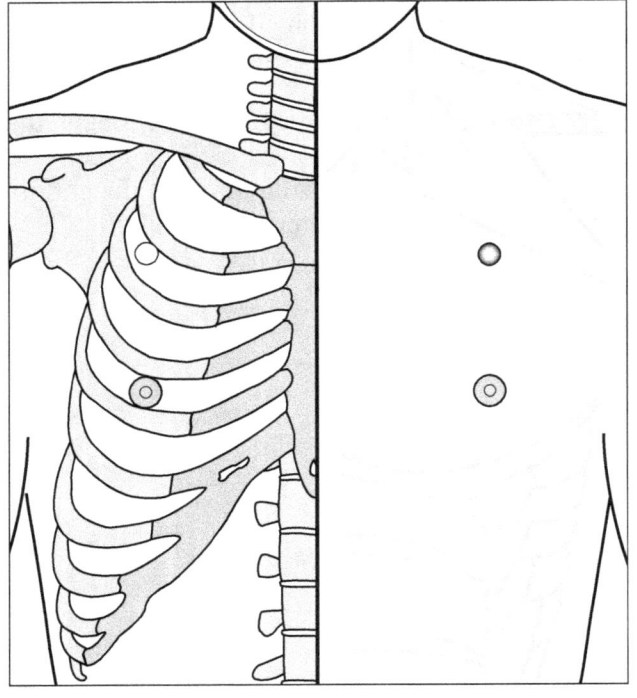

Location: On the chest, in the 2nd intercostal space, 4 cun lateral to the anterior midline.

Functions: Descends rebellious Qi, opens the chest, benefits the breasts.

Indications: Cough, asthma, chest distention, pain in the chest and hypochondrium, acute mastitis.

Notes

Point Combinations

ST 16
YINGCHUANG

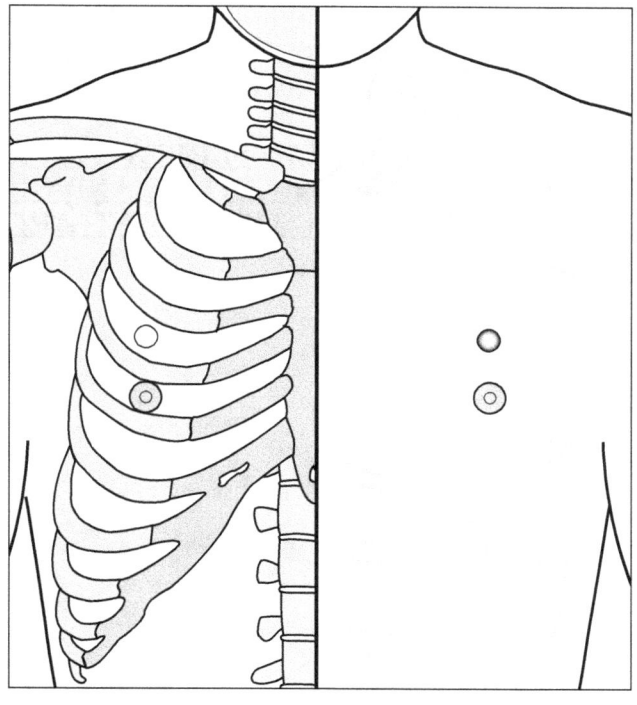

Location: On the chest, in the 3rd intercostal space, 4 cun lateral to the anterior midline.

Functions: Descends rebellious Qi, opens the chest, benefits the breasts.

Indications: Cough, asthma, chest distention, pain in the chest and hypochondrium, acute mastitis.

Notes

Point Combinations

ST 17
RUZHONG

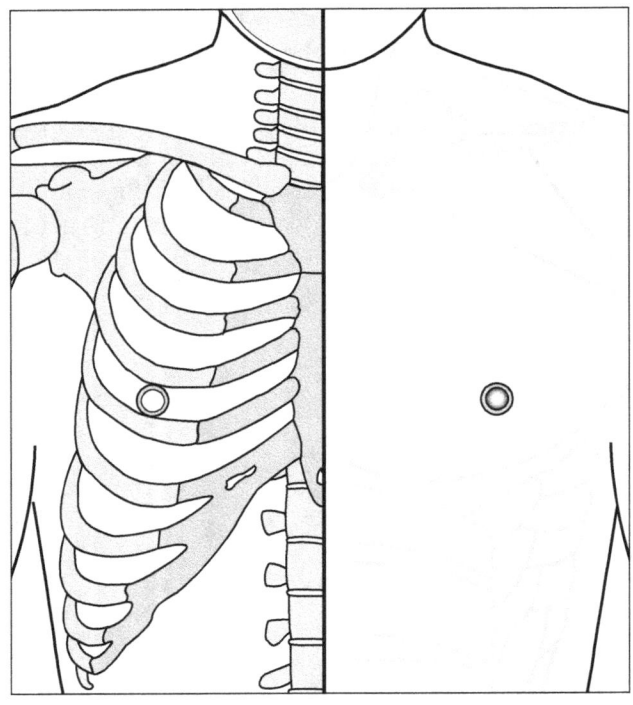

Location: On the chest, in the 4th intercostal space, in the center of the nipple, 4 cun lateral to the anterior midline.

THIS POINT ONLY SERVES AS A LANDMARK, ACUPUNCTURE AND/OR MOXIBUSTION ON THIS POINT ARE CONTRAINDICATED

Notes

Point Combinations

ST 18
RUGEN

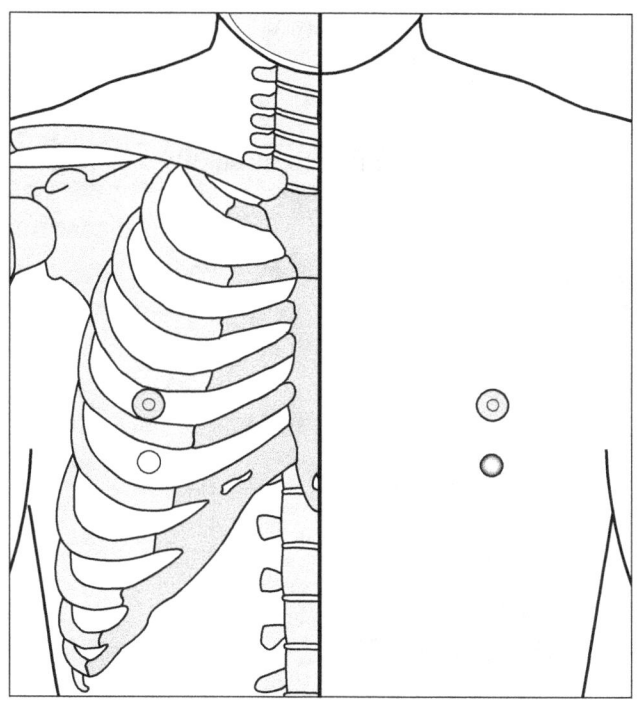

Location: On the chest, in the 5th intercostal space, directly below the nipple, on the lower border of the breast, 4 cun lateral to the anterior midline.

Functions: Opens the chest, benefits the breasts, regulates Lung Qi.

Indications: Cough, asthma, chest pain, insufficient lactation, acute mastitis, wheezing.

Notes

Point Combinations

ST 19
BURONG

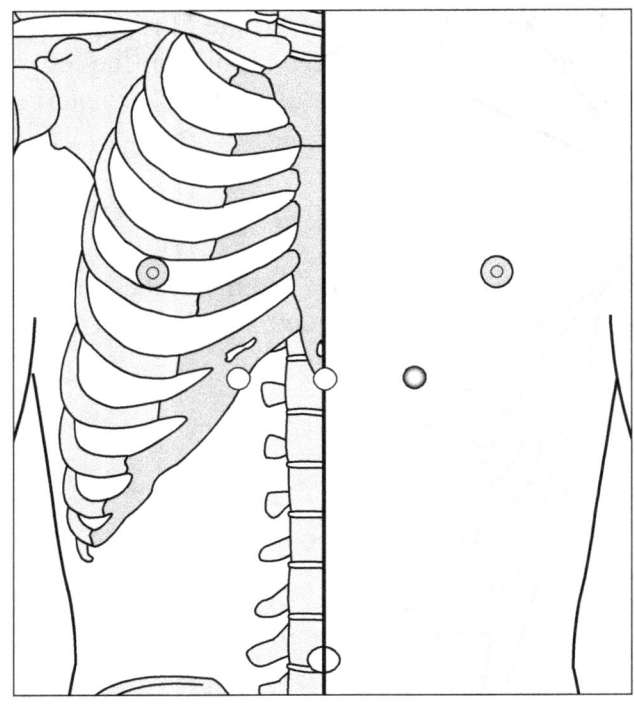

Location: On the abdomen, 6 cun above the center of the umbilicus, 2 cun lateral to the anterior midline.

Functions: Descends rebellious Qi, harmonizes the middle jiao.

Indications: Gastric pain, abdominal distention, vomiting, poor digestion, anorexia.

Notes
_____
_____
_____
_____
_____
_____
_____
_____

Point Combinations
_____
_____
_____
_____
_____
_____
_____

ST 20
CHENGMAN

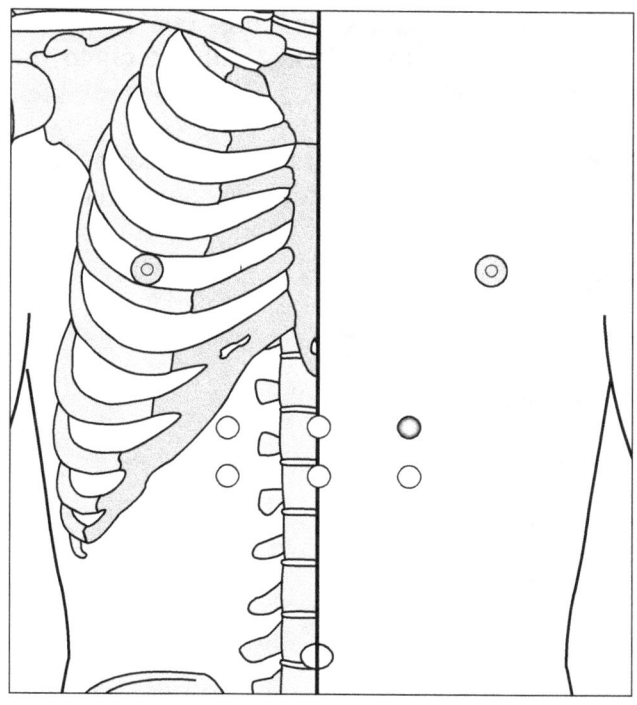

Location: On the abdomen, 5 cun above the center of the umbilicus, 2 cun lateral to the anterior midline.

Functions: Descends rebellious Qi, harmonizes the middle jiao.

Indications: Gastric pain, abdominal distention, vomiting, poor appetite, anorexia.

Notes

Point Combinations

ST 21
LIANGMEN

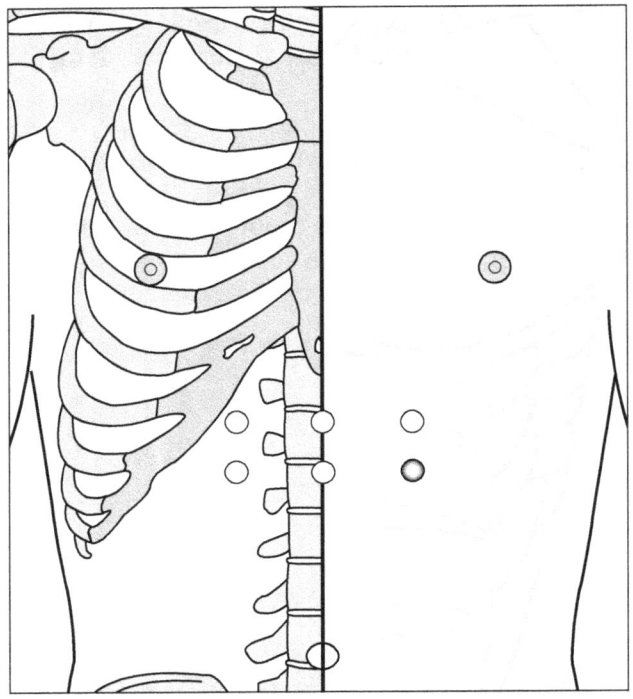

Location: On the abdomen, 4 cun above the center of the umbilicus, 2 cun lateral to the anterior midline.

Functions: Harmonizes and descends rebellious Qi, harmonizes the middle jiao, stops diarrhea.
Indications: Gastric pain, abdominal distention, vomiting, poor appetite, diarrhea.

Notes

Point Combinations

ST 22
GUANMEN

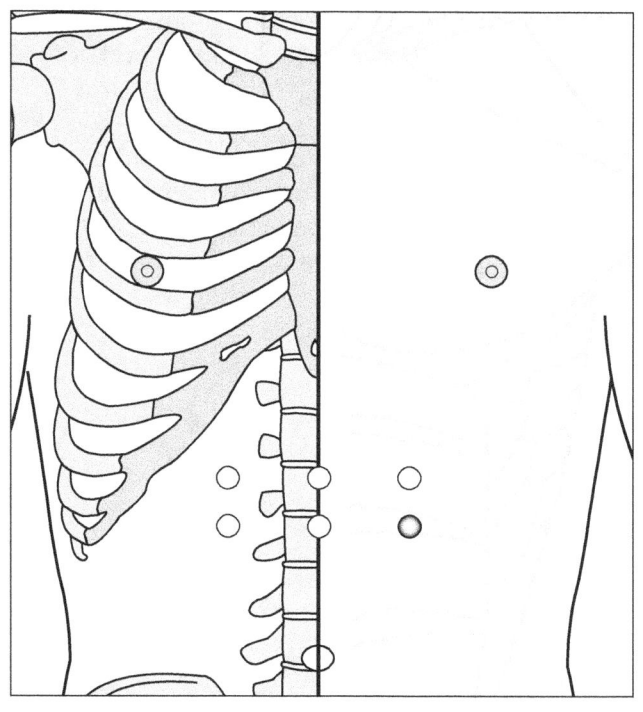

Location: On the abdomen, 3 cun above the center of the umbilicus, 2 cun lateral to the anterior midline.

Functions: Regulates Qi, regulates the Intestines, promotes urination.

Indications: Abdominal distention and pain, diarrhea, borborygmus, edema.

Notes
_____
_____
_____
_____
_____
_____
_____
_____

Point Combinations
_____
_____
_____
_____
_____
_____

ST 23
TAIYI

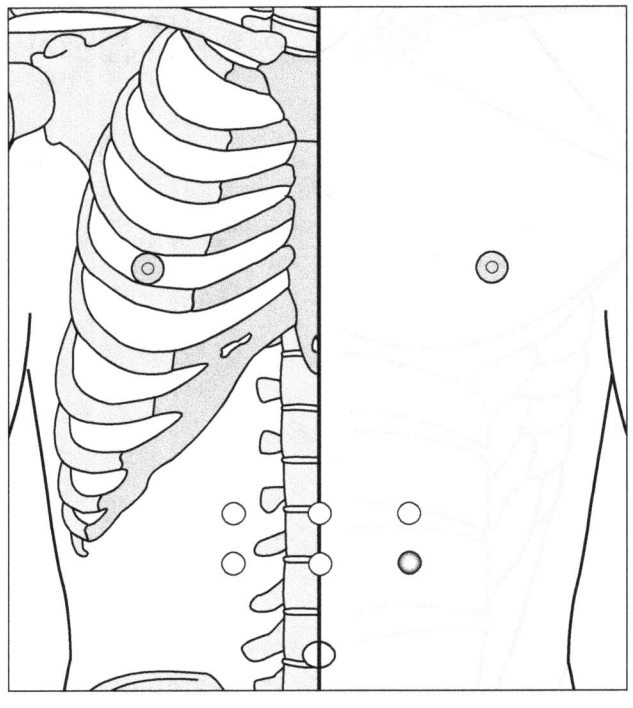

Location: On the abdomen, 2 cun above the center of the umbilicus, 2 cun lateral to the anterior midline.

Functions: Harmonizes the middle jiao, fortifies Spleen and harmonizes Stomach, calms shen, transforms phlegm, calms the spirit.

Indications: Gastric pain, indigestion, mania, psychosis, irritability, protruding tongue.

Notes

_____
_____
_____
_____
_____
_____
_____
_____

Point Combinations

_____
_____
_____
_____
_____
_____
_____

ST 24
HUAROUMEN

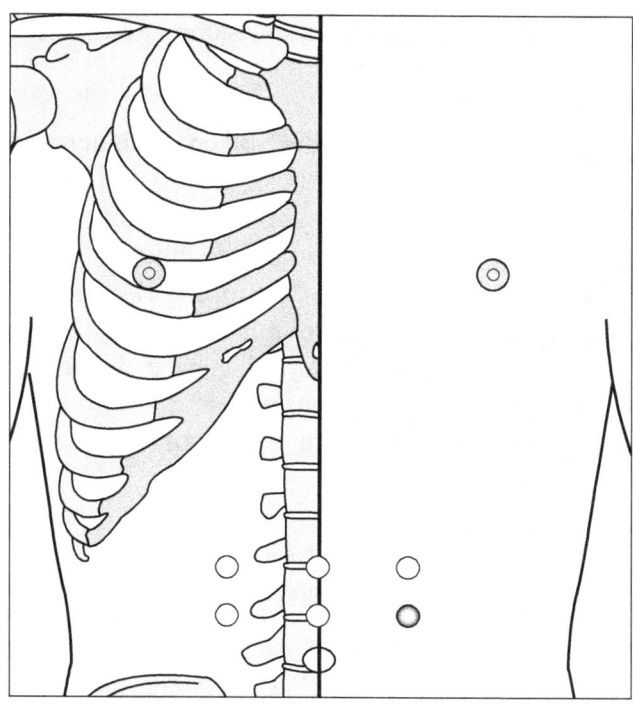

Location: On the abdomen, 1 cun above the center of the umbilicus, 2 cun lateral to the anterior midline.

Functions: Harmonizes the middle jiao, fortifies Spleen and harmonizes Stomach, calms shen, transforms phlegm, calms the spirit.

Indications: Gastric pain, indigestion, mania, psychosis, irritability, protruding tongue, stiff tongue.

Notes

_____

_____

_____

_____

_____

_____

_____

_____

_____

Point Combinations

_____

_____

_____

_____

_____

_____

_____

ST 25
TIANSHU

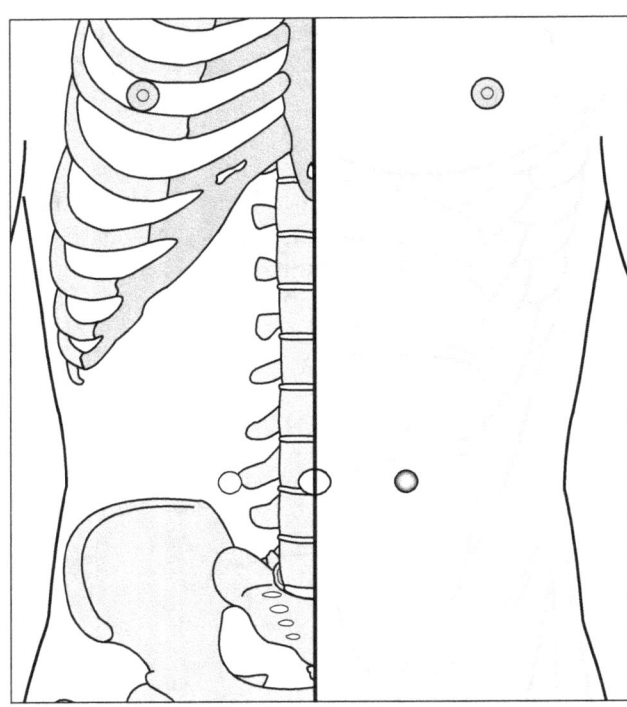

Location: On the abdomen, 2 cun lateral to the center of the umbilicus.

Functions: Regulates the Spleen, Stomach and Intestines, dispels dampness, dispels damp heat, regulates Qi and blood, food accumulation.

Indications: Abdominal distention, pain around umbilicus, constipation, borborygmus, diarrhea, dysentery, irregular menses, female infertility, edema, milky discharge, intestinal parasites, abdominal masses.

Attributes: Front Mu point of the Large Intestine channel.

Notes

_____
_____
_____
_____
_____
_____
_____
_____
_____

Point Combinations

_____
_____
_____
_____
_____
_____
_____

ST 26
WAILING

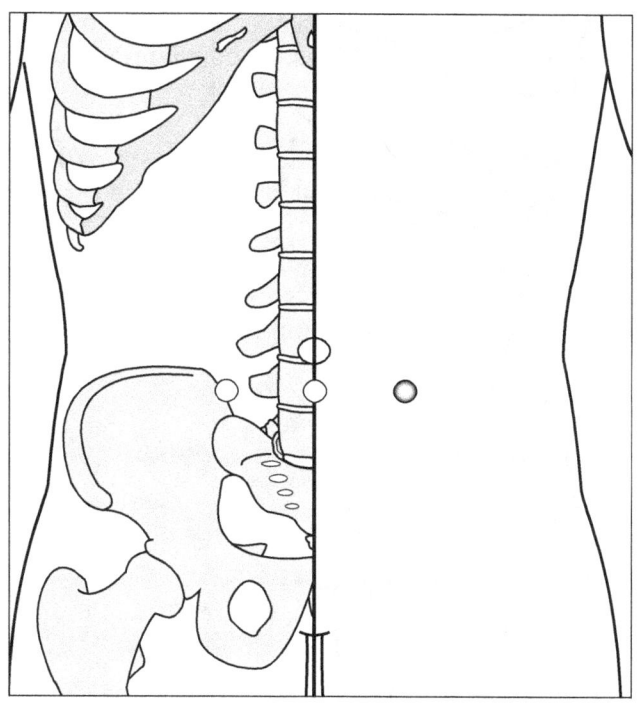

Location: On the abdomen, 1 cun below the center of the umbilicus, 2 cun lateral to the anterior midline.

Functions: Regulates Qi, relieves pain.
Indications: Abdominal pain, hernia, dysmenorrhea.

Notes

_____

_____

_____

_____

_____

_____

_____

_____

Point Combinations

_____

_____

_____

_____

_____

_____

ST 27
DAJU

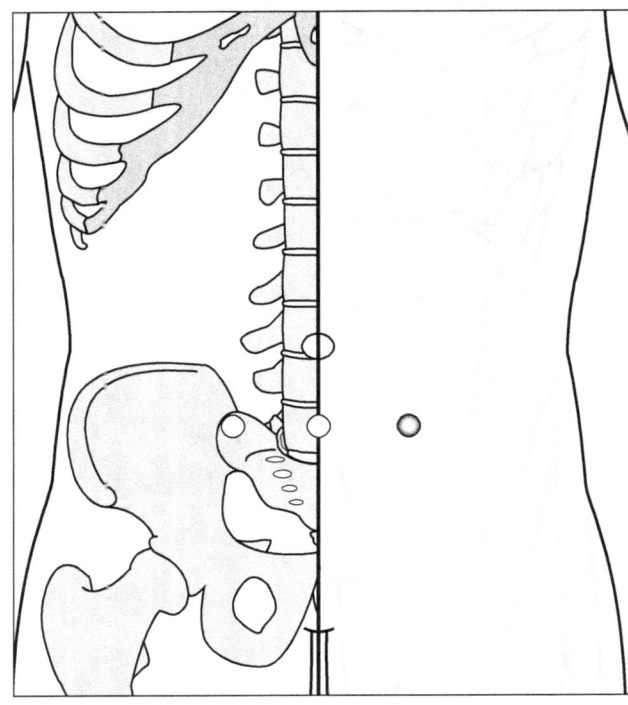

Location: On the abdomen, 2 cun below the center of the umbilicus, 2 cun lateral to the anterior midline.

Functions: Tonifies essence and strengthens Kidneys, regulates Stomach Qi, promotes urination.

Indications: Lower abdominal pain and distention, hernia, dysuria, spermatorrhea, premature ejaculation, impotence.

Notes

Point Combinations

ST 28
SHUIDAO

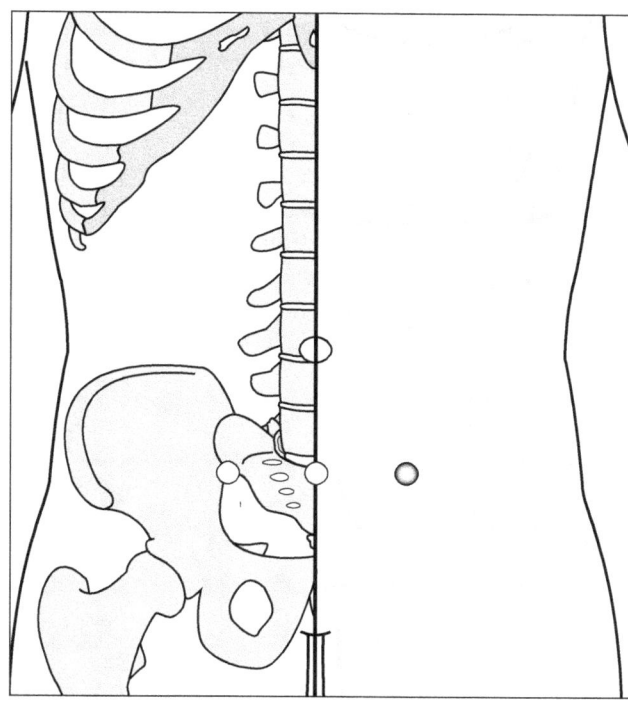

Location: On the abdomen, 3 cun below the center of the umbilicus, 2 cun lateral to the anterior midline.

Functions: Regulates the lower jiao, opens up the water passages, promotes urination, removes stagnation, benefits the bladder and uterus.

Indications: Lower abdominal pain and distention, dysuria, dysmenorrhea, infertility, hernia, constipation, edema, sterility.

Notes

_____

_____

_____

_____

_____

_____

_____

_____

_____

Point Combinations

_____

_____

_____

_____

_____

_____

_____

ST 29
GUILAI

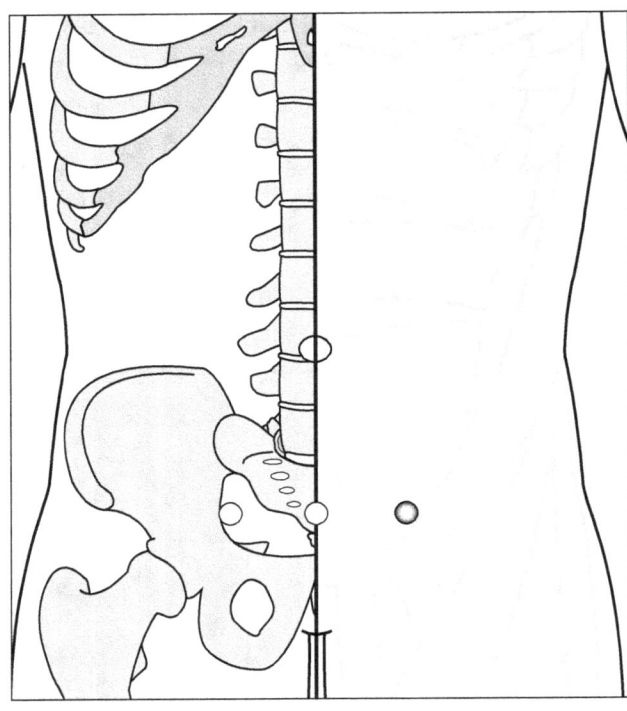

Location: On the abdomen, 4 cun below the center of the umbilicus, 2 cun lateral to the anterior midline.

Functions: Warms the lower jiao, regulates menstruation and removes blood stagnation.

Indications: Irregular menstruation, amenorrhea, leukorrhea, hernia, abdominal pain, prolapse uterus.

Notes

Point Combinations

ST 30
QICHONG

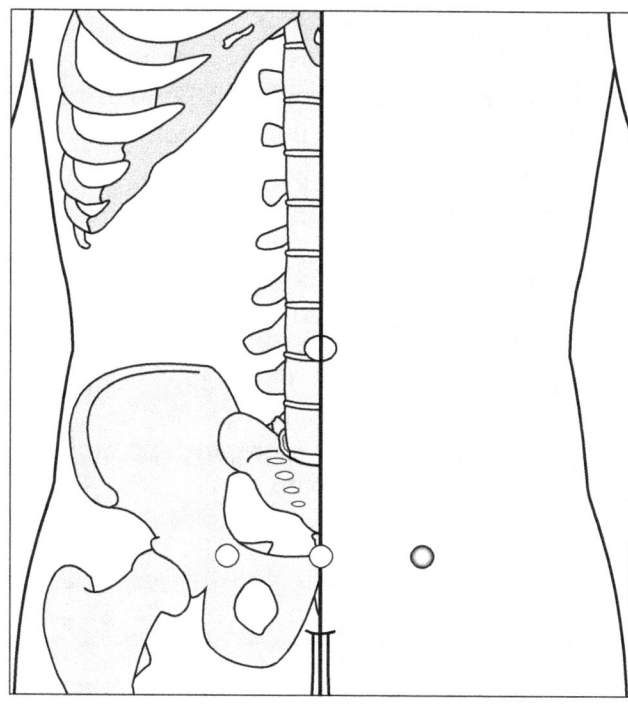

Location: On the abdomen, 5 cun below the center of the umbilicus, 2 cun lateral to the anterior midline, level with the superior border of the pubic symphysis.

Functions: Regulates the Pentrating Vessel and the lower jiao, subdues running piglet syndrome.

Indications: Abdominal pain, borborygmus, hernia, pain and swelling of the external genitalia, impotence, dysmenorrhea, irregular menstruation.

Notes

_____

_____

_____

_____

_____

_____

_____

_____

_____

Point Combinations

_____

_____

_____

_____

_____

_____

ST 31
BIGUAN

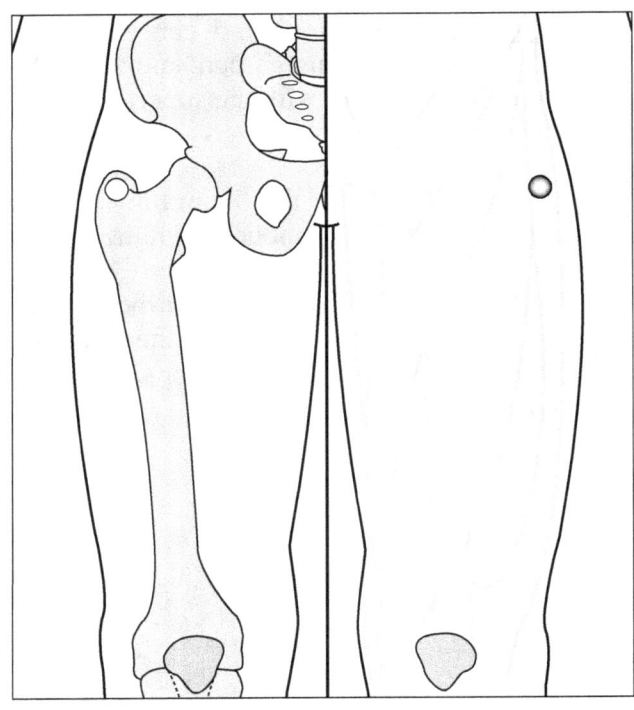

Location: On the anterior side of the thigh, on the line connecting the antero-superior iliac spine and the superolateral corner of the patella, at the level of the perineum when the thigh is flexed, in the depression lateral to the sartorius muscle.

Functions: Expels wind-damp, relieves pain, activates the channel and unblocks obstructions in the channel.

Indications: Pain in the thigh, weakness, coldness, numbness and pain in lower extremities, muscular atrophy, hemiplegia, apoplexy, lower back pain.

Notes

Point Combinations

ST 32
FUTU

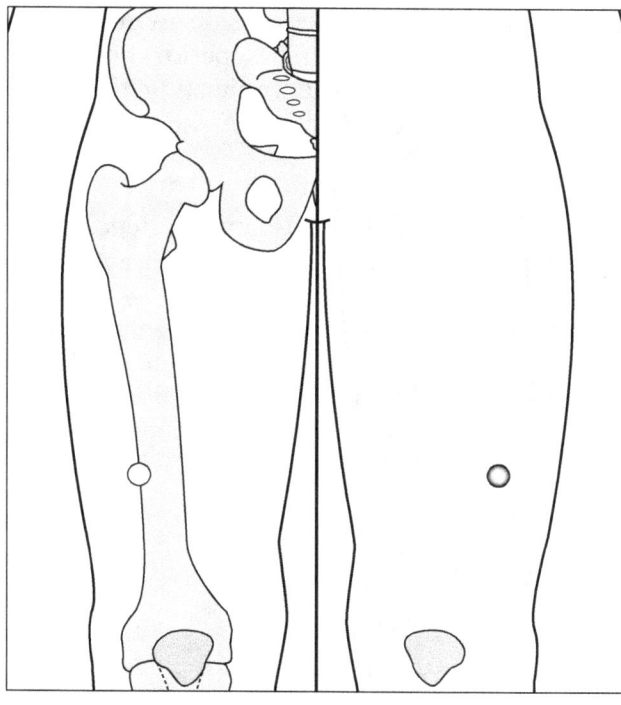

Location: On the anterior side of the thigh, 6 cun above the lateral superior border of the patella, on the line connecting the ASIS (anterior superior iliac spine) and the lower border of the patella.

Functions: Expels wind-damp, relieves pain, activates the channel and unblocks obstructions in the channel.

Indications: Paralysis and motor impairment, pain in the lumbar and iliac region, coldness, numbness and pain in lower extremities.

Notes

Point Combinations

ST 33
YINSHI

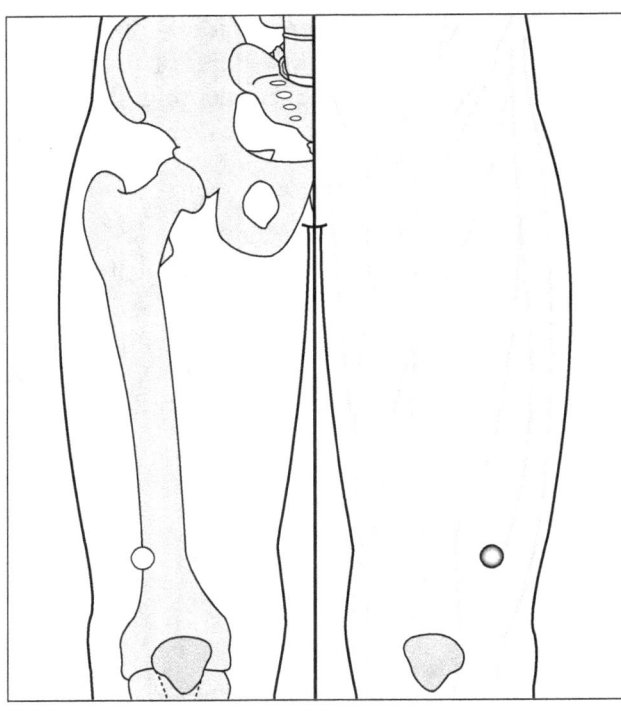

Location: On the anterior side of the thigh, 3 cun above the lateral superior border of the patella, on the line connecting the ASIS (anterior superior iliac spine) and the lower border of the patella.

Functions: Expels wind-damp, relieves pain, activates the channel, unblocks obstructions in the channel.

Indications: Paralysis and motor impairment, pain in the lumbar and iliac region, coldness, numbness and pain in lower extremities, hernia, abdominal pain and distention.

Notes

Point Combinations

ST 34
LiangQiu

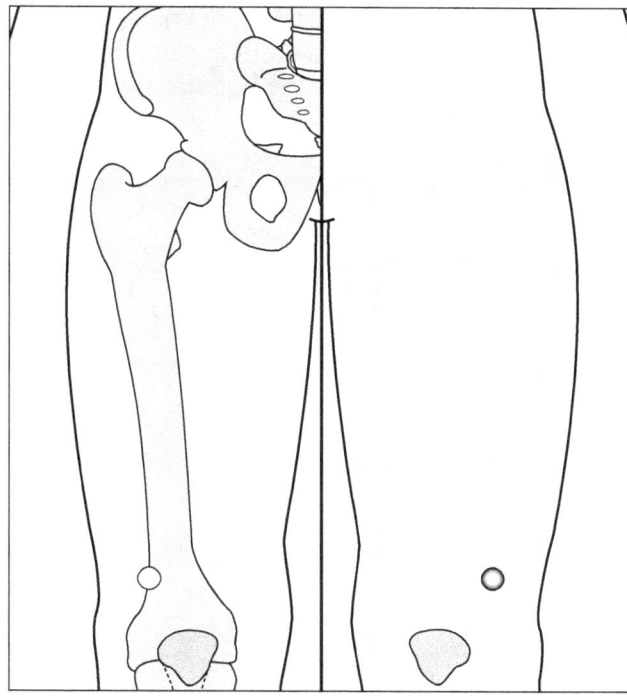

Location: With the knee flexed, on the anterior side of the thigh and on the line connecting the anterior-superior iliac spine and the supero-lateral corner of the patella, 2 cun above this corner.

Functions: Harmonizes the stomach, subdues rebellious Qi, activates the channel and relieves pain, relieves acute conditions.

Indications: Swelling of the knee, paralysis or weakness of the lower extremities, acute gastric pain, acute mastitis.

Attributes: Xi-Cleft point.

Notes

_____
_____
_____
_____
_____
_____
_____
_____
_____

Point Combinations

_____
_____
_____
_____
_____
_____
_____

ST 35
DUBI

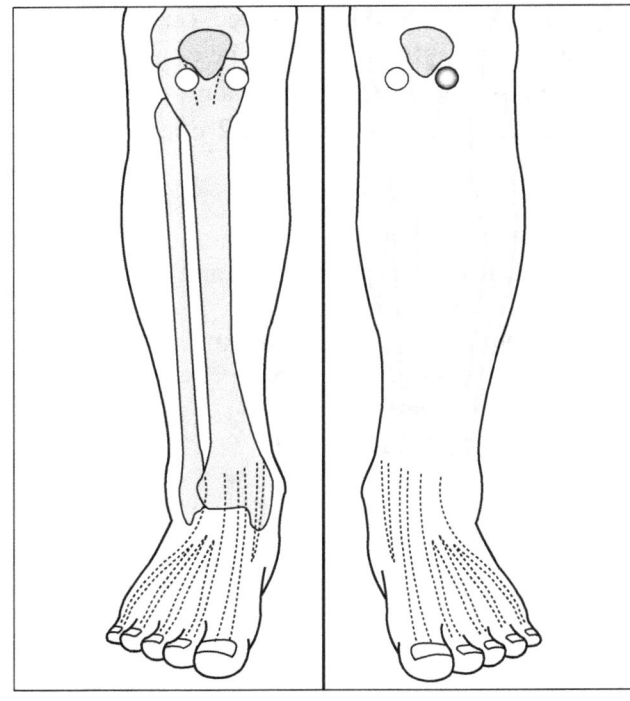

Location: On the knee, with the knee flexed, in the depression below the lateral inferior border of the patella, lateral to the patellar ligament.

Functions: Expels wind-damp, reduces swelling, activates the channel and relieves pain.

Indications: Swelling and pain of the knee joint, limited range of motion of the knees, beriberi.

Notes
_____
_____
_____
_____
_____
_____
_____
_____

Point Combinations
_____
_____
_____
_____
_____
_____

ST 36
ZUSANLI

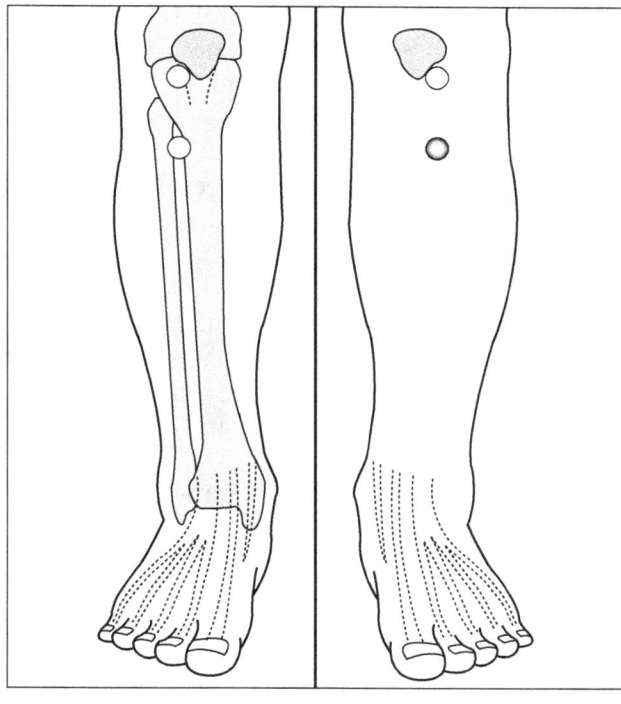

Location: On the antero-lateral side of the leg, 3 cun below ST-35 Dubi, one finger breadth (middle finger) from the anterior crest of the tibia.

Functions: Harmonizes the Spleen and Stomach, tonifies Qi and nourishes blood and yin, strengthens the Spleen and resolves dampness, strengthens the body and Wei Qi, clears fire and calms the spirit, revives yang and restores consciousness, activates the channel and relieves pain.

Indications: Gastric pain, vomiting, abdominal pain and distention, dysphagia, borborygmus, diarrhea, dysentery, enteritis, constipation, indigestion, acute mastitis, shortness of breath, emaciation due to general deficiency, poor appetite, lassitude, lethargy, dizziness, palpitations, insomnia, cough and asthma, pain in the knee joint, apoplexy, hemiplegia, edema, beriberi, depression, psychosis, mania.

Attributes: Earth point, He-Sea point, command point of the abdomen, point of the Sea of Water and Grain.

Notes

_____
_____
_____
_____
_____
_____
_____
_____

Point Combinations

_____
_____
_____
_____
_____
_____
_____

ST 37
SHANGJUXU

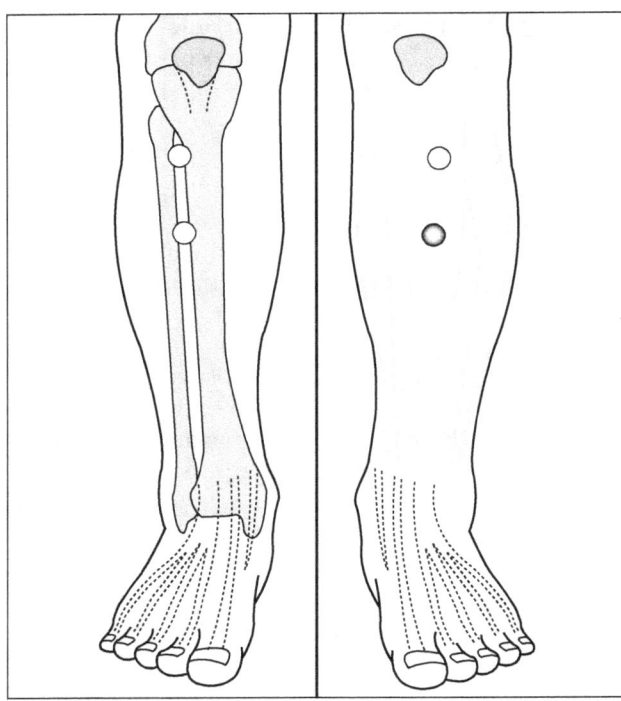

Location: On the antero-lateral side of the leg, 6 cun below ST-35 Dubi, one finger breadth (middle finger) from the anterior crest of the tibia.

Functions: Regulates the Spleen and Stomach, regulates the intestines and moves stagnation, clears damp heat, relieves diarrhea and dysenteric disorder, relieves pain.

Indications: Abdominal pain, acute appendicitis, constipation, diarrhea, borborygmus, muscular atrophy, paralysis due to stroke, weakness, numbness and pain of the lower extremities, beriberi.

Attributes: Lower He-Sea point of the Large Intestine, point of the Sea of Blood.

Notes

Point Combinations

ST 38
TIAOKOU

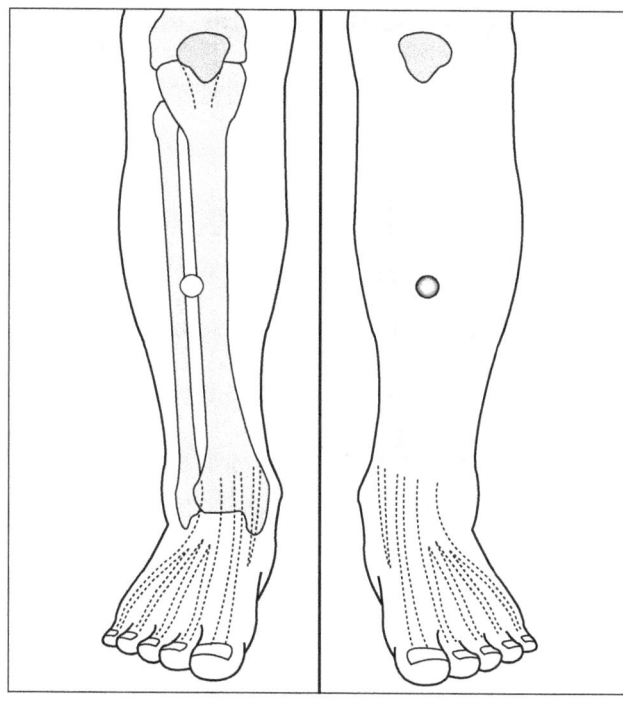

Location: On the antero-lateral side of the leg, 8 cun below ST-35 Dubi, one finger breadth (middle finger) from the anterior crest of the tibia.

Functions: Expels wind-damp, relieves pain, benefits the shoulder, unblocks obstructions in the channel.

Indications: Coldness, pain, weakness of the shoulder, muscular atrophy, weakness, numbness and pain of the lower extremities, swelling of the foot, spasms, motor impairment of the foot, motor impairment of the shoulder, abdominal pain.

Notes

Point Combinations

ST 39
XIAJUXU

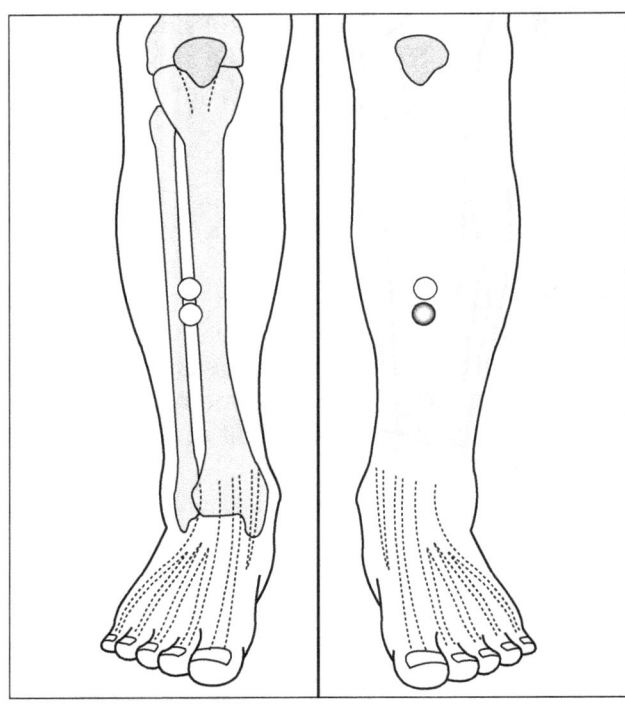

Location: On the antero-lateral side of the leg, 9 cun below ST-35 Dubi, one finger breadth (middle finger) from the anterior crest of the tibia.

Functions: Regulates the Qi of the Small Intestine, harmonizes the Intestines, resolves damp-heat, activates the channel, resolves stagnation, relieves pain.

Indications: Lower abdominal pain, back pain referring into the testis, mastitis, numbness and paralysis of the lower extremities, diarrhea, dysentery.

Attributes: Lower He-Sea point of the Small Intestine, point of the Sea of Blood.

Notes

_____
_____
_____
_____
_____
_____
_____
_____

Point Combinations

_____
_____
_____
_____
_____
_____
_____

ST 40
FENGLONG

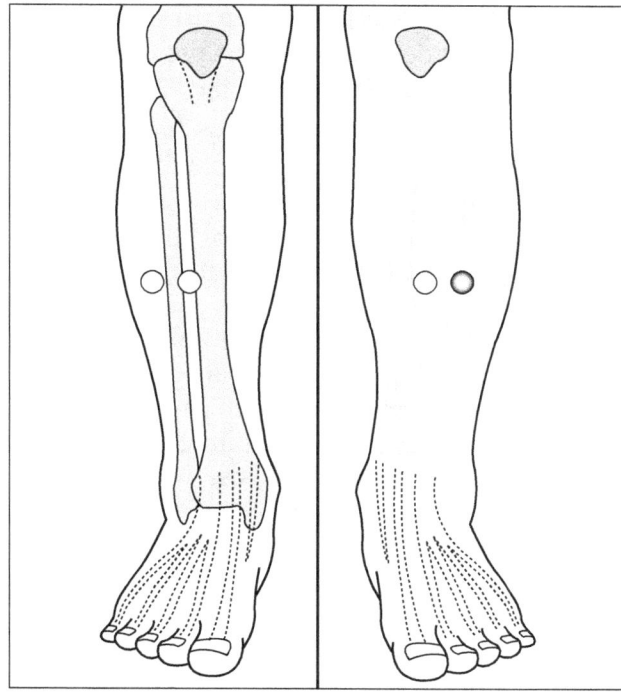

Location: On the anterolateral side of the leg, 8 cun above the tip of the external malleolus, lateral to ST-38 Tiaokou, and two finger breadths (middle finger) from the anterior crest of the tibia.

Functions: Transforms phlegm and dampness, benefits the chest, clears phlegm from the lungs and relieves cough and wheezing, activates the channel and relieves pain, clears phlegm from the Heart and calms the spirit.

Indications: Cough, excessive phlegm, asthma, headaches, dizziness, vertigo, mania, psychosis, epilepsy, paralysis or weakness of the lower extremities, constipation.

Attributes: Luo-Connecting point.

Notes

_____
_____
_____
_____
_____
_____
_____
_____

Point Combinations

_____
_____
_____
_____
_____
_____

ST 41
JIEXI

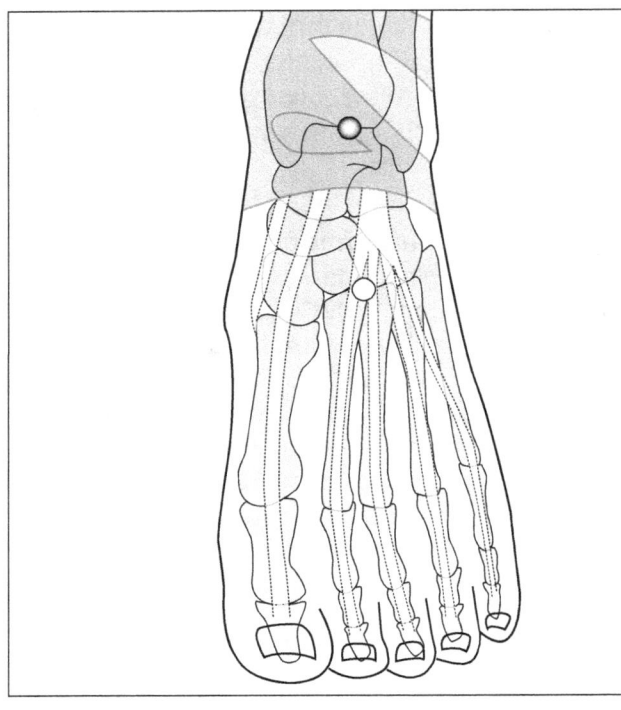

Location: On the transverse crease of the ankle, in the central depression of the crease between the dorsum of the foot and leg, between the tendons of the long extensor muscle of the great toe and the long extensor muscle of the toes.

Functions: Clears heat from the Stomach channel, calms the spirit, activates the channel, unblocks obstructions, relieves pain.

Indications: Pain of the ankle joint, muscular atrophy, motor impairment, pain and paralysis of the lower extremities, epilepsy, headaches, dizziness, vertigo, abdominal distention, constipation, mania, psychosis.

Attributes: Fire point, Jing River point, Tonifying point.

Notes

Point Combinations

ST 42
CHONGYANG

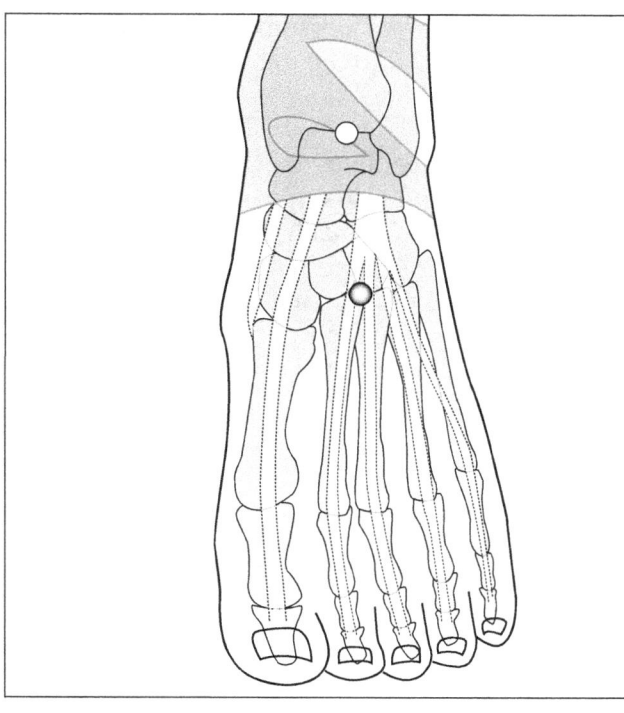

Location: On the dorsum of the foot (at the highest point), between the tendons of the long extensor muscle of the great toe and the long extensor muscle of the toes (between the 2nd and 3rd metatarsal bones.

Functions: Clears heat from the Stomach channel, harmonizes the Stomach, calms the spirit, activates the channel and relieves pain.
Indications: Gastric pain, abdominal distention, redness, swelling and pain around the dorsum of the foot, muscular atrophy and motor impairment of the foot, swelling of the face, facial paralysis, toothaches, activates the channel, stops pain.
Attributes: Yuan Source point, Exit point.

Notes

Point Combinations

ST 43
XIANGU

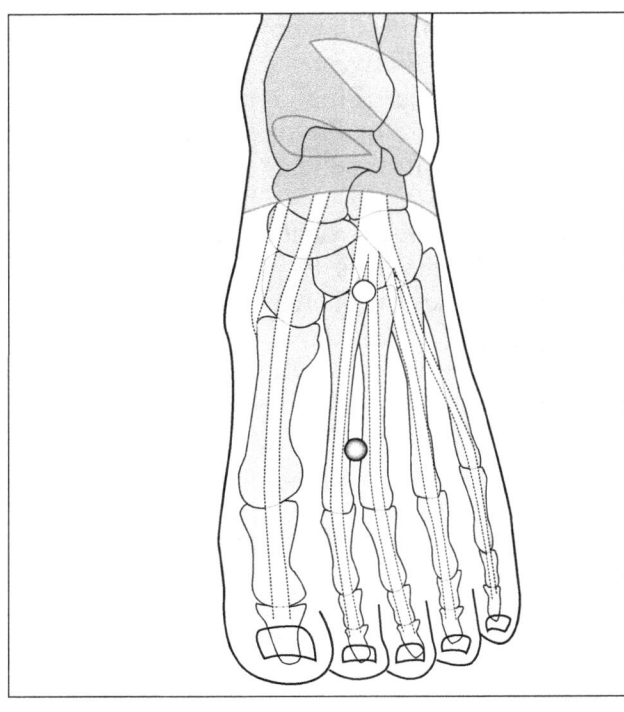

Location: On the dorsum of the foot, in the depression distal to the junction of the 2nd and 3rd metatarsal bones.

Functions: Regulates the Spleen and dispels edema, resolves dampness, regulates and harmonizes the Stomach and Intestines.

Indications: Abdominal pain, general or facial edema, myasthenia of the upper eyelid, difficulty opening the eyes, borborygmus, swelling and pain of the dorsum of the foot.

Attributes: Wood point, Shu Stream point.

Notes

Point Combinations

ST 44
NEITING

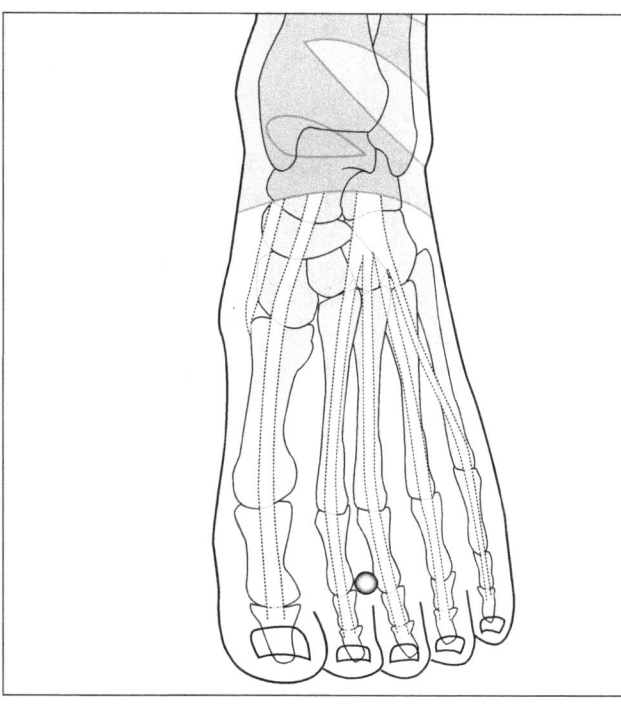

Location: On the dorsum of the foot, at the junction of the red and white skin 0.5 cun proximal to the margin of the web between the 2nd and 3rd metatarsal bones.

Functions: Clears heat from the Stomach channel, harmonizes the intestines, resolves damp heat in the Intestines, calms the spirit, relieves pain.

Indications: Toothache, pain in the face, sore throat, deviation of the mouth, epistaxis, febrile diseases, gastric pain, acid reflux, abdominal distention, diarrhea, dysentery, constipation, swelling and pain in the dorsum of the foot.

Attributes: Water point, Ying Spring point,

Notes

_____

_____

_____

_____

_____

_____

_____

_____

Point Combinations

_____

_____

_____

_____

_____

_____

ST 45
LIDUI

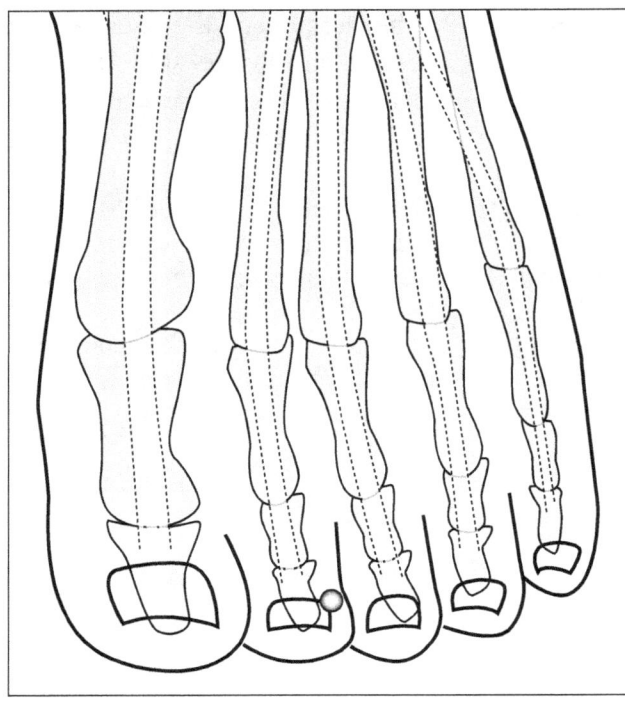

Location: On the lateral side of the distal segment of the 2nd toe, 0.1 cun from the corner of the nail.

Functions: Clears heat from the Stomach channel, calms the spirit and revives consciousness.

Indications: Swelling of the face, deviation of the mouth, toothache, febrile disease, sore throat, hoarse voice, epistaxis, dream disturbed sleep, mania, psychosis, abdominal distention, coldness in the leg and foot.

Attributes: Metal point, Jing Well point, Sedating point.

Notes

Point Combinations

SP 1
YINBAI

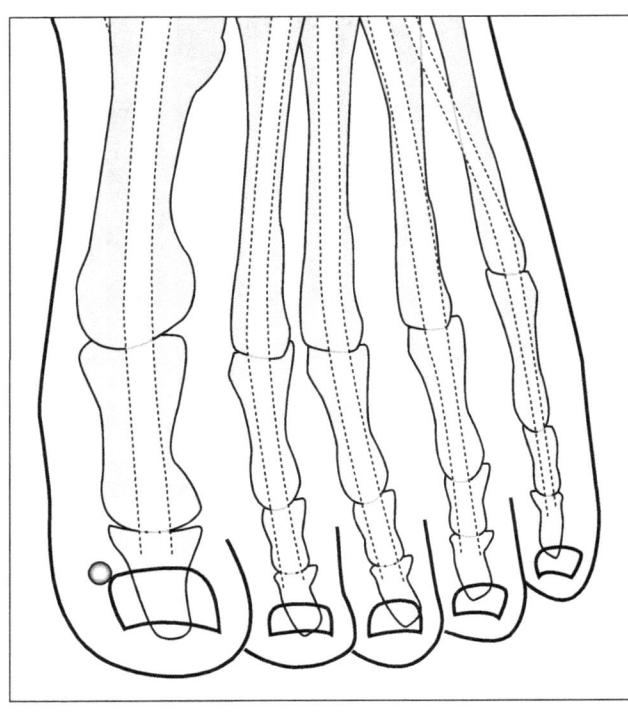

Location: On the medial side of the distal segment of the big toe, 0.1 cun from the corner of the toenail.

Functions: Regulates blood stasis especially in the uterus, warms yang, supports and strengthens Spleen, unblocks the chest, calms the Heart and shen.

Indications: Bleeding disorders seen in stool, urine, menstruation and nostrils, abdominal distension, dream disturbed sleep, mental disorders, convulsions.

Attributes: Wood point, Entry point, Jing Well point, Ghost point.

Notes

_____

_____

_____

_____

_____

_____

_____

_____

Point Combinations

_____

_____

_____

_____

_____

_____

SP 2
DADU

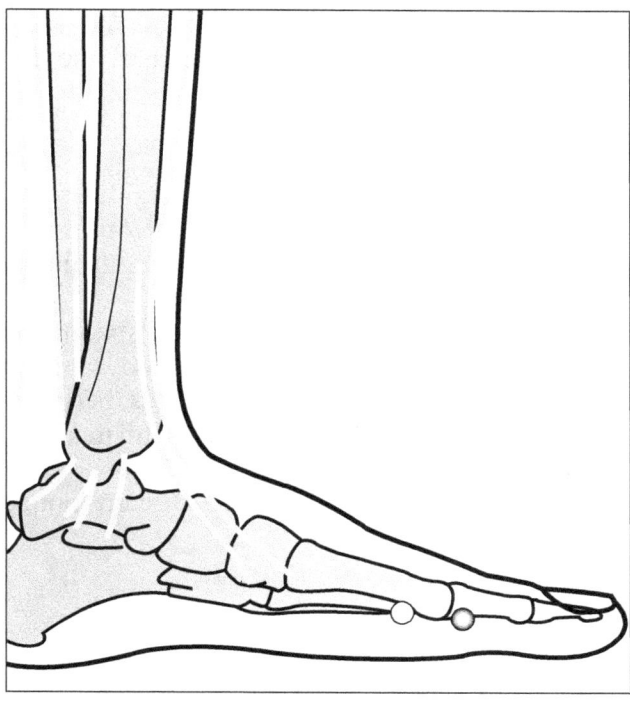

Location: On the medial side of the foot, in the depression anterior and inferior to the 1st metatarsaldigital joint of the big toe and the junction of the red and white skin.

Functions: Strengthens Spleen and balances Stomach, restores yang, clears heat, transforms damp and damp heat, promotes digestion.

Indications: Constipation, abdominal distension, gastric pain, cold feet, foot pain, lumbar pain with limited range of motion, febrile disease with absence of sweating, local point for gout.

Attributes: Fire point, Ying Spring point, Tonifying point.

Notes
_____
_____
_____
_____
_____
_____
_____
_____

Point Combinations
_____
_____
_____
_____
_____
_____
_____

SP 3
TAIBAI

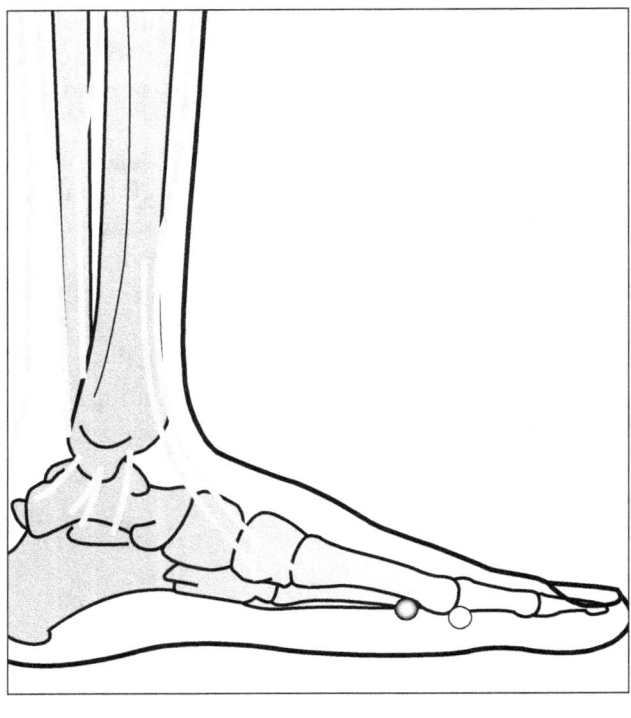

Location: On the medial side of the foot, proximal and inferior to the head of the 1st metatarsalphalangeal joint and the junction of the red and white skin.

Functions: Tonifies the Spleen, regulates Qi, transforms damp and damp heat, balances Spleen and Stomach, supports, strengthen and straightens the spine.

Indications: Constipation, abdominal distension, gastric pain, diarrhea, dysentery, vomiting, borborygmus, sluggishness, beriberi, mental obsessions, febrile disease with inability to lie down.

Attributes: Earth point, Shu Stream point, Yuan Source point.

Notes

Point Combinations

SP 4
GONGSUN

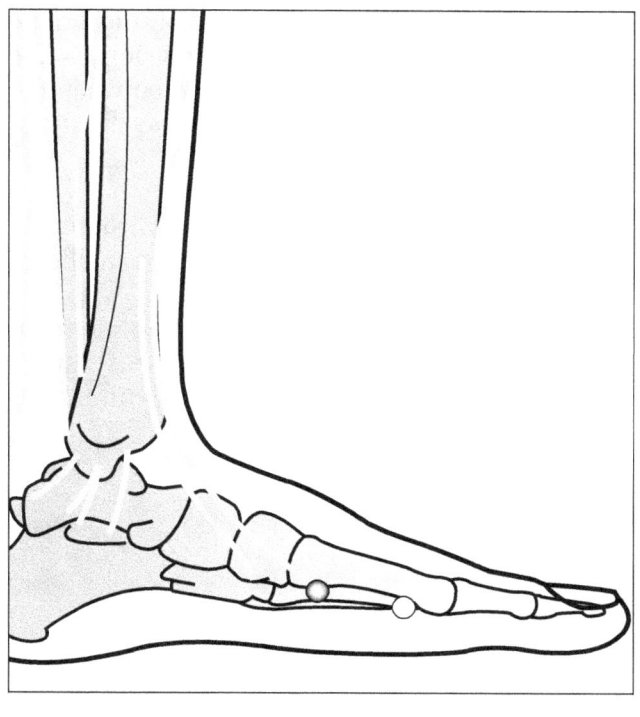

Location: On the medial side of the foot, anterior and inferior to the proximal end of the 1st metatarsal bone.

Functions: Tonifies Spleen and Stomach and balances middle jiao, manages Qi and transforms damp, assists Heart and chest, manages Penetrating Vessel and regulates menstruation and stops bleeding, manages Ren and synchronizes Du.

Indications: Abdominal distension, gastric pain, diarrhea, dysentery, undigested food in stools, vomiting, borborygmus, enteritis, endometriosis, amenorrhea, epilepsy, mania.

Attributes: Luo-Connecting point, Confluent point of the Penetrating Vessels, Master point of Pentrating Vessel.

*Great point for stomachache and gynecological issues.

Notes

_____

_____

_____

_____

_____

_____

_____

_____

Point Combinations

_____

_____

_____

_____

_____

_____

SP 5
SHANGQIU

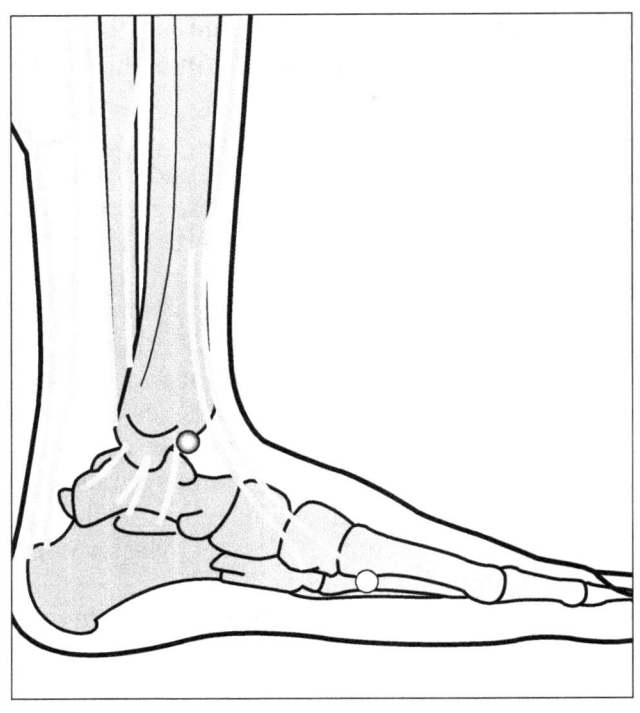

Location: On the medial side of the ankle, in the depression distal and inferior to the medial malleolus, at the midpoint between the tuberosity of the navicular bone and the tip of the medial malleolus.

Functions: Tonifies Spleen and Stomach, transforms damp and assists bones and tendons, calms shen.

Indications: Constipation, abdominal distension, borborygmus, diarrhea, ankle and knee pain, impaired speech, infertility, hemorrhoids.

Attributes: Metal point, Jing River point, Sedation point.

Notes

Point Combinations

SP 6
SANYINJIAO

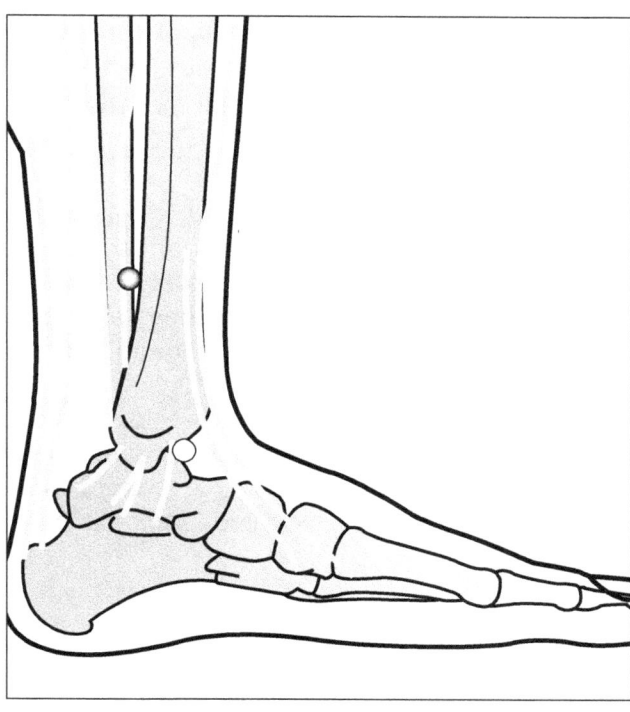

Location: On the medial side of the leg, 3 cun above the tip of the medial malleolus, in the depression posterior to the medial border of the tibia.

Functions: Tonifies the Spleen, Stomach and Kidneys, supports blood and yin, transforms damp, synchronizes the Liver and lower jiao and removes blockages in Qi of the Liver, manages menstruation and urination, assists the genitals, calms shen, cools and courses blood, stimulates the channel, reduces pain, induces labor.

Indications: Abdominal distension, gastric pain, diarrhea, dysentery, borborygmus, irregular menses or uterine bleeding, uterine prolapse, any issues involving sexual/reproductive organs and external genitalia, muscular atrophy, paralysis, motor impairment, and pain of the lower limbs, insomnia, vertigo, dizziness, eczema.

Attributes: Intersecting point of three Yin channels of the leg (Spleen, Liver, and Kidney)
*Contraindicated in pregnancy.

Notes

Point Combinations

SP 7
LOUGU

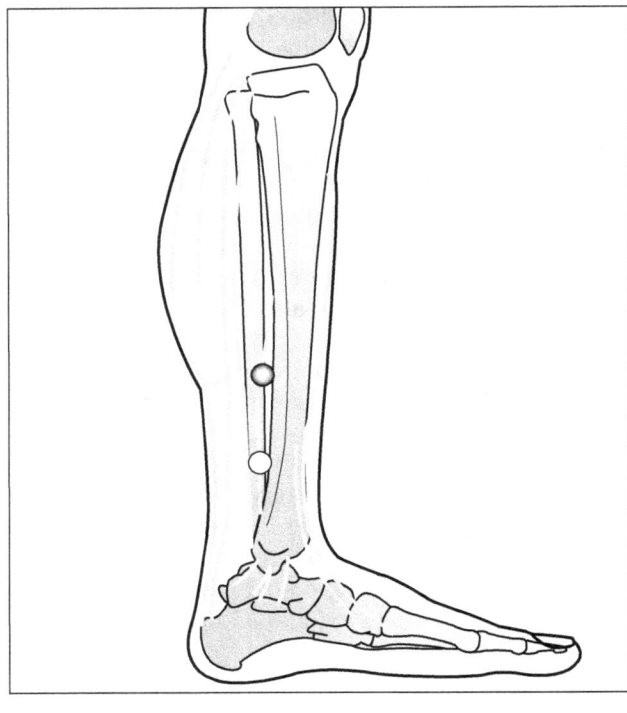

Location: On the medial side of the leg, 6 cun above the medial malleolus,on the line connecting the tip of the medial malleolus and SP-9 Yinlingquan.

Functions: Tonifies Spleen and synchronizes Spleen and Stomach, transforms damp, manages menses, manages Qi and blood, moves blood and reduces swelling, promotes urination, unblocks the channels and courses the connecting vessels.

Indications: Abdominal distension, borborygmus, bloody stools, numbness, paralysis of the knee and leg, convulsions, coldness, dreamed disturbed sleep, mental disorders.

Notes

_____

_____

_____

_____

_____

_____

_____

_____

Point Combinations

_____

_____

_____

_____

_____

_____

SP 8
DIJI

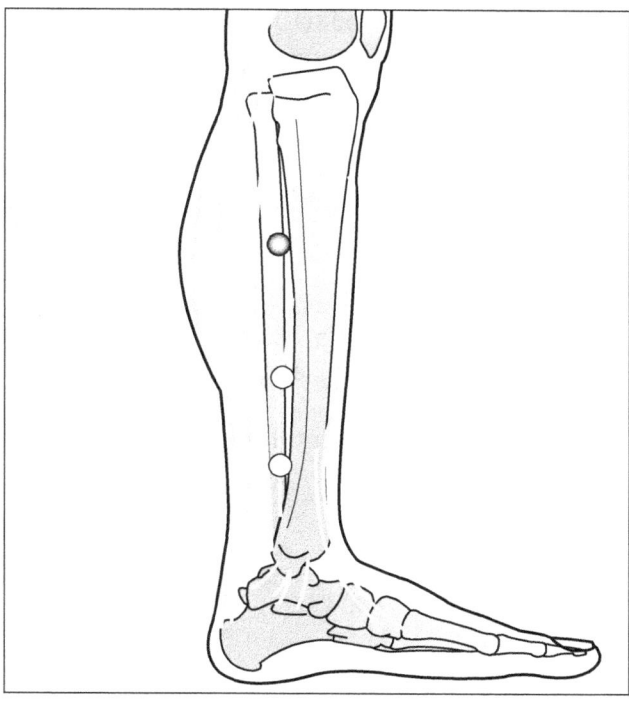

Location: On the medial side of the leg, 3 cun below Yinlingquan SP-9, on the line connecting the tip of the medial malleolus and SP-9 Yinlingquan.

Functions: Synchronizes the Spleen, removes blockages from the channel to reduce pain, manages uterus, manages Qi and blood.

Indications: Abdominal distension, gastric pain, dysuria, diarrhea, nocturnal emissions, irregular or painful menstruation, edema of abdomen or legs, emotional blockages.

Attributes: Xi-Cleft point.

Notes

_____
_____
_____
_____
_____
_____
_____
_____
_____

Point Combinations

_____
_____
_____
_____
_____
_____
_____

SP 9
YINLINGQUAN

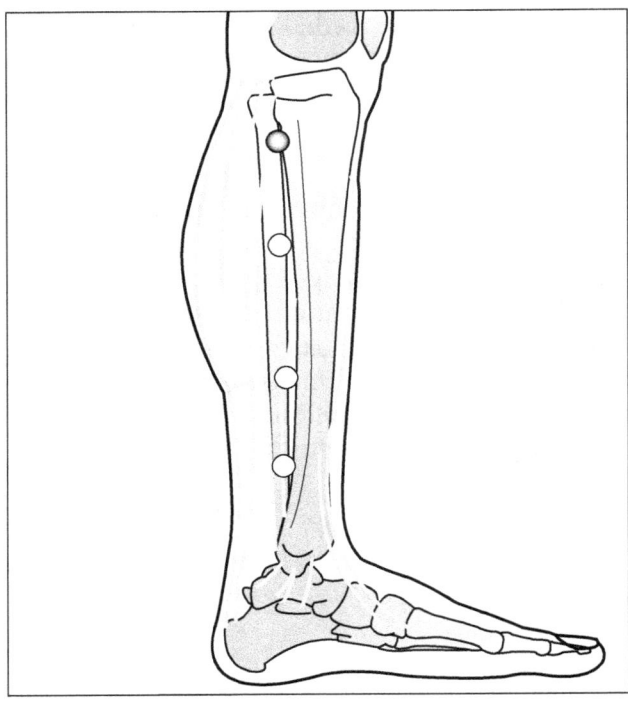

Location: On the medial side of the leg, in the depression posterior and inferior to the medial condyle of the tibia.

Functions: Clears damp from lower jiao, courses and warms middle jiao, assists lower jiao, assists urination, unblocks channel, reduces pain.

Indications: Abdominal distension and pain, pain in genitals, edema, ascites, incontinence or retention of urine, loose stool with undigested food.

Attributes: Water point, He-Sea point
* Good point for leukorrhea.

Notes

Point Combinations

SP 10
XUEHAI

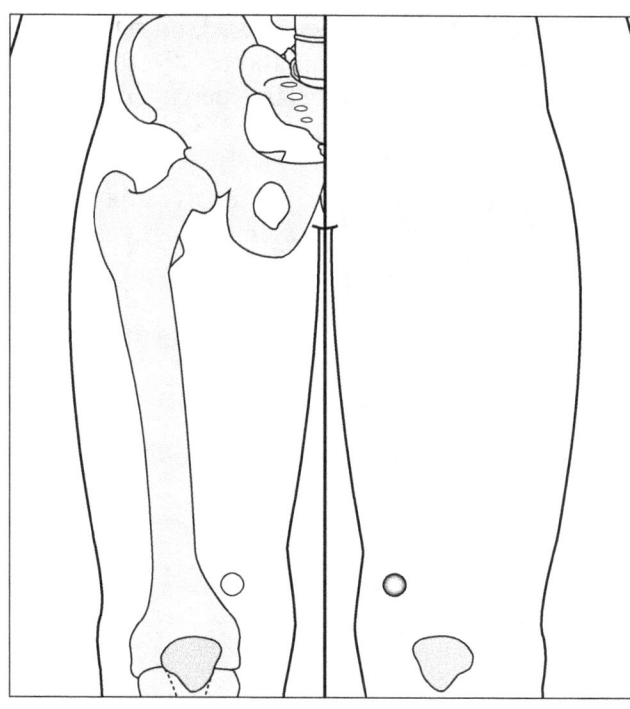

Location: With the knee flexed, on the medial side of the thigh, 2 cun above the superior medial corner of the patella, on the prominence of the medial head of the quadriceps muscle of the thigh.

Functions: Manages, courses and tonifies blood, removes stasis, cools blood, manages menstruation, supports lower jiao.

Indications: Amenorrhea, irregular menses, dysmenorrhea, uterine bleeding, any skin disease, urticarial, pain of the medial thigh.

Notes

Point Combinations

SP 11
JIMEN

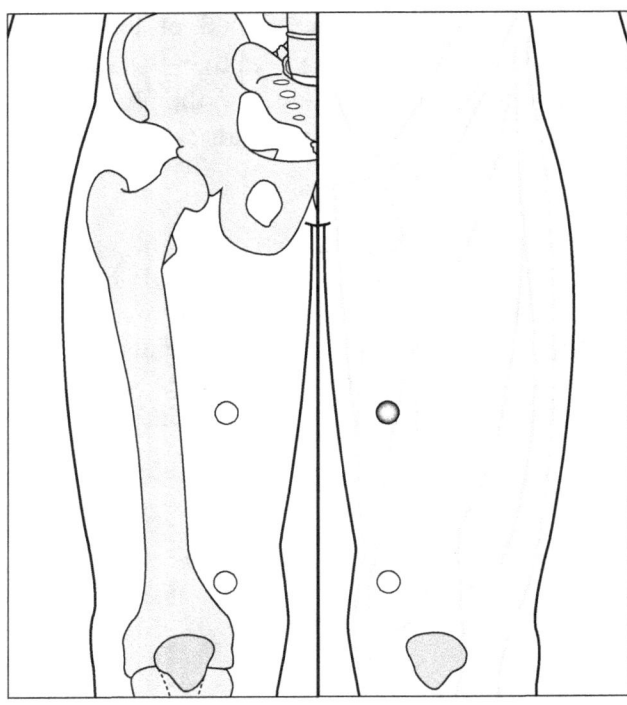

Location: With the knee flexed, on the medial side of the thigh, 6 cun above SP-10 Xuehai, on the line joining SP-10 Xuehai and SP-12 Chongmen.

Functions: Manages urine, resolves damp and clears heat, unblocks water passageways and calms shen.

Indications: Pain, paralysis, motor impairment, and muscular atrophy of the lower extremities.

Notes

Point Combinations

SP 12
CHONGMEN

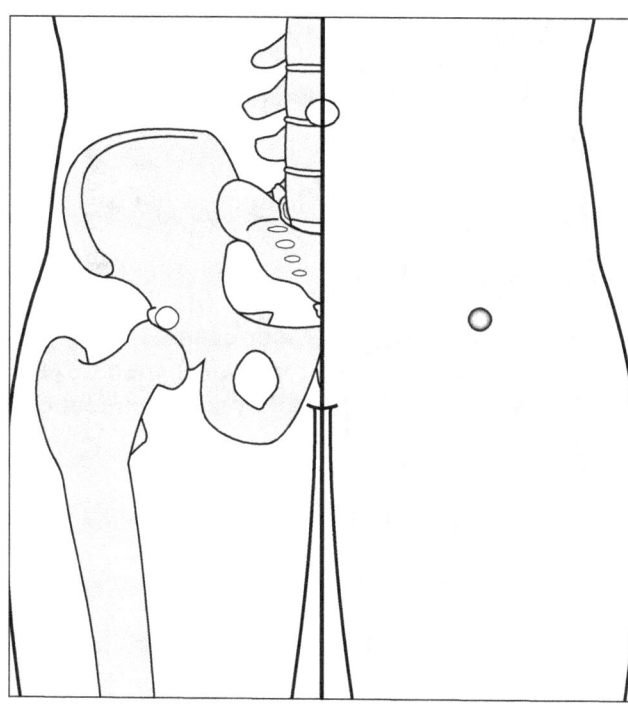

Location: On the abdomen, at the lateral end of the inguinal groove, 3.5 cun lateral to the anterior midline (level with the pubic symphysis).

Functions: Builds yin, removes channel blockages, manages Qi and clears heat and resolves damp.

Indications: Hernia, abdominal pain, hemorrhoid related pain, difficult lactation, dysuria.

Attributes: Meeting point for the Yin Linking Vessel and Spleen and Liver channels.

*Caution: may puncture the femoral artery in a medial direction and the femoral nerve in a lateral direction.

Notes

Point Combinations

SP 13
FUSHE

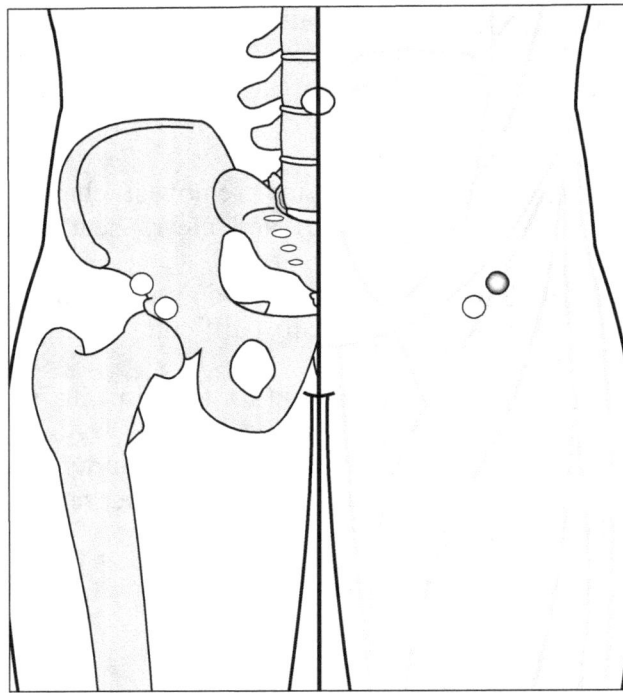

Location: On the abdomen, 4.3 cun below the center of the umbilicus, 2 cun lateral to the anterior midline. (0.7 laterosuperior to SP-12 Chongmen)

Functions: Courses Qi and sedates Liver, reduces pain.
Indications: Hernia, lower abdominal pain.
Attributes: Meeting point for the Yin Linking Vessel and Spleen and Liver channels.
*Caution: Deep needling can penetrate the peritoneal cavity, especially on thin patients.

Notes

Point Combinations

SP 14
FUJIE

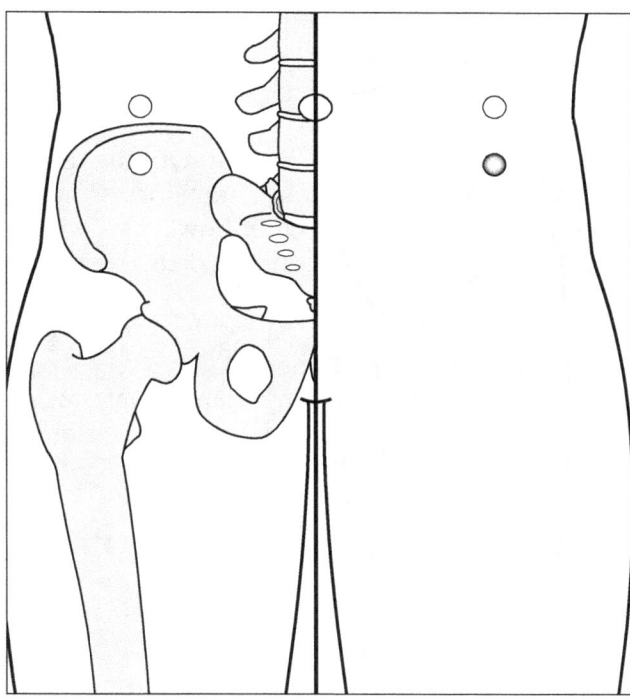

Location: On the abdomen, on the lateral side of the rectus abdominis muscle, 4 cun lateral to the anterior midline (1.3 cun below SP-15 Daheng).

Functions: Warms the middle and drives out cold, corrects Qi, courses counterflow downward.

Indications: Hernia, abdominal distention, pain in umbilical region, constipation, diarrhea.

Attributes: *Caution: Deep needling can penetrate the peritoneal cavity, especially on thin patients.

Notes
_____
_____
_____
_____
_____
_____
_____
_____

Point Combinations
_____
_____
_____
_____
_____
_____

SP 15
DAHENG

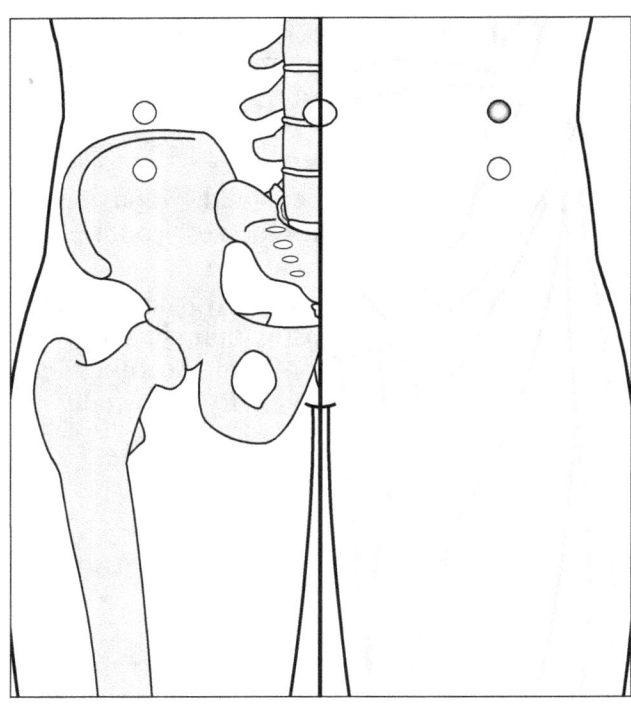

Location: On the abdomen, on the lateral side of the rectus abdominis muscle, 4 cun lateral to the center of the umbilicus.

Functions: Nourishes Spleen Qi, the limbs and function of Intestines, transforms damp, reduces pain, unblocks Qi of bowels.

Indications: Constipation, diarrhea, dysentery, abdominal distention and pain.

Attributes: Meeting point for the Yin Linking Vessel and Spleen channel.

*Caution: Deep needling can penetrate an enlarged Spleen or Liver, or the peritoneal cavity, especially on thin patients.

Notes

Point Combinations

SP 16
FUAI

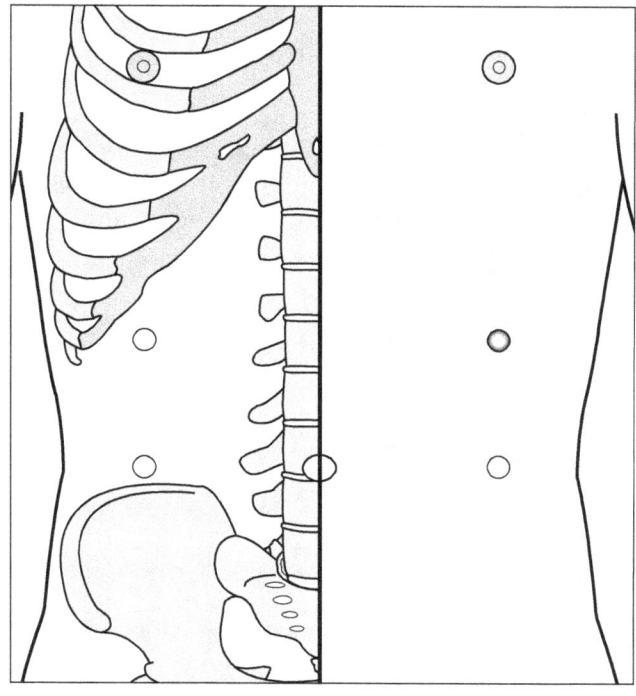

Location: On the abdomen, 3 cun above the center of the umbilicus, 4 cun lateral to the anterior midline.

Functions: Manages the function of Intestines, transforms damp and clears heat, unblocks Qi of bowels.

Indications: Constipation, diarrhea, dysentery and abdominal pain.

Attributes: Meeting point for the Yin Linking Vessel and Spleen channel.

Notes
_____
_____
_____
_____
_____
_____
_____
_____
_____

Point Combinations
_____
_____
_____
_____
_____
_____
_____

SP 17
SHIDOU

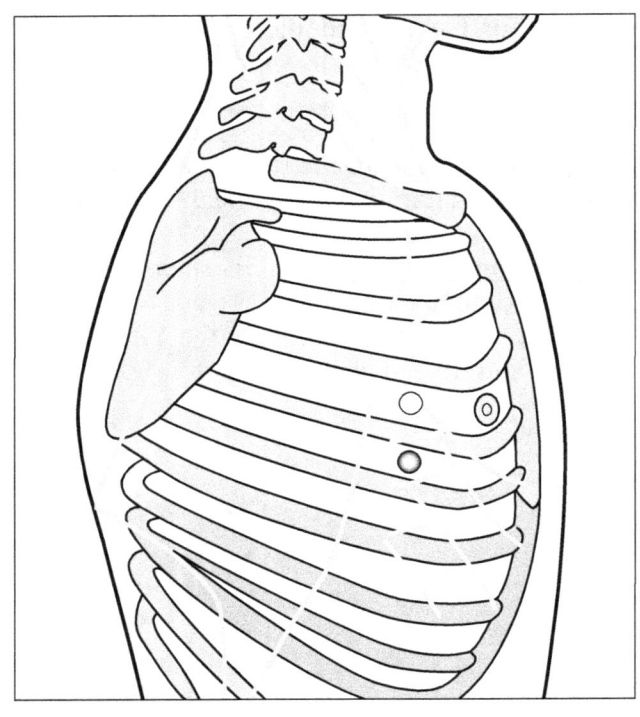

Location: On the chest, in the 5th intercostal space, 6 cun lateral to the anterior midline.

Functions: Correct Qi, unblocks water passageways, remove blockages from the 3 jiaos, assist digestion and dislodge food stasis.
Indications: Chest and hypochondrium pain and fullness.

Notes

Point Combinations

SP 18
TIANXI

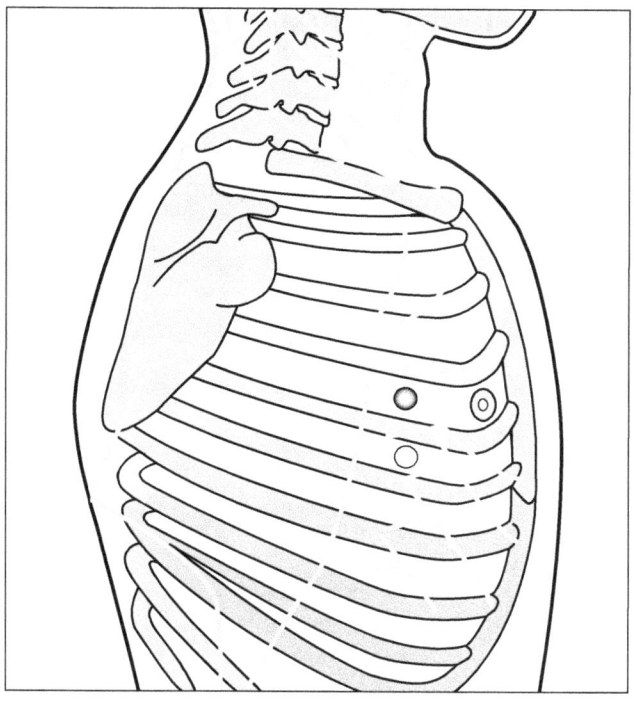

Location: On the chest, in the 4th intercostal space, 6 cun lateral to the anterior midline.

Functions: Unbinds the chest, assists the breast and lactation, corrects Qi and courses counterflow downward, reduces cough.

Indications: Chest and hypochondrium pain and fullness, hiccup, cough, mastitis.

Notes

_____
_____
_____
_____
_____
_____
_____
_____
_____

Point Combinations

_____
_____
_____
_____
_____
_____
_____

SP 19
XIONGXIANG

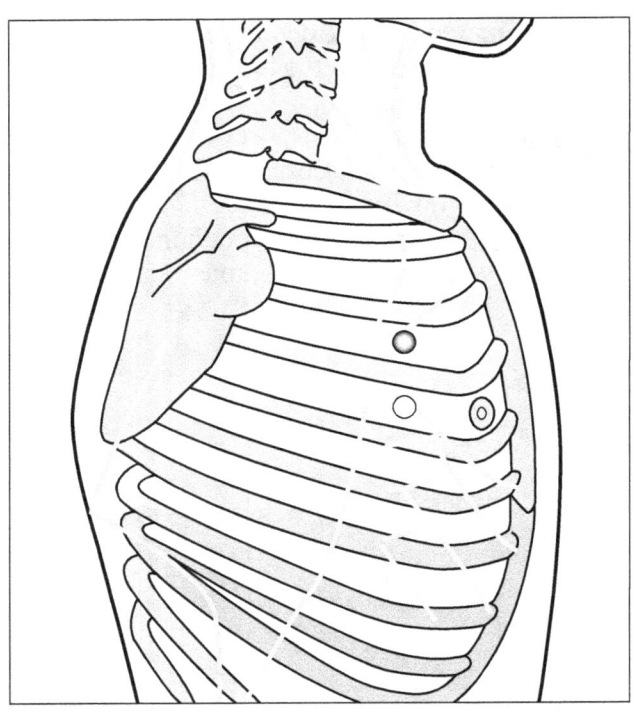

Location: On the chest, in the 3rd intercostal space, 6 cun lateral to the anterior midline.

Functions: Manages Qi and courses counterflow, directs Qi of Lung downward.

Indications: Chest and hypochondrium pain and fullness, dyspnea, cough.

Notes

Point Combinations

SP 20
ZHOURONG

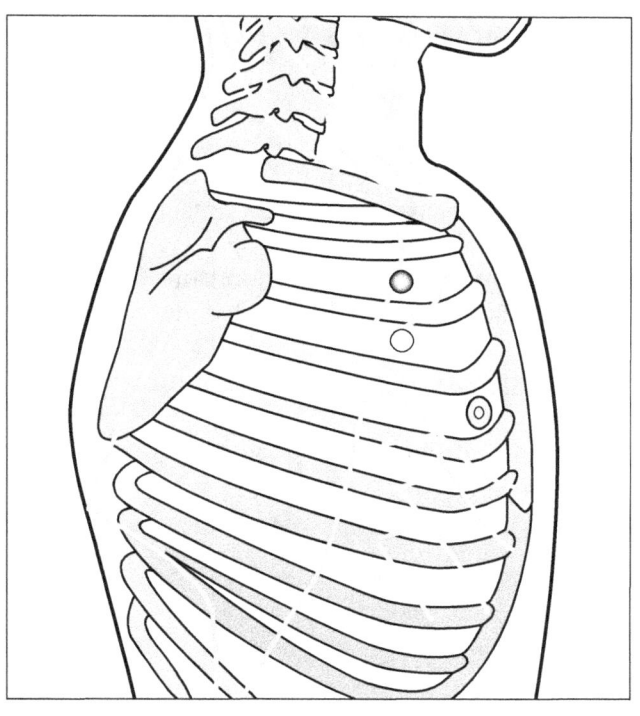

Location: On the chest, in the 2nd intercostal space, 6 cun lateral to the anterior midline.

Functions: Unbinds the chest, manages Qi and courses counterflow, directs Qi of Lung downward.

Indications: Chest, hypochondrium, and lateral costal pain and fullness, hiccup, cough.

Notes

_____
_____
_____
_____
_____
_____
_____
_____
_____

Point Combinations

_____
_____
_____
_____
_____
_____
_____

SP 21
DABAO

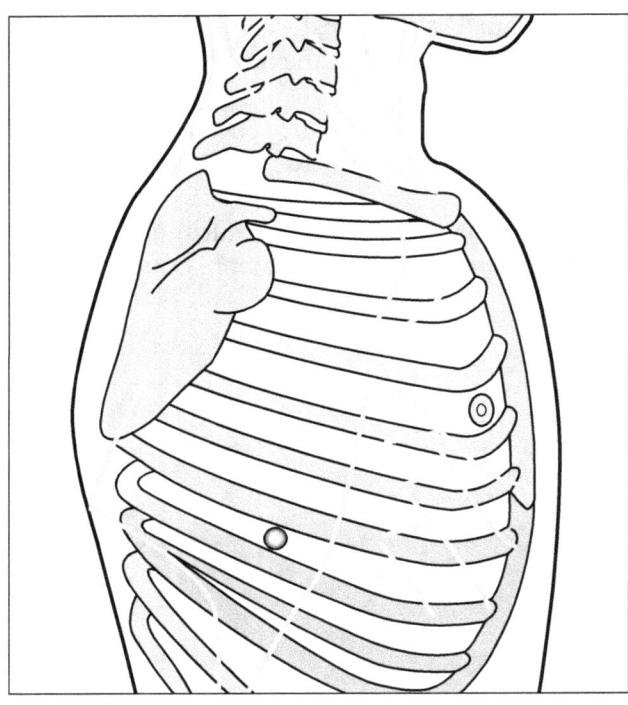

Location: On the lateral side of the chest and on the middle axilary line, in the 6th intercostal space.

Functions: Manages Qi and blood, courses blood in the channels, assist muscles, tendons, joints and ligaments.

Indications: Chest, hypochondrium, and lateral costal pain, body aches and general soreness and weakness, cough, asthma.

Attributes: Great Luo-Connecting point, Exit point.

*Caution of inducing a pneumothorax.

Notes

Point Combinations

HT 1
JIQUAN

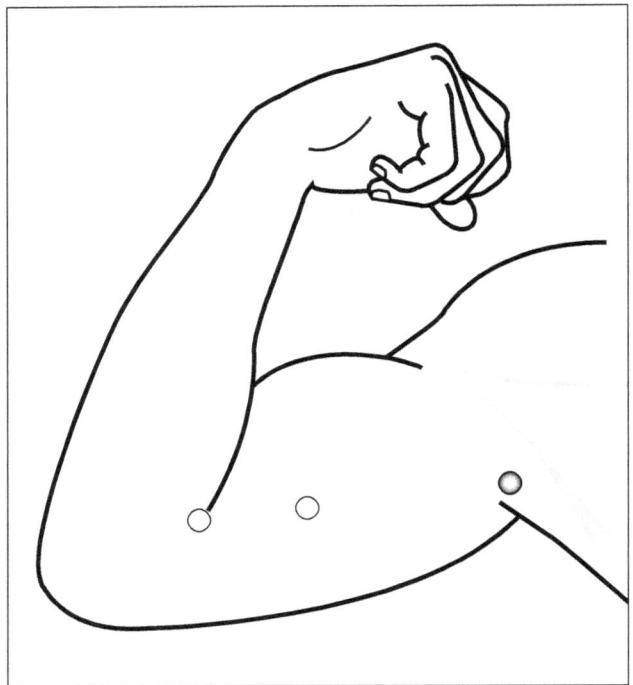

Location: In the center of the axilla, on the radial side of the axillary artery.

Functions: Supports yin of the Heart, sedates deficient heat.

Indications: Issues relating to the armpit.

Notes

Point Combinations

HT 2
QINGLING

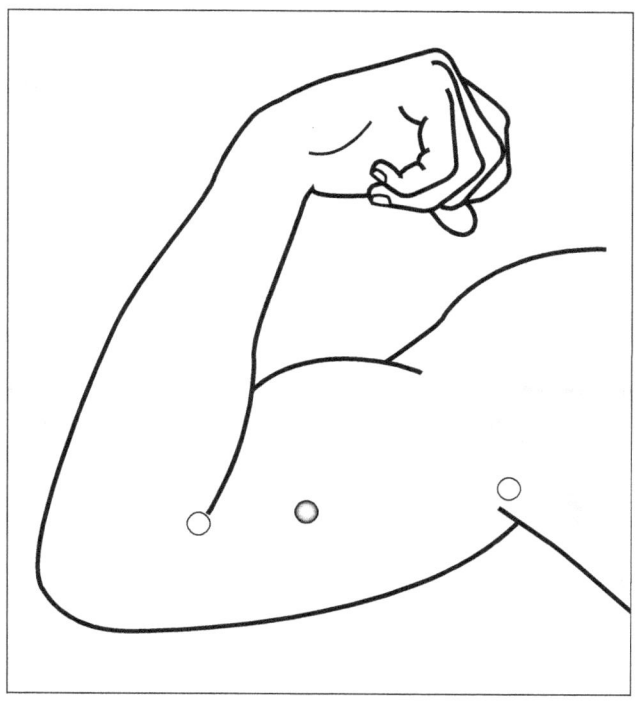

Location: On the medial side of the arm, 3 cun above the transverse cubital crease, on the line joining HT-1 Jiquan and HT-3 Shaohai (in the groove medial to biceps brachii muscle).

Functions: Manages Qi and blood, removes blockages from the channel, reduces pain, stimulates the Ren channel.

Indications: Pain in the cardiac, shoulder, arm and hypochondrium areas.

Notes

_____
_____
_____
_____
_____
_____
_____
_____

Point Combinations

_____
_____
_____
_____
_____
_____

HT 3
SHAOHAI

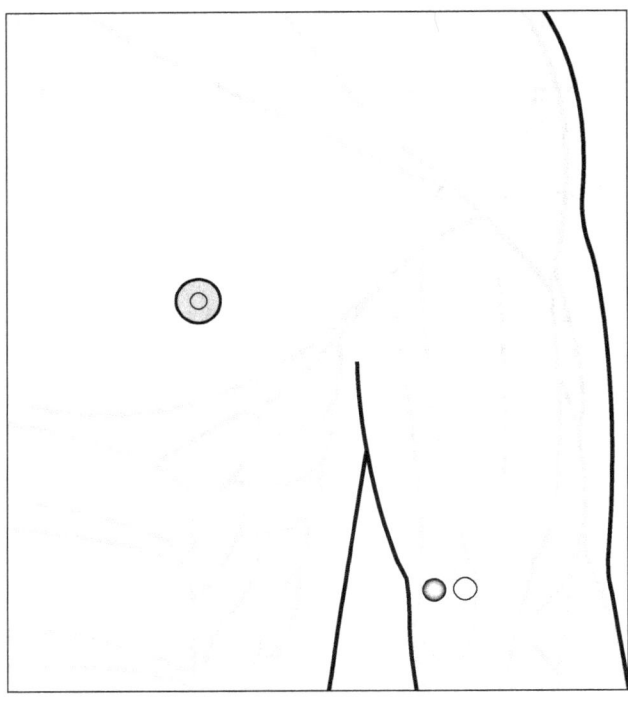

Location: With the elbow flexed, the point is at the midpoint on the line connecting the ulnar end of the cubital crease and the medial epicondyle of the humerus.

Functions: Remove blockages from the channel, calms shen, clears heat, deficient Heart heat and Heart fire, moves and manages Heart Qi and blood, unblocks Pericardium, rectify drooling.

Indications: Cardiac, hypochondrium region and axilla pain, spasm and numbness of upper extremity, scrofula, tremor on the hand.

Attributes: Water point, He-Sea point

*Good point for shaking and trembling from Parkinson's.

Notes

_____

_____

_____

_____

_____

_____

_____

_____

Point Combinations

_____

_____

_____

_____

_____

_____

_____

HT 4
LINGDAO

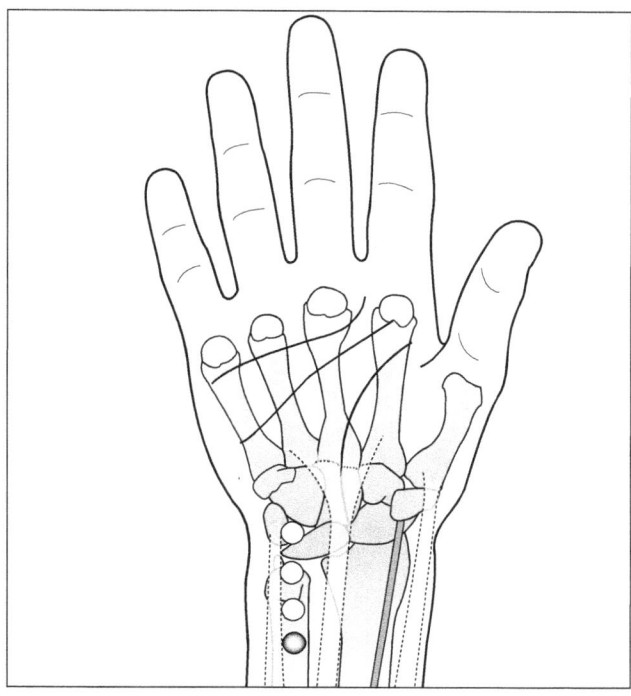

Location: On the palmar side of the forearm and on the radial side of the tendon of the ulnar flexor muscle of the wrist, 1.5 cun proximal to the crease of the wrist.

Functions: Remove blockages from the channel, stimulates the connecting vessel, tendons and ligaments, calms shen.

Indications: Bradycardia, aphasia, emotionally related stuttering, anxiety, cardiac, arm and elbow pain, arthritis.

Attributes: Metal point, Jing River point
* Main point for difficulty in speaking.

Notes

Point Combinations

HT 5
TONGLI

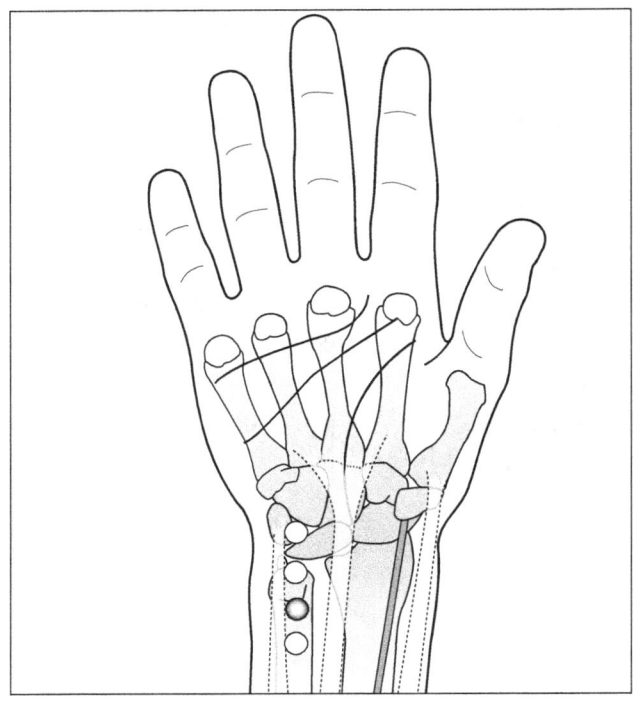

Location: On the palmar side of the forearm and on the radial side of the tendon of the ulnar flexor muscle of the wrist, 1 cun proximal to the crease of the wrist.

Functions: Supports Qi of Heart, calms shen, assists bladder, opens the tongue.

Indications: Sore throat, blurred vision, dizziness, aphasia and tongue stiffness, palpitations, elbow and wrist pain.

Attributes: Luo-Connecting point.

*Main point for building Heart Qi.

Notes

_____

_____

_____

_____

_____

_____

_____

Point Combinations

_____

_____

_____

_____

_____

HT 6
YINXI

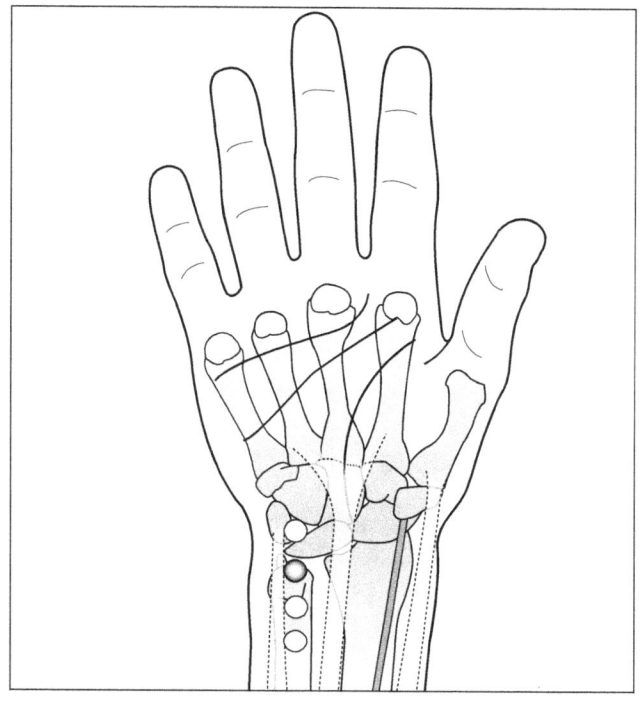

Location: On the palmar side of the forearm and on the radial side of the tendon of the ulnar flexor muscle of the wrist, 0.5 cun proximal to the crease of the wrist.

Functions: Sedates heat and Heart fire, supports yin of the Heart, restricts sweating, calms shen.

Indications: Night sweats, epistaxis, hemoptysis, aphasia, hysteria, cardiac pain.

Attributes: Xi-Cleft point.

Notes

_____
_____
_____
_____
_____
_____
_____
_____
_____

Point Combinations

_____
_____
_____
_____
_____
_____

HT 7
SHENMEN

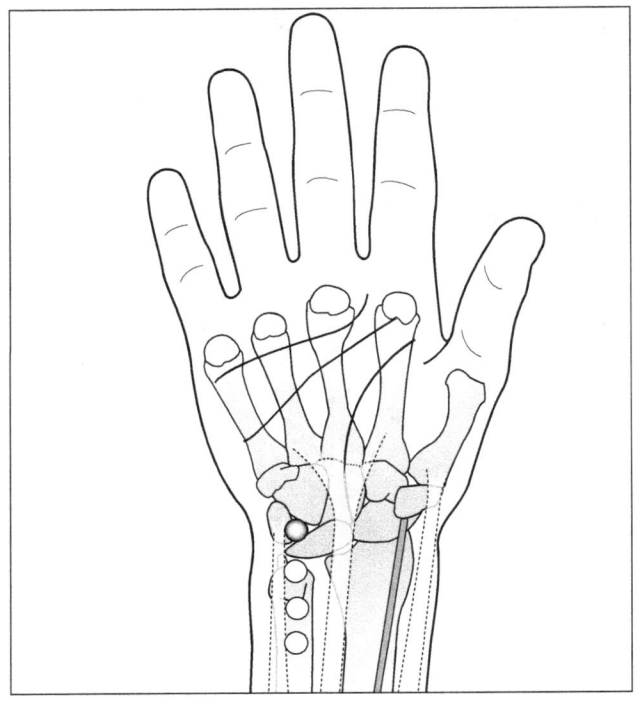

Location: On the wrist, at the ulnar end of the crease of the wrist, in the depression on the radial side of the tendon of the ulnar flexor muscle of the wrist.

Functions: Builds blood of the Heart, manages counterflow of Qi, relaxes Heart and calms shen and sedates heat and fire.

Indications: Insomnia, irritability, dementia, hysteria, epilepsy, mania, amnesia, cardiac pain and palpitations, yellowing of the eyes, sweaty palms.

Attributes: Earth point, Shu Stream point, Yuan source point.

Notes

Point Combinations

HT 8
SHAOFU

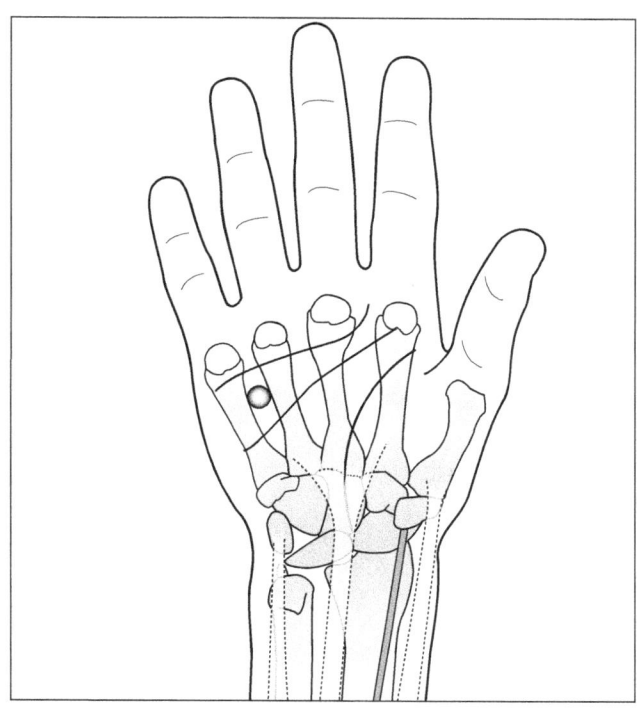

Location: In the palm, between the 4th and 5th metacarpal bones, at the part of the palm touching the tip of the little finger when a fist is made.

Functions: Sedates fire, phlegm fire, and deficient heat of the Heart, relaxes Heart and shen.

Indications: Itching of groin, ulcers of the tongue, sweaty palms, dark urine, dysuria, enuresis, chest pain and palpitations, mental restlessness, spasm in little finger.

Attributes: Ying Spring point.

Notes

_____
_____
_____
_____
_____
_____
_____
_____
_____

Point Combinations

_____
_____
_____
_____
_____
_____
_____

HT 9
SHAOCHONG

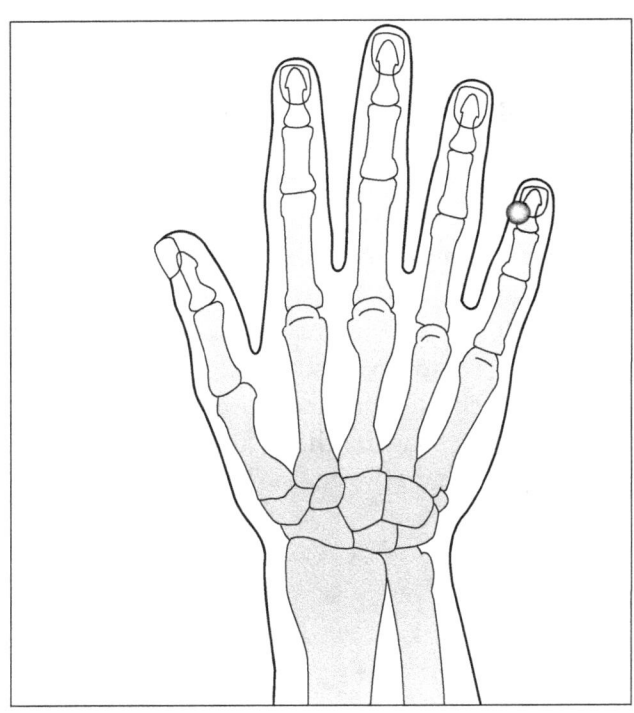

Location: On the radial side of the distal segment of the little finger, 0.1 cun from the corner of the nail.

Functions: Opens the Heart, sedates wind, heat and pathogenic heat, restores consciousness, rcalms shen.

Indications: Cardiac, chest, and hypochondrium region pain and palpitations, fever, mania, coma.

Attributes: Wood point, Jing Well point, Exit point.

*Resuscitation point.

Notes

_____
_____
_____
_____
_____
_____
_____
_____

Point Combinations

_____
_____
_____
_____
_____
_____

SI 1
SHAOZE

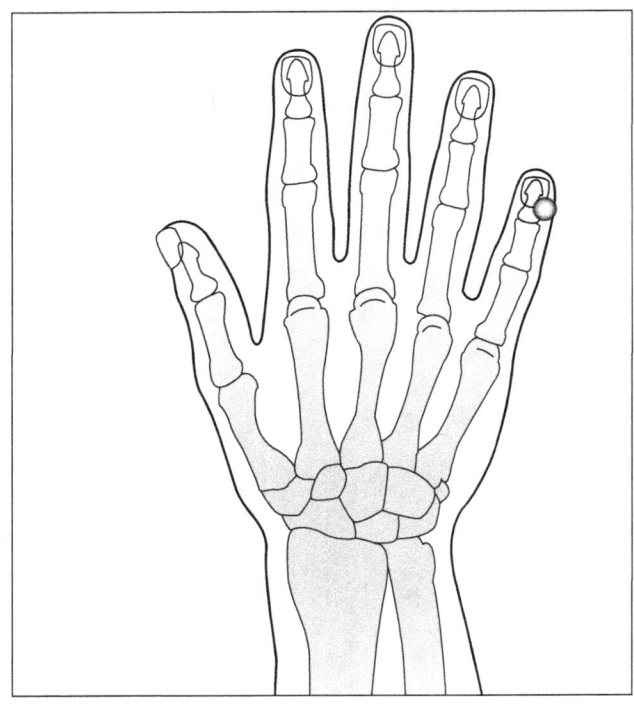

Location: On the ulnar side of the distal segment of the little finger, 0.1 cun from the corner of the nail.

Functions: Expels wind-heat, settles wind, promotes lactation, removes blockages in the channel, clears Heart fire, opens orifices.

Indications: Loss of consciousness, headache, febrile disease, fore throat, red eyes, cloudiness of the cornea, insufficient lactation.

Attributes: Metal point, Jing Well point, Entry point.
*Resuscitation point.

Notes
_____
_____
_____
_____
_____
_____
_____
_____

Point Combinations
_____
_____
_____
_____
_____
_____

SI 2
QIANGU

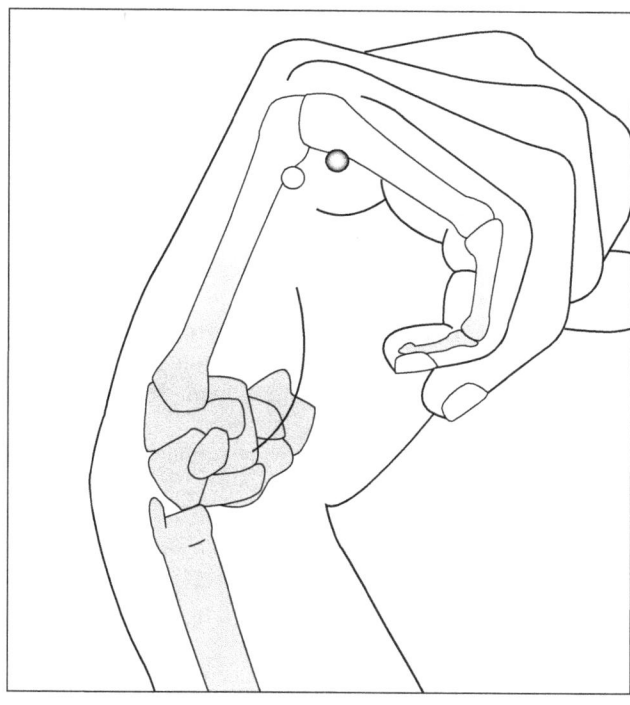

Location: On the ulnar side of the little finger, at the junction of the red and white skin along the ulnar border of the hand, at the ulnar end of the crease distal to the 5th metacarpophalangeal joint when a loose fist is made.

Functions: Sedates heat.

Indications: Febrile disease, tinnitus, red urine or burning sensation during urination, numbness of the fingers.

Attributes: Water point, Ying Spring point.

Notes

Point Combinations

SI 3
HOUXI

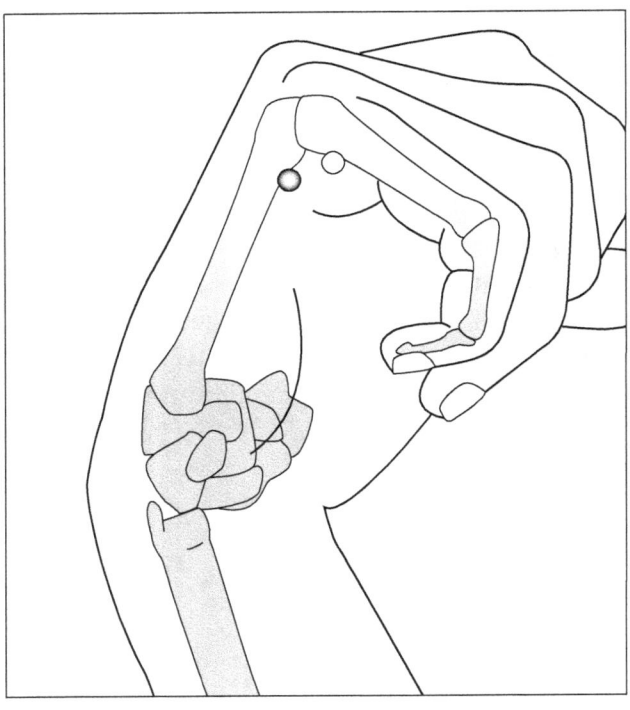

Location: On the ulnar side of the little finger, at the junction of the red and white skin along the ulnar border of the hand, at the ulnar end of the distal palmar crease, proximal to the 5th metacarpophalangeal joint when a loose fist is made.

Functions: Extinguishes exterior wind, extinguishes interior wind from Du channel, sedates interior heat, resolves damp, relieves pain, relieves the exterior, relaxes and benefits tendons and ligaments, calms shen.

Indications: Deafness, tinnitus, sore throat, stiff neck, seizures, mania, psychosis, low back pain, febrile disease, numb fingers, contracted fingers, pain in shoulder or elbow, malaria, night sweats, jaundice.

Attributes: Wood point, Shu Stream point, and Tonification point.

*Master point of Du Mai.

** Great point for whiplash and frozen shoulder.

Notes

Point Combinations

SI 4
WANGU

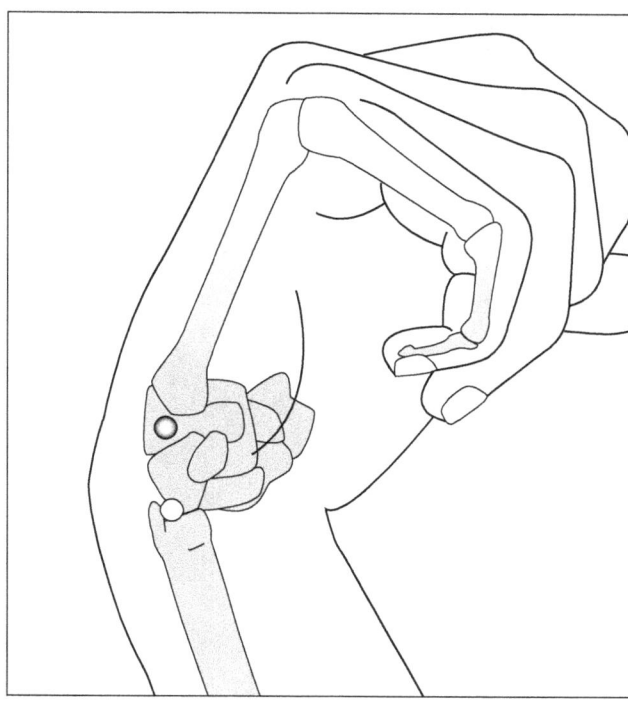

Location: On the ulnar border of the hand, in the depression between the proximal end of the 5th metacarpal bone and hamate bone, and at the junction of the red and white skin.

Functions: Resolves damp, clears heat, opens channels.

Indications: Occipital headache, neck stiffness, contracture of the fingers, pain in the wrist, headache, febrile disease with out perspiration, jaundice.

Attributes: Yuan source point.

Notes

_____
_____
_____
_____
_____
_____
_____
_____
_____

Point Combinations

_____
_____
_____
_____
_____
_____
_____

SI 5
YANGGU

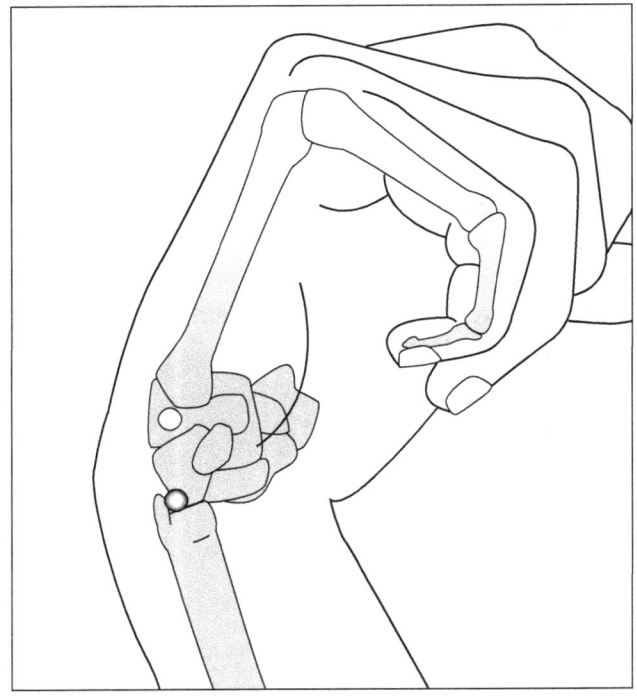

Location: On the ulnar side of the tranverse wrist crease, in the depression between the styloid process of the ulna and the triquetral bone.

Functions: Opens the channel, clears and focuses the mind, extinguishes exterior damp heat and swelling, clears wind heat.

Indications: Febrile disease, pain of the hand and wrist.

Attributes: Fire point, Jing River point, Horary point.

Notes

_____

_____

_____

_____

_____

_____

_____

_____

Point Combinations

_____

_____

_____

_____

_____

_____

SI 6
YANGLAO

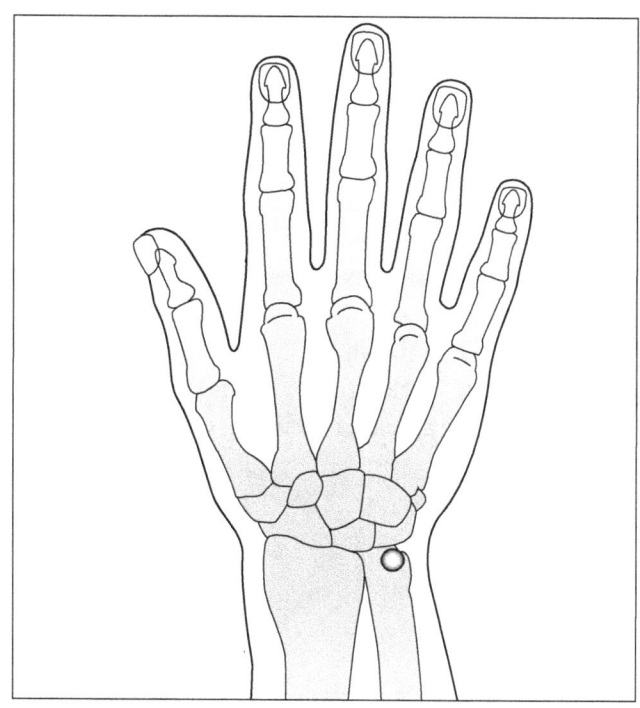

Location: On the dorsal, ulnar aspect of the forearm, in the depression on the radial side of the styloid process of the ulna.

Functions: Removes blockages from the channel, relaxes and benefits the muscles, brightens the eyes, benefits joints.

Indications: Acute low back pain, whiplash, arthritis, pain of the shoulder, elbow or arm, hernia, blurred vision.

Attributes: Xi-cleft point.

Notes

_____

_____

_____

_____

_____

_____

_____

_____

Point Combinations

_____

_____

_____

_____

_____

_____

SI 7
ZHIZHENG

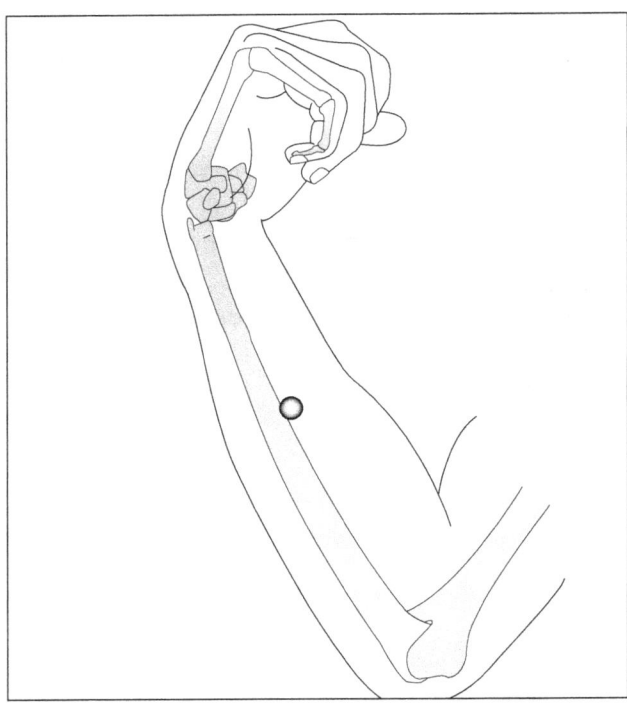

Location: On the dorsal, ulnar aspect of the forearm, 5 cun above the tranverse wrist crease of the wrist, on the line joining SI-5 Yanggu and SI-8 Xiaohai.

Functions: Clears the mind, calms the Heart, removes blockages from the channel, clears exterior heat and extinguishes wind, induces perspiration.

Indications: Pain and spasm of the elbow and fingers, stiff neck, mania, depression, anxiety, headache, dizziness, febrile disease.

Notes

_____

_____

_____

_____

_____

_____

_____

Point Combinations

_____

_____

_____

_____

_____

_____

SI 8
XIAOHAI

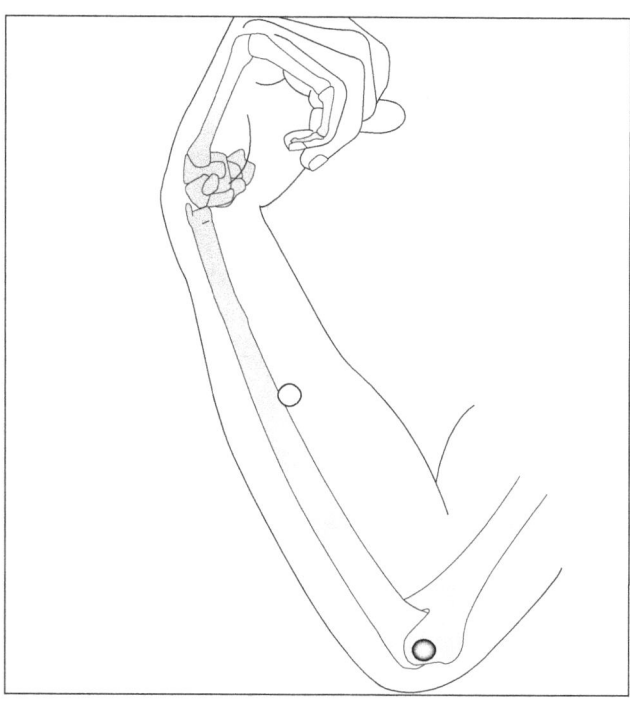

Location: With the elbow flexed, the point is on the medial side of the elbow, in the depression between the olecranon of the ulna and the medial epicondyle of the humerus.

Functions: Clears heat from the Small Intestine and tai yang, drains damp and clears heat.

Indications: Headache, swelling of the cheek or jaw, pain in neck, nape, shoulder, arm, elbow, nerve pain or numbness of the ulnar nerve, psychosis, epilepsy, seizures.

Attributes: Earth point, He-Sea point, Sedation point.

Notes

_____
_____
_____
_____
_____
_____
_____
_____
_____

Point Combinations

_____
_____
_____
_____
_____
_____

SI 9
JIANZHEN

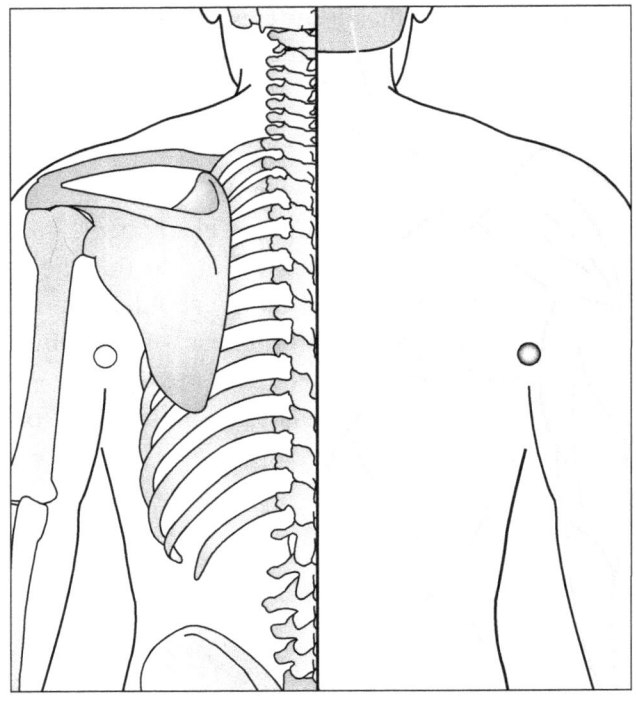

Location: With the arm abducted, on the back, 1 cun above the posterior end of the axillary fold, posterior and inferior to the shoulder joint.

Functions: Benefits the shoulder and scapula, removes blockages from the channel to treat pain locally, extinguishes wind.

Indications: Pain of the scapula.

Notes

Point Combinations

SI 10
NAOSHU

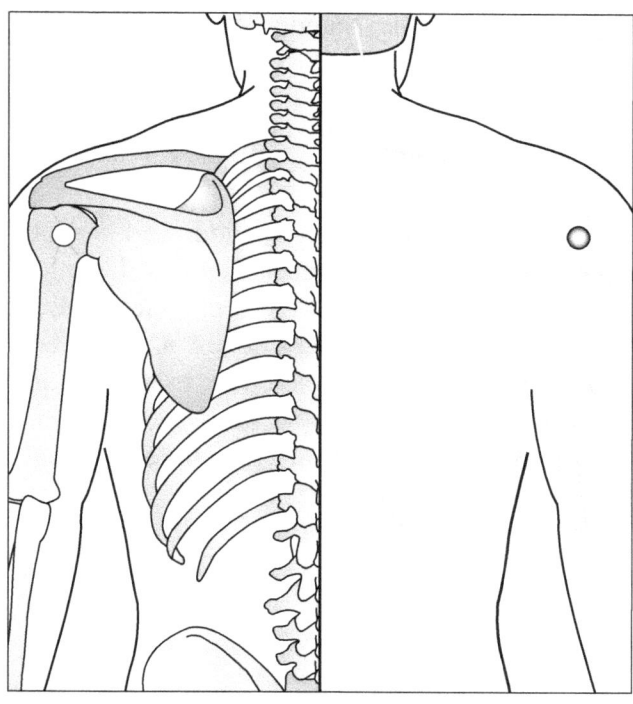

Location: With the arm abducted, on the shoulder, directly above the posterior end of the axillary fold, in the depression inferior to the spine of the scapula.

Functions: Benefits the tendons of the shoulder, moves Qi and blood, removes blockages from the channel to treat pain locally, relaxes muscles, extinguishes wind, dissolves masses.

Indications: Swelling, pain, achiness and weakness of the shoulder or arm.

Attributes: Point of intersection between the Small Intestine, Yang Wei, and Yin Qiao vessels.

Notes

Point Combinations

SI 11
TIANZONG

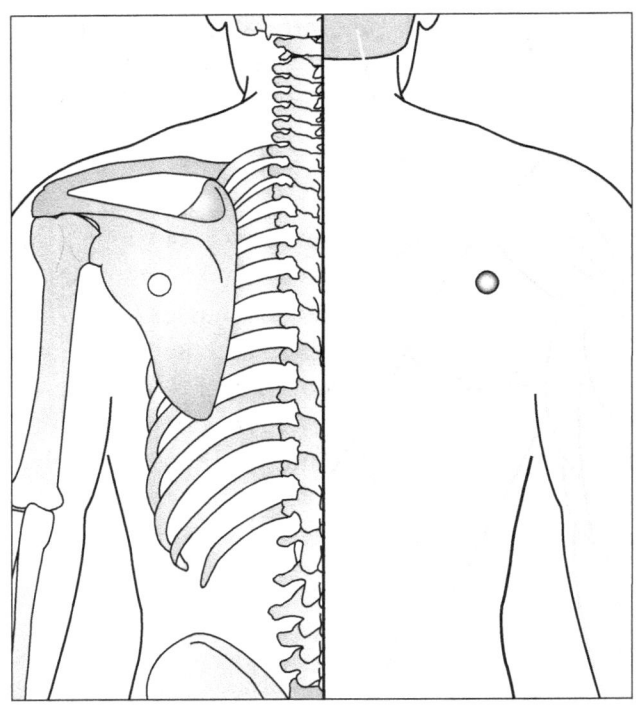

Location: On the scapula, in the depression in the center of the infrascapular fossa, at the junction of the upper and middle third of the scapula between the lower scapular spine and the inferior angle of the scapula.

Functions: Benefits the shoulder and scapula, benefits the breasts and promotes lactation, removes blockages from the channel to treat pain locally, stimulates, moves and corrects rebellious Qi, expands the chest, treats tai yang syndromes.

Indications: Pain in the shoulder, scapula and upper arm, swelling of the cheek and jaw, asthma, insufficient lactation.

Notes

Point Combinations

SI 12
BINGFENG

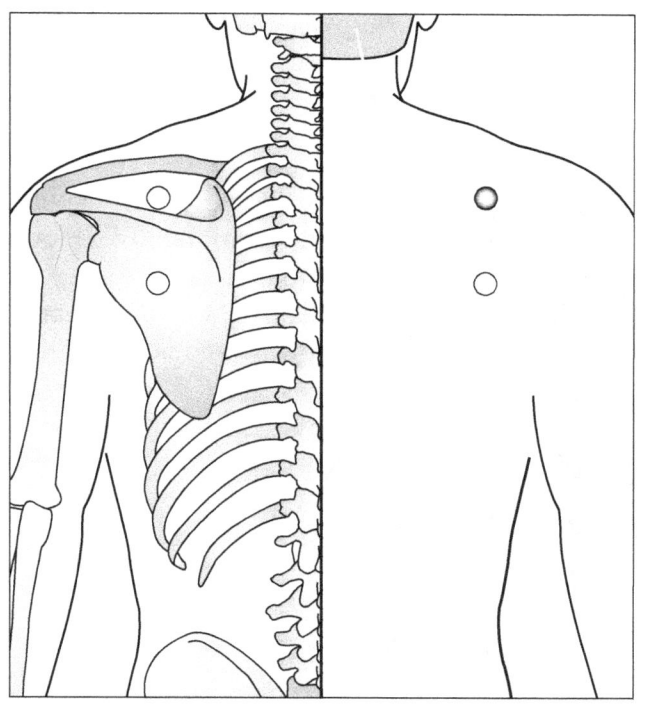

Location: With the arm abducted, on the scapula, in the depression in the center of the suprascapular fossa, directly above SI-11 Tianzhong.

Functions: Benefits the shoulder and scapula, removes blockages from the channel, extinguishes wind.

Indications: Pain, motor impairment, numbness and achiness of the shoulder, scapula and upper arm.

Attributes: Point of intersection between Small Intestine, Gall Bladder, San Jiao and Large Intestine.

Notes

Point Combinations

SI 13
QUYUAN

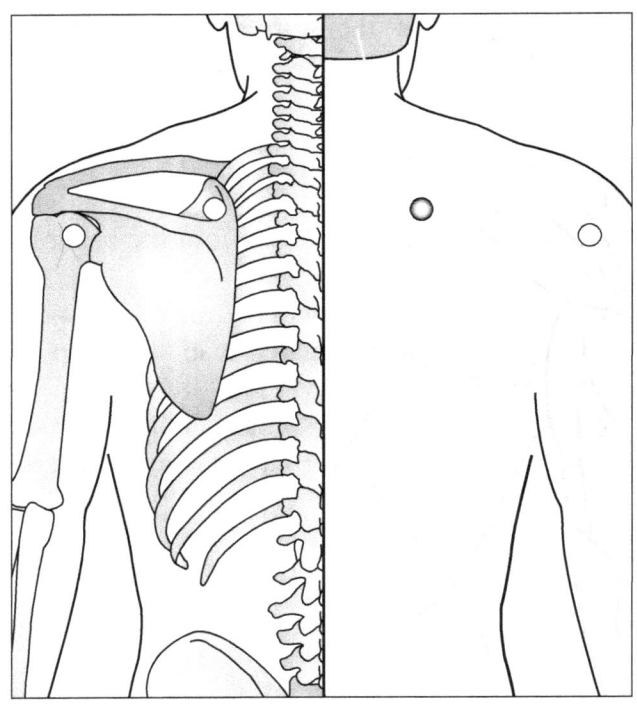

Location: On the scapula, at the medial extremity of the suprascapular fossa, midway on the line joining SI-10 Naoshu and the spinous process of 2nd thoracic vertebra.

Functions: Benefits the shoulder and scapula, relaxes the muscles and tendons, removes blood stasis from the channel to treat pain.

Indications: Pain and stiffness of the scapula region and soft tissue of the shoulder, muscle spasm.

Notes _____

_____

_____

_____

_____

_____

_____

_____

Point Combinations _____

_____

_____

_____

_____

_____

_____

SI 14
JIANWAISHU

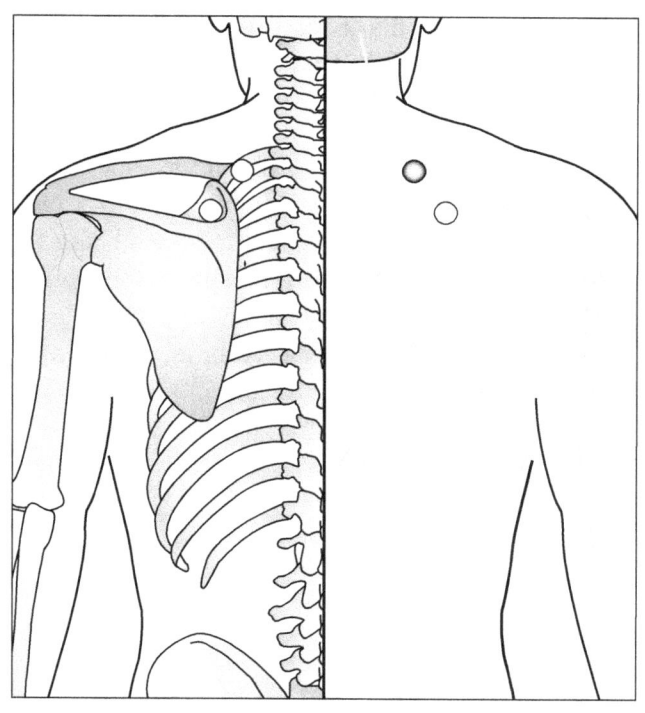

Location: On the back, below the spinous process of the 1st thoracic vertebra, 3 cun lateral to the posterior midline.

Functions: Benefits the shoulder and scapula, expels cold, warms the channel, extinguishes wind and relieves pain.

Indications: Shoulder, scapula, and back pain, neck pain and stiffness.

Notes

Point Combinations

SI 15
JIANZHONGSHU

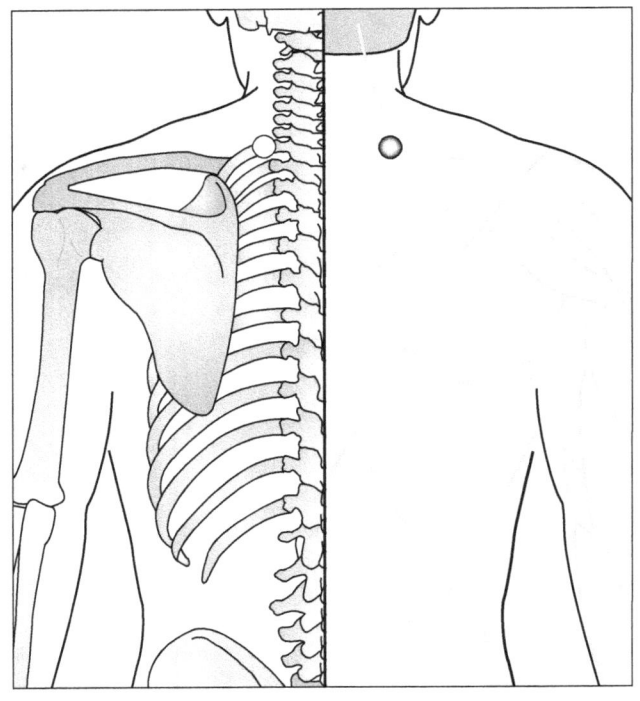

Location: On the back, below the spinous process of the 7th cervical vertebra, 2 cun lateral to the posterior midline.

Functions: Benefits the shoulder, opens the lung, transforms phlegm, removes blockages from the channel, clears heat, courses Lung Qi downwards, relieves pain, brightens the eyes.

Indications: Pain in shoulder and back, stiff neck, cough, hemoptysis, asthma, fever with chills, bronchitis, blurred vision.

Notes _____

_____

_____

_____

_____

_____

_____

_____

Point Combinations _____

_____

_____

_____

_____

_____

_____

SI 16
TIANCHUANG

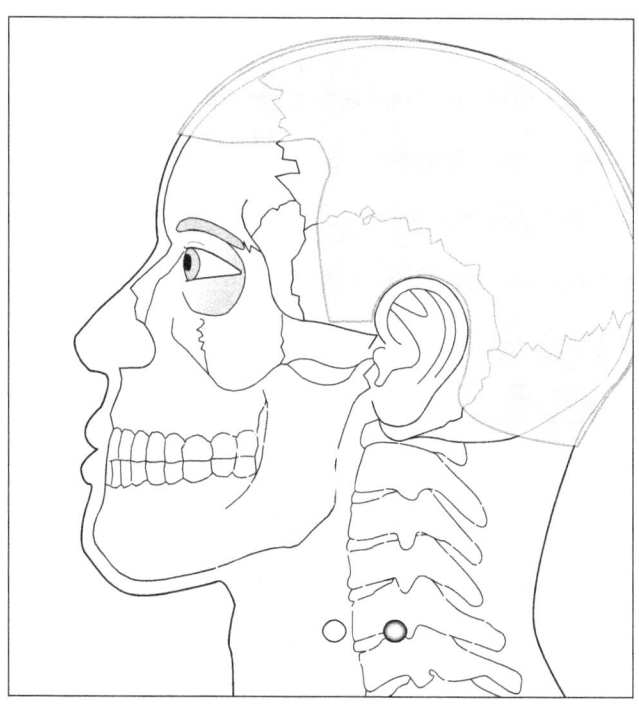

Location: On the lateral side of the neck, on the posterior border of the sternocleidomastoid muscle (posterior to LI-18 Futu, level with the laryngeal protuberance).

Functions: Removes blockages from the channel, benefits the ear, throat and voice, clears heat, relieves pain.

Indications: Goiter, sudden loss of voice, deafness, tinnitus, sore throat, stiff neck.

Attributes: Window of the Sky point.

Notes

Point Combinations

SI 17
TIANRONG

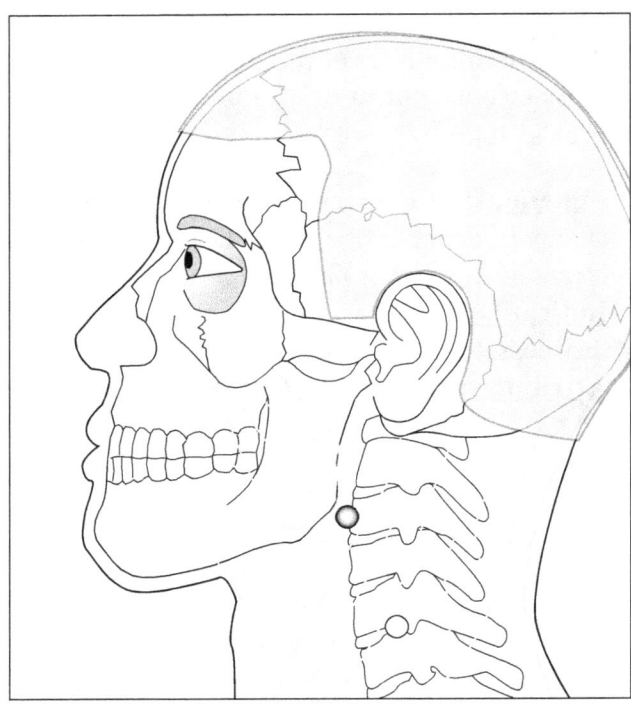

Location: On the lateral aspect of the neck, posterior to the angle of the mandible, in the depression on the anterior border of the sternocleidomastoid muscle.

Functions: Reduces swelling, dissipates hard masses, expels damp-heat and fire toxins.

Indications: Deafness, tinnitus, asthma, severe cough, pharyngitis, tonsillitis, sore throat, soreness or neck distention, sensation of foreign body in throat, goiter, swelling of the cheek.

Attributes:
*Main point for tonsillitis.

Notes
_____

_____

_____

_____

_____

_____

_____

_____

Point Combinations
_____

_____

_____

_____

_____

_____

SI 18
QUANLIAO

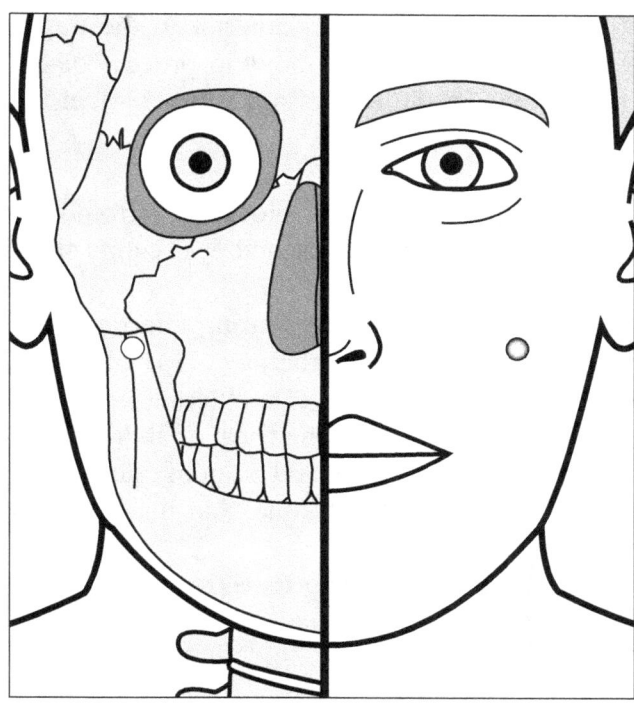

Location: On the face, directly below the outer canthus, in the depression below the zygomatic bone.

Functions: Removes blockages from the channel, clears heat, relieves pain, expels wind.

Indications: Yellow sclera, pain in the face, toothache in upper jaw, spasmodic facial muscles, swelling of the cheek, facial paralysis, trigeminal neuralgia.

Attributes: Meeting point of the three yang channels of the leg. Point of intersection between Small Intestine and San Jiao channels.

Notes
_____
_____
_____
_____
_____
_____
_____
_____
_____

Point Combinations
_____
_____
_____
_____
_____
_____

SI 19
TINGGONG

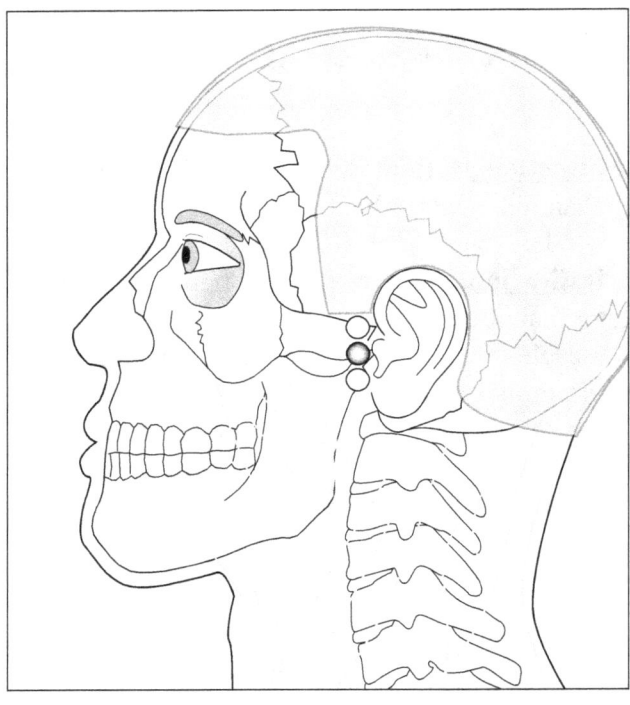

Location: On the face, anterior to the tragus and posterior to the condyloid process of the mandible, in the depression formed when the mouth is opened.

Functions: Removes blockages from the channel, benefits the ear and eye, calms shen, relieves pain.

Indications: Difficulty hearing and deafness, otitis media, issues of the jaw (TMJ), tinnitus, toothache, pus in the ear, external ear canal inflammation, pain in the chest or abdomen.

Attributes: Exit point and point of intersection between the Small Intestine, San Jiao and Gall Bladder.

*Main point for hearing issues.

Notes
_____
_____
_____
_____
_____
_____
_____
_____

Point Combinations
_____
_____
_____
_____
_____
_____

UB 1
TIANZONG

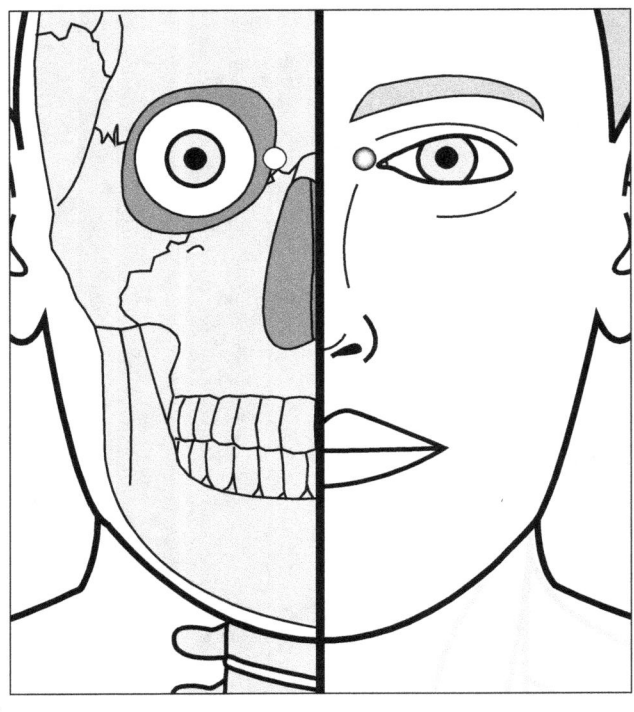

Location: On the face, in the depression 0.1 cun above the inner canthus.

Functions: Benefits the eyes, treats all eye disorders, clears heat, extinguishes wind.

Indications: Blurred vision, myopia, night blindness, pterygium, cataract, redness, swelling pain of the eye, lacrimation, itching, twitching, acute lumbar pain, infantile convulsion, nebula, visual dizziness, color blindness.

Attributes: Meeting point of the Urinary Bladder, Small Intestine, Stomach, Yin Qiao and Yang Qiao.

Notes
_____

_____

_____

_____

_____

_____

_____

_____

Point Combinations
_____

_____

_____

_____

_____

_____

_____

UB 2
BingFeng

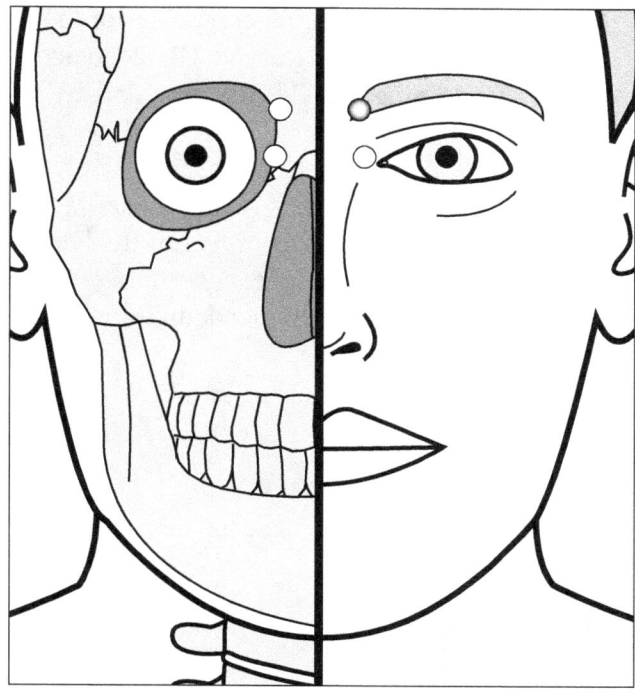

Location: On the face, in the depression at the medial end of the eyebrow, at the supraorbital notch.

Functions: Benefits the eyes, clears heat, extinguishes wind.

Indications: Pain in the supraorbital region, sinus congestion, headache, blurred vision, redness, swelling, itchiness, pain of the eye, watery eyes, hiccups, spasms of the diaphragm, twitching of the eyelid, allergic rhinitis, high blood pressure, night blindness.

Notes

Point Combinations

UB 3
MEICHONG

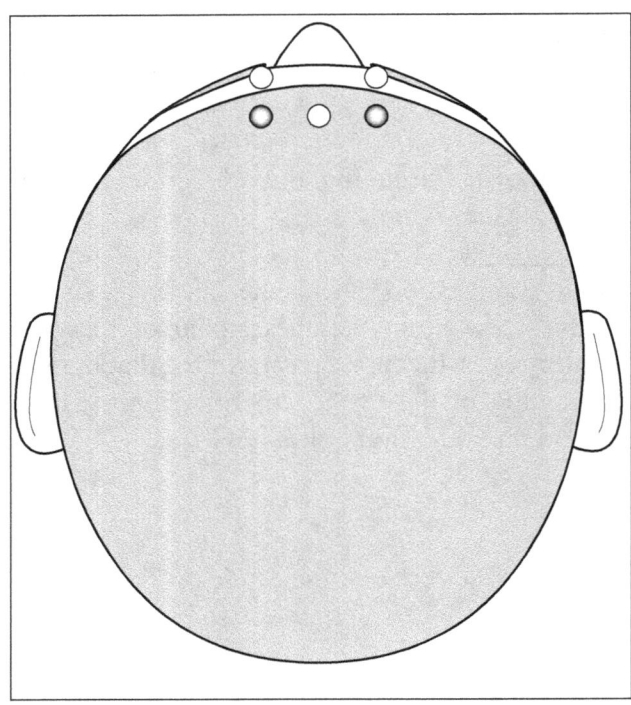

Location: On the head, 0.5 cun posterior to the anterior hairline, directly above BL-2 Cuanzhu on the line joining DU-24 Shenting and BL -4 Qucha.

Functions: Extinguishes wind, benefits the eyes and nose, treats all disorders of the head.
Indications: Headache, vertigo, nasal congestion, epilepsy, light headedness.

Notes
_____
_____
_____
_____
_____
_____
_____
_____
_____

Point Combinations
_____
_____
_____
_____
_____
_____
_____

UB 4
QUCHAI

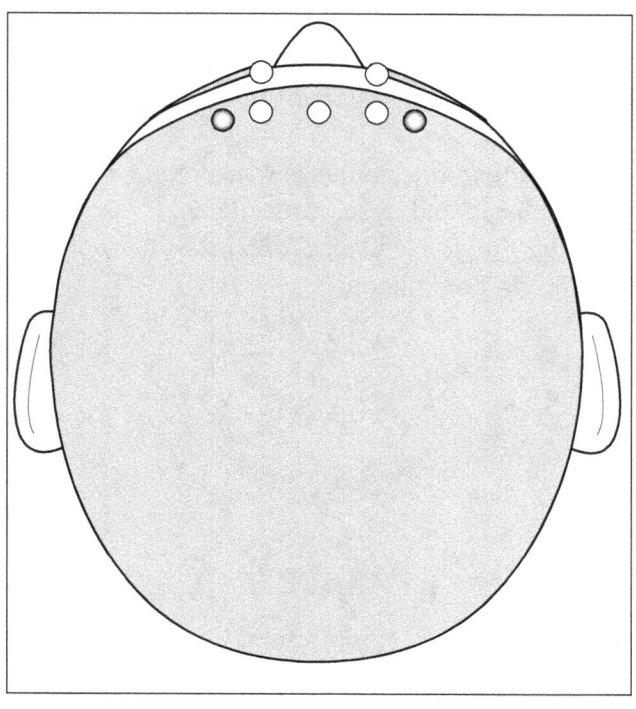

Location: On the head, 0.5 cun inside the anterior hairline, 1.5 cun lateral to the anterior midline at the junction of the medial third and lateral two-thirds of the distance between DU -24 Shenting and ST-8 Touwei.

Functions: Extinguishes wind, benefits the eyes and nose, treats all disorders of the head.
Indications: Headache, nasal congestion, epistaxis, blurred vision.

Notes

Point Combinations

UB 5
WUCHU

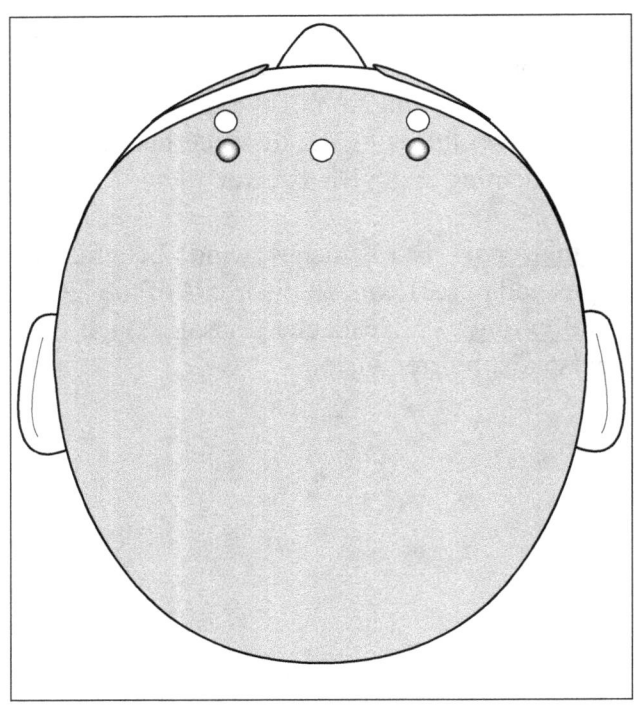

Location: On the head, 1 cun posterior to the anterior hairline, 1.5 cun lateral to the anterior midline (0.5 cun posterior to BL-4 Qucha).

Functions: Extinguishes wind, treats disorders of the head and nose, resuscitates.

Indications: Headache, dizziness, hemiplegia, epilepsy, convulsion.

Notes

_____

_____

_____

_____

_____

_____

_____

_____

Point Combinations

_____

_____

_____

_____

_____

_____

_____

UB 6
CHENGGUANG

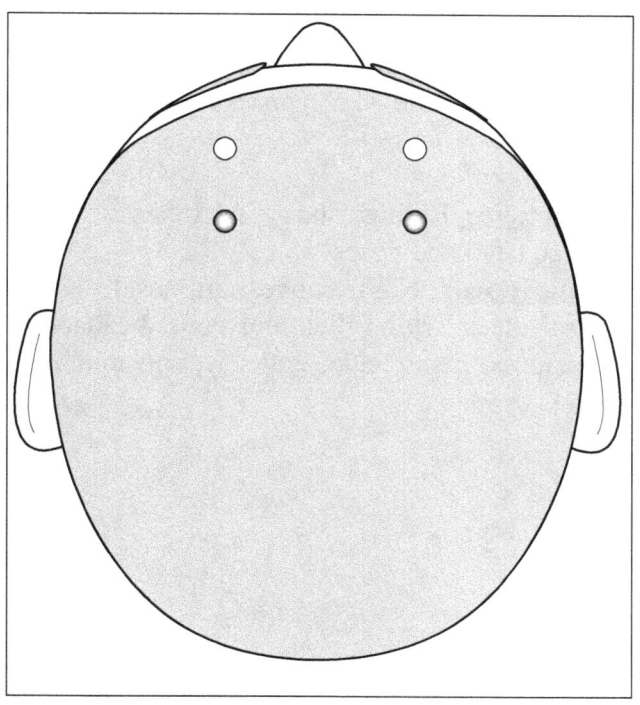

Location: On the head, 2.5 cun posterior to the anterior hairline, 1.5 cun lateral to the anterior midline (1.5 cun posterior to BL-5 Wuchu).

Functions: Extinguishes wind, clears heat, treats disorders of the head, nose and eyes.

Indications: Blurred vision, hemiplegia, epilepsy, dizziness.

Notes

Point Combinations

UB 7
TONGTIAN

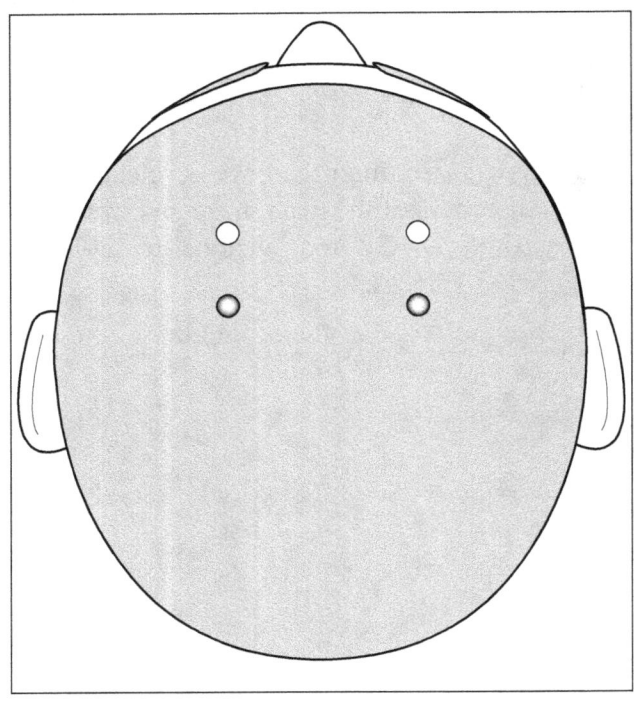

Location: On the head, 4 cun posterior to the anterior hairline, 1.5 cun lateral to the anterior midline (1.5 cun posterior to BL-6 Chengguang).

Functions: Extinguishes wind, treats disorders of the head and nose.

Indications: Nasal congestion, nasal polyps, nasal ulcers, rhinorrhea, epistaxis, headaches, dizziness, hemiplegia, epilepsy, anosmia, stiff neck, dyspnea.

Notes

_____

_____

_____

_____

_____

_____

_____

_____

Point Combinations

_____

_____

_____

_____

_____

_____

_____

UB 8
LUOQUE

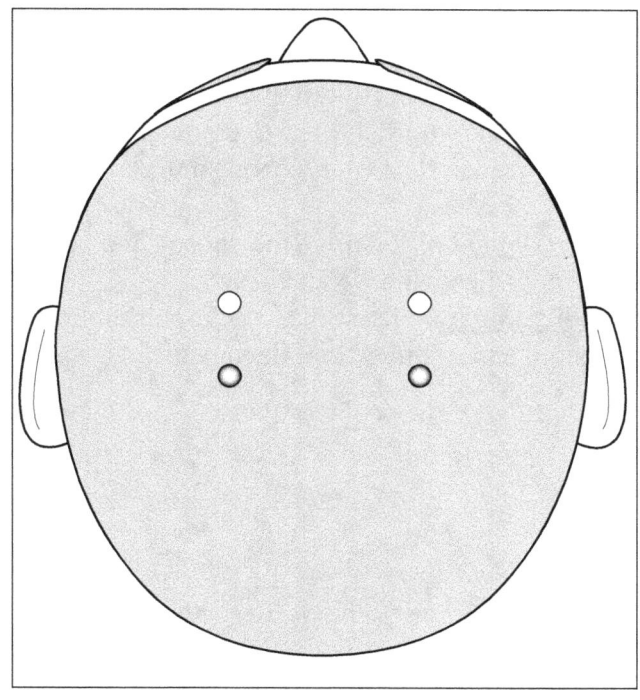

Location: On the head, 5.5 cun posterior to the anterior hairline, 1.5 cun lateral to the anterior midline (1.5 cun posterior to BL-7 Tongtian).

Functions: Benefits the eyes, extinguishes wind, transforms phlegm, treats disorders of the head.

Indications: Blurred vision, hemiplegia, epilepsy, tinnitus, mania.

Notes

_____

_____

_____

_____

_____

_____

_____

_____

Point Combinations

_____

_____

_____

_____

_____

_____

UB 9
YUZHEN

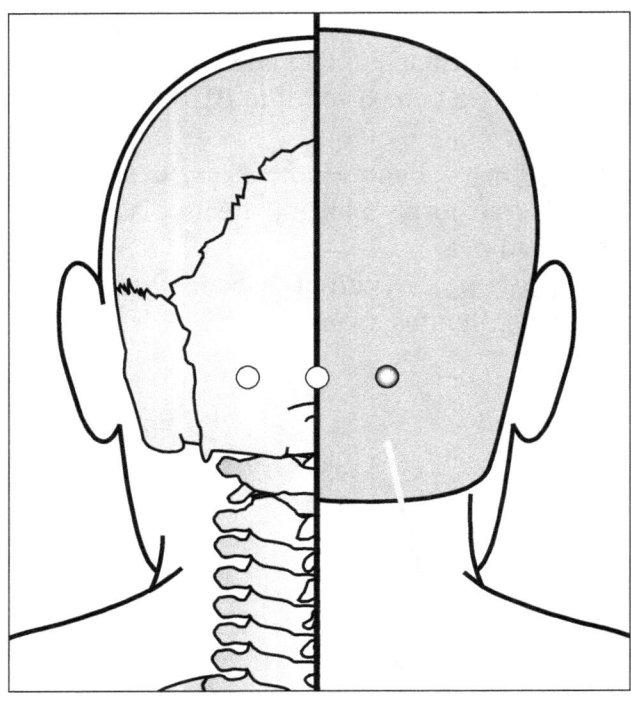

Location: On the posterior aspect of the head, 2.5 cun superior to the posterior hairline, 1.3 cun lateral to the posterior midline, level with the superior border of the external occipital protuberance (or DU-17 Zhongshui).

Functions: Benefits the nose and eyes, extinguishes wind, relieves pain.

Indications: Headache, neck pain, blurred vision, nasal congestion, tinea pedis.

Notes
_____
_____
_____
_____
_____
_____
_____
_____

Point Combinations
_____
_____
_____
_____
_____
_____
_____

UB 10
TIANZHU

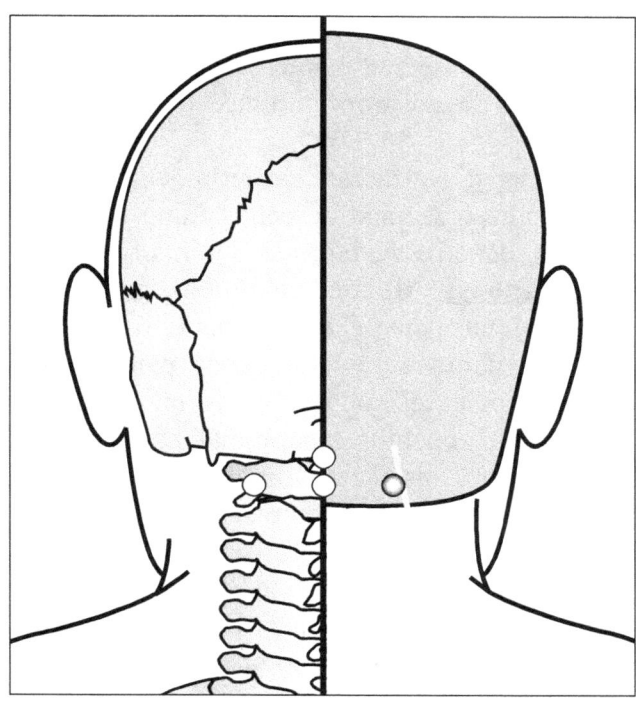

Location: On the nape, in the depression of the lateral border of the trapezius muscle and 1.3 cun lateral to the midpoint of the posterior hairline.

Functions: Extinguishes wind, activates the channel, soothes the sinews, disorders of the head, relieves pain, opens the orifices.

Indications: Dizziness, headache, neck stiffness, pain in the shoulders and back, nasal congestion, sore throat, excessive lacrimation, infantile convulsions, epilepsy, common cold.

Attributes: Sea of Qi point, Window of the Sky point.

Notes

_____
_____
_____
_____
_____
_____
_____
_____
_____

Point Combinations

_____
_____
_____
_____
_____
_____
_____

UB 11
TIANZHU

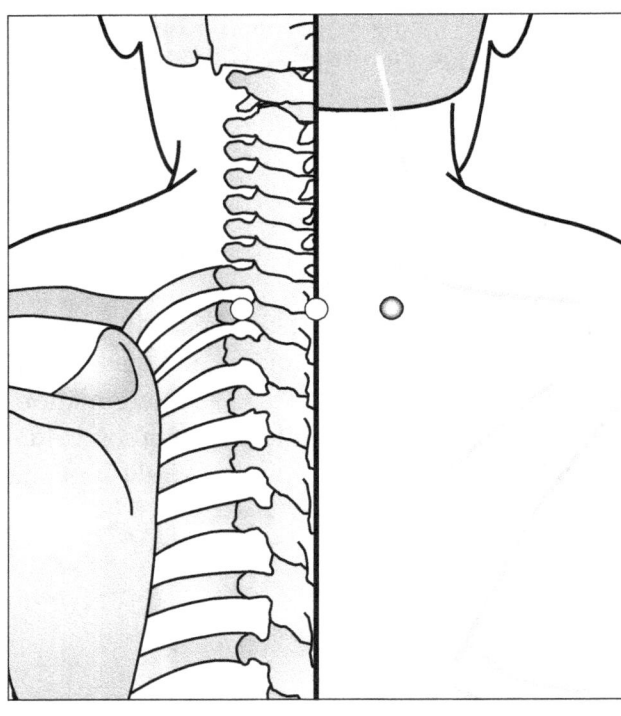

Location: On the back, below the spinous process of the 1st thoracic vertebra, 1.5 cun lateral to the posterior midline.

Functions: Releases the exterior, extinguishes wind, disperses and descends Lung Qi, stops cough, benefits the bones and joints.

Indications: All bone conditions, pain in the bone, joint pain, shoulder pain, back pain, lumbar pain, sacral pain, knee pain, cough, headache, nasal congestion, fever, tonsillitis, pleurisy, bronchitis, abdominal pain, blurred vision, paralysis of extremities, inguinal hernia, madness, muscular contracture, cannot turn around.

Attributes: Converging point of bone, meeting point of the Urinary Bladder and Small Intestine, Sea of Blood point.

Notes

Point Combinations

UB 12
FENGMEN

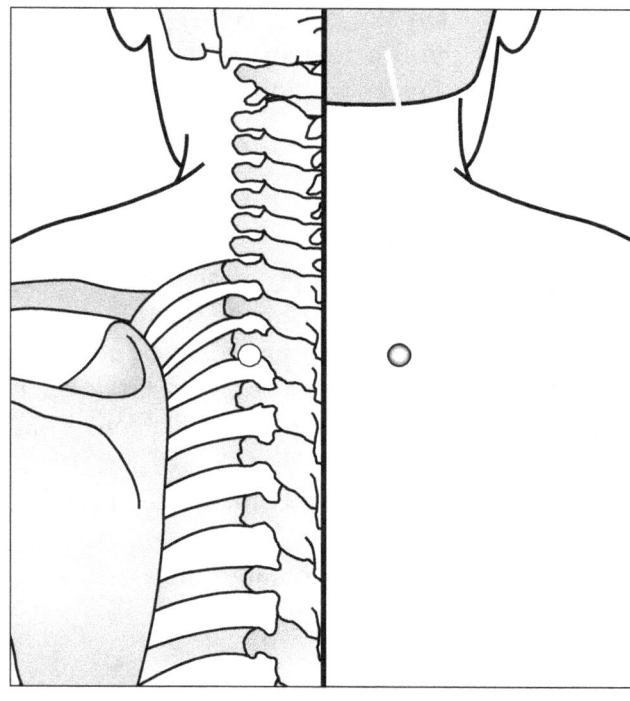

Location: On the back, below the spinous process of the 2nd thoracic vertebra, 1.5 cun lateral to the posterior midline.

Functions: Releases the exterior, strengthens Wei Qi, disperses Lung Qi, regulates Ying and Wei Qi.

Indications: Common cold, cough, fever, headache, stiff neck, pain in the back and chest, nasal obstruction, abscess on the back, jaundice, heavy eye, sneezing, tonsillitis, infantile malnutrition, hemiplegia, quadriplegia.

Attributes: Meeting point of the Urinary Bladder and DU channels.

Notes

Point Combinations

UB 13
FEISHU

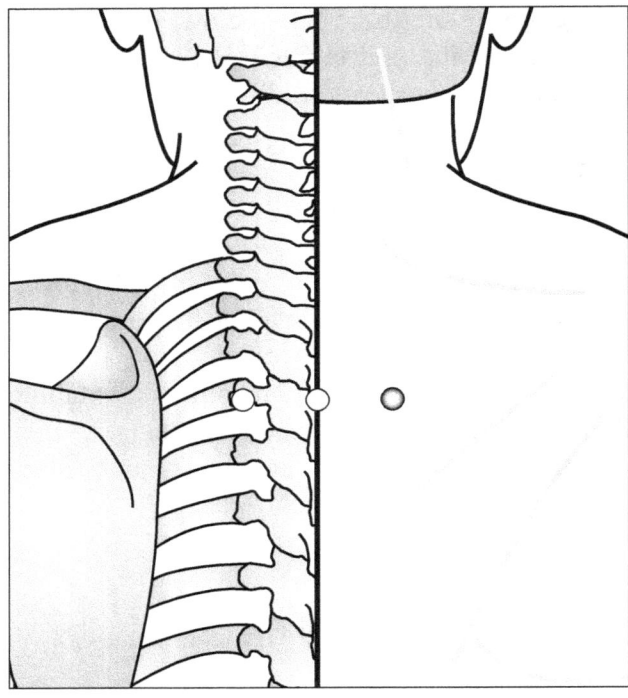

Location: On the back, below the spinous process of the 3rd thoracic vertebra, 1.5 cun lateral to the posterior midline.

Functions: Releases the exterior, strengthens Wei Qi, disperse and descends Lung Qi, regulates Ying and Wei Qi.

Indications: Hemoptysis/spitting blood, asthma, cough/bronchitis, bone steaming fever, night sweats, pulmonary tuberculosis, common cold, cough, fever, headache, stiff neck, pain in the back and chest, pneumonia, tonsillitis, goiter, skin disorders, diseases of the nose, stomatitis, endocarditis, convulsions, insanity, vomiting, no sweating.

Attributes: Back Shu point of the Lung.

Notes

_____

_____

_____

_____

_____

_____

_____

_____

Point Combinations

_____

_____

_____

_____

_____

_____

UB 14
JUEYINSHU

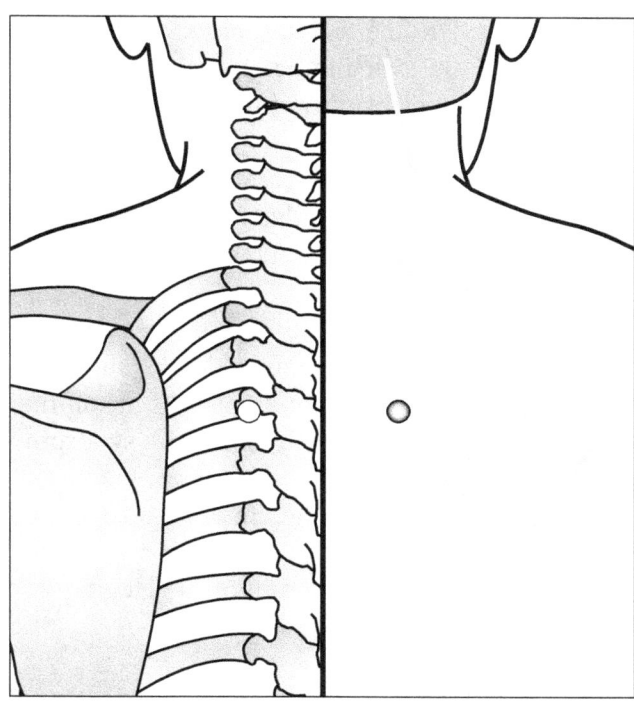

Location: On the back, below the spinous process of the 4th thoracic vertebra, 1.5 cun lateral to the posterior midline.

Functions: Regulates the Heart, soothes Liver Qi, opens the chest.

Indications: Cardiac pain, palpitations, cough, chest congestion, toothache, vomiting.

Attributes: Back Shu point of the Pericardium.

Notes

_____
_____
_____
_____
_____
_____
_____
_____
_____

Point Combinations

_____
_____
_____
_____
_____
_____
_____

UB 15
XINSHU

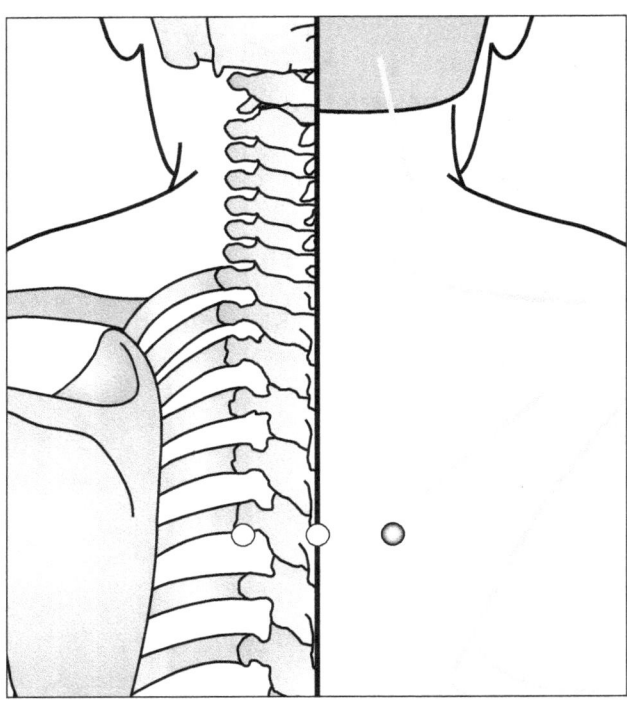

Location: On the back, below the spinous process of the 5th thoracic vertebra, 1.5 cun lateral to the posterior midline.

Functions: Strengthens and nourishes the Heart, calms shen, regulates Heart Qi, opens the chest, resolves blood stagnation, clears Heart heat/fire.

Indications: Cardiac pain, hemoptysis, palpitations, chest congestion, shortness of breath, cough, hematemesis, insomnia, psychosis, irritability, arrhythmia, lin syndrome (UTI), poor memory, epilepsy, nocturnal emission, night sweating, muteness, 5 palms heat.

Attributes: Back Shu point of the Heart.

Notes

Point Combinations

UB 16
JUEYINSHU

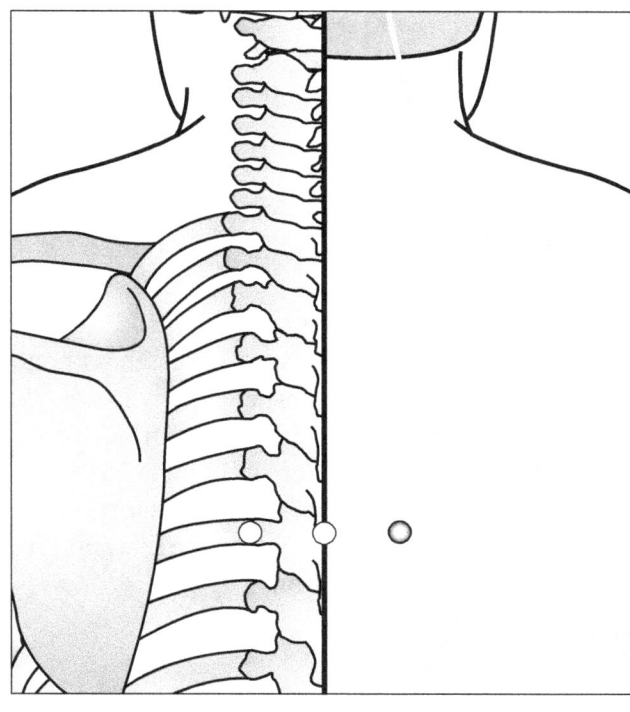

Location: On the back, below the spinous process of the 6th thoracic vertebra, 1.5 cun lateral to the posterior midline.

Functions: Invigorates the blood, opens the chest, regulates the Qi in the chest and abdomen.

Indications: Cardiac pain, chest congestion, borborygmus, gastric pain, abdominal pain, cough, asthma, alopecia, mastitis, intercostal neuralgia, pruritus, psoriasis.

Attributes: Back Shu point of the Du channel.

Notes
_____
_____
_____
_____
_____
_____
_____
_____
_____

Point Combinations
_____
_____
_____
_____
_____
_____
_____

UB 17
GESHU

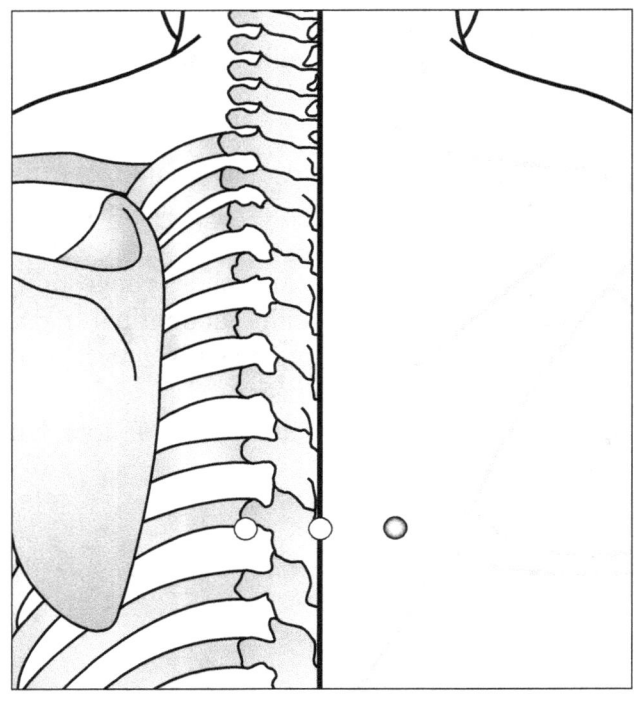

Location: On the back, below the spinous process of the 7th thoracic vertebra, 1.5 cun lateral to the posterior midline.

Functions: Invigorates the blood, cools the blood, nourishes the blood, stops bleeding, descends rebellious Qi, harmonizes the diaphragm, calms shen.

Indications: Acute epigastric pain, hiccup, dysphagia, blood in the stools, cough asthma, hematemesis, hectic fever and night sweating, difficulty swallowing, bone steaming fever, cardiac inflammation, stomach cancer, enteritis, abdominal distention, lassitude, lethargy.

Attributes: Back Shu point of the Diaphragm, meeting point of the blood.

*Main point for hiccups.

Notes

_____
_____
_____
_____
_____
_____
_____
_____

Point Combinations

_____
_____
_____
_____
_____
_____

UB 18
GANSHU

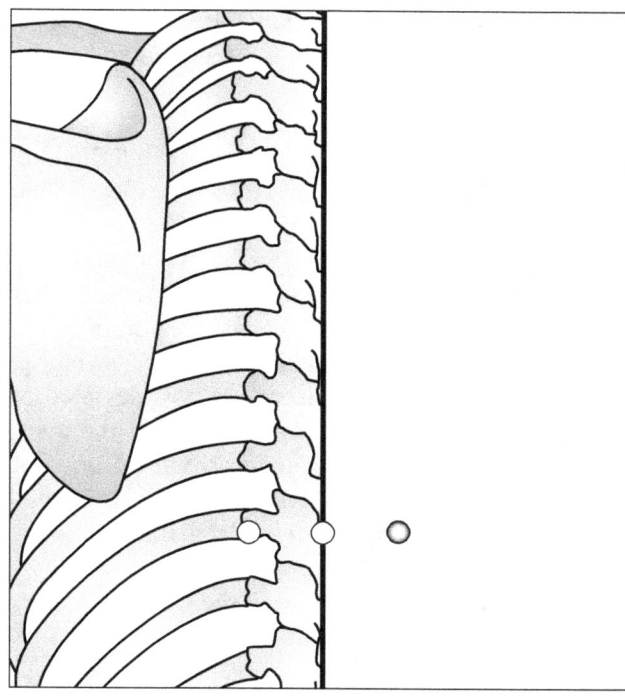

Location: On the back, below the spinous process of the 9th thoracic vertebra, 1.5 cun lateral to the posterior midline.

Functions: Moves Liver Qi, nourishes and regulates Liver blood, resolves damp-heat, benefits the eyes and the sinews, extinguishes wind.

Indications: Pain in the hypochondrium, jaundice, diseases of the eyes, vomiting, epistaxis, mania, psychosis, back pain, jaundice, night blindness, epilepsy, gastric diseases, painful masses in chest and abdomen, bitter taste in mouth, cerebral hemorrhage, scrofula, insomnia, shortness of breath, diabetes, irregular menstruation, genital disorders lassitude, lethargy.

Attributes: Back Shu point of the Liver.

Notes

Point Combinations

UB 19
DANSHU

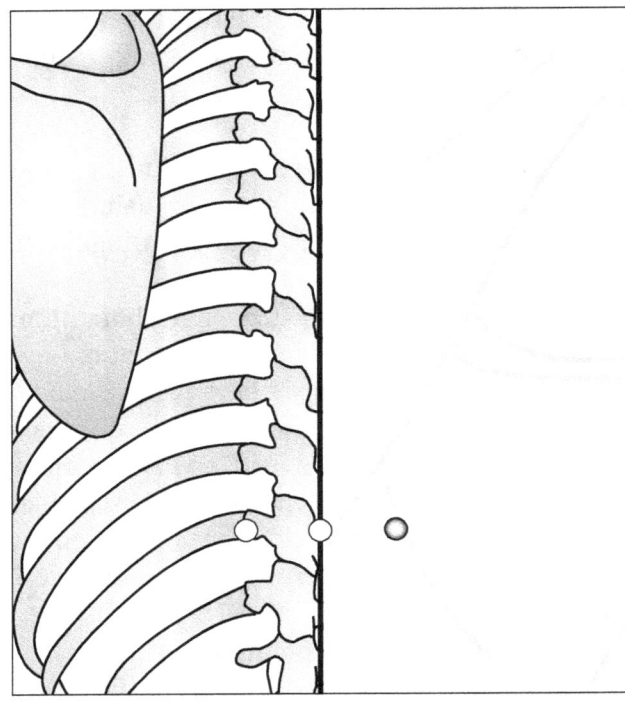

Location: On the back, below the spinous process of the 10th thoracic vertebra, 1.5 cun lateral to the posterior midline.

Functions: Regulates and strengthens Gall Bladder, resolves Gall Bladder/Liver damp-heat, clears Shao Yang syndromes.

Indications: Jaundice, pain in the hypochondrium, pulmonary tuberculosis, bone steaming fever, bitter taste in mouth, hepatitis, cholecystitis, vomiting/dry heaves, sore throat, irritability, axillary swelling, sperm in urine, all eye disorders, eyes deviated or rolled back, pain in eyebrows, blood in the eyes, pleurisy, coughing fits, madness with fear, fear if dying, apoplexy due to Liver, gastritis, cramps in calf, tuberculosis of lymph glands, osseous tuberculosis.

Attributes: Back Shu point of the Gall Bladder.

Notes

_____
_____
_____
_____
_____
_____
_____
_____

Point Combinations

_____
_____
_____
_____
_____
_____
_____

UB 20
PISHU

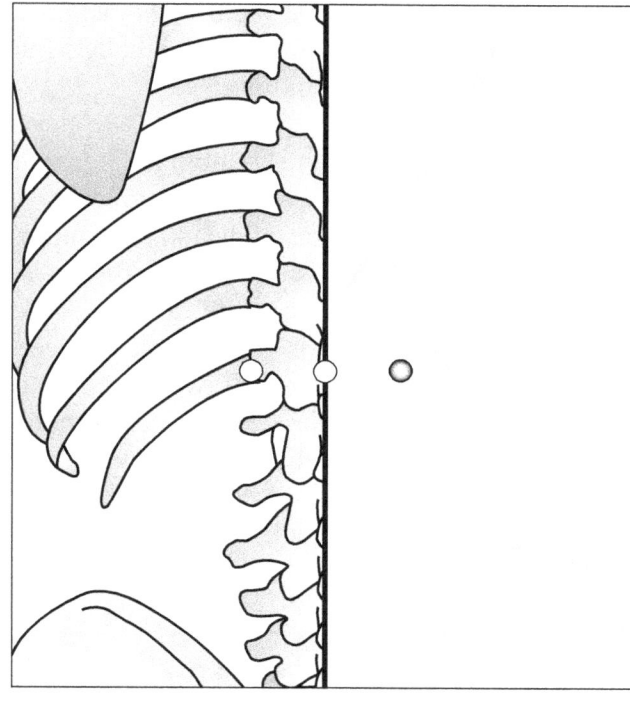

Location: On the back, below the spinous process of the 11th thoracic vertebra, 1.5 cun lateral to the posterior midline.

Functions: Tonifies and regulates Spleen Qi/Stomach Qi, tonifies yang, nourishes blood, resolves damp.

Indications: Abdominal distention, Jaundice, vomiting, diarrhea, dysentery, blood in the stool, edema, poor digestion, poor appetite, stomach prolapse, blood in stool, difficulty swallowing, gastritis, epigastric pain, excessive appetite with diabetes, back pain, masses in chest and abdomen, enlargement of Liver or Spleen, anemia, lethargy, lassitude, borborygmus, abundant stools, constipation, heavy menstruation, prolapse uterus.

Attributes: Back Shu point of the Spleen.

Notes

_____
_____
_____
_____
_____
_____
_____
_____
_____

Point Combinations

_____
_____
_____
_____
_____
_____
_____
_____

UB 21
WEISHU

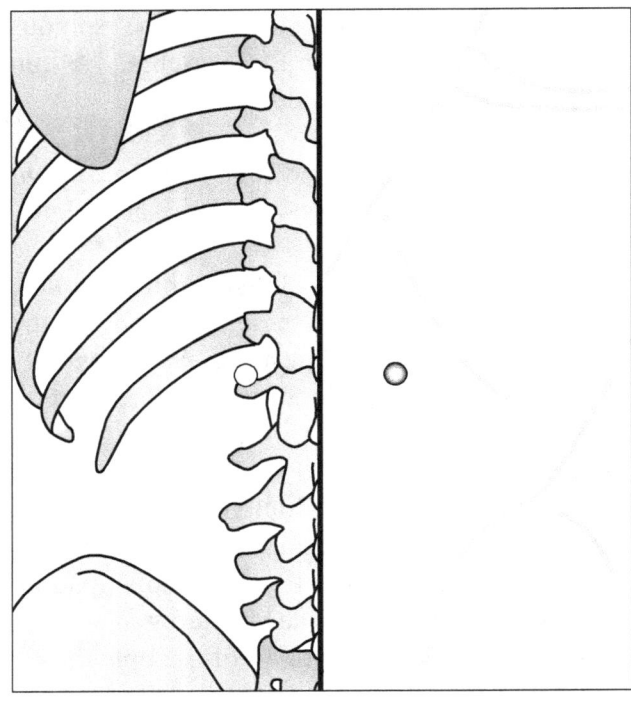

Location: On the back, below the spinous process of the 12th thoracic vertebra, 1.5 cun lateral to the posterior midline.

Functions: Regulates and harmonizes Stomach Qi, resolves damp, removes food stagnation.

Indications: Epigastric pain and distention, vomiting, abdominal distention, borborygmus, poor digestion, poor appetite, pain in the chest, gastric spasms, gastritis, gastric ulcer, enlarged Liver, difficulty swallowing, intestinal parasitosis, night blindness, jaundice, insomnia, prolapses stomach, gastrointestinal disorders, prolapse of the rectum.

Attributes: Back Shu point of the Stomach.

Notes _____

_____

_____

_____

_____

_____

_____

_____

Point Combinations _____

_____

_____

_____

_____

_____

UB 22
SANJIAOSHU

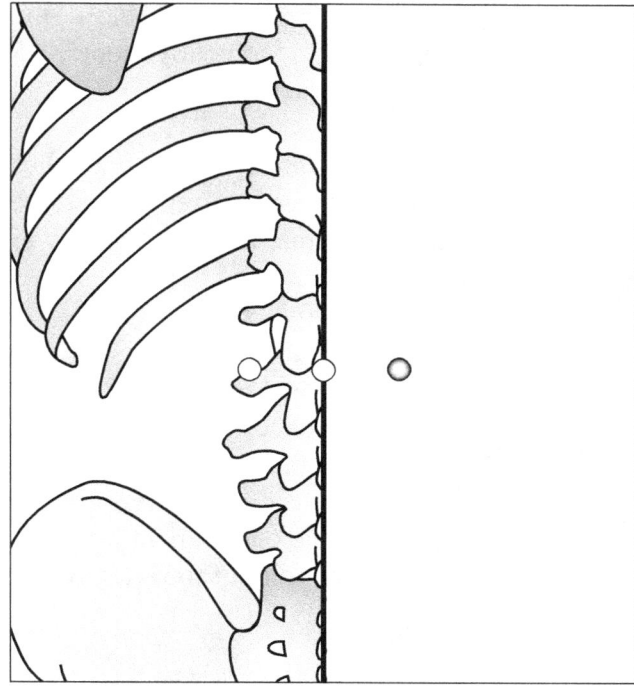

Location: On the lower back, below the spinous process of the 1st lumbar vertebra, 1.5 cun lateral to the posterior midline.

Functions: Opens and regulates water passages, benefits urination, resolves damp, regulates and moves the San Jiao.

Indications: Edema, dysuria, dysentery, diarrhea, abdominal distention, borborygmus, weakness is in the knees, vomiting, pain and stiffness in the low back, indigestion, jaundice, visual dizziness, headache, enuresis, nephritis, headaches, neurasthenia, stomach ache, spasms of the stomach and intestine, urinary retention, impotence, alternating chills and fever.

Attributes: Back Shu point of San Jiao.

Notes

Point Combinations

UB 23
SHENSHU

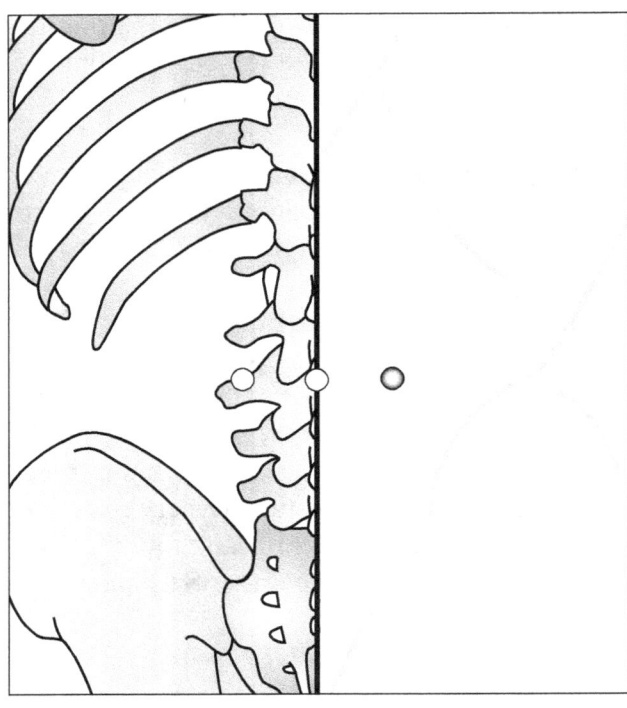

Location: On the lower back, below the spinous process of the 2nd lumbar vertebra, 1.5 cun lateral to the posterior midline.

Functions: Tonifies Kidney yang, nourishes Kidney yin and essence, strengthens the Kidneys, strengthens the Kidneys ability to grasp Qi, benefits the ears and bones, resolves damp, strengthens the low back.

Indications: Seminal emission, edema, enuresis, dysuria, leukorrhea, irregular menstruation, impotence, spermatorrhea, deafness, tinnitus, asthma, cough, hemiplegia, lumbar pain, bone disease, hematuria, blurred vision, nephritis, asthma, genital pain.

Attributes: Back Shu point of the Kidney.

Notes

_____

_____

_____

_____

_____

_____

_____

_____

Point Combinations

_____

_____

_____

_____

_____

_____

UB 24
QIHAISHU

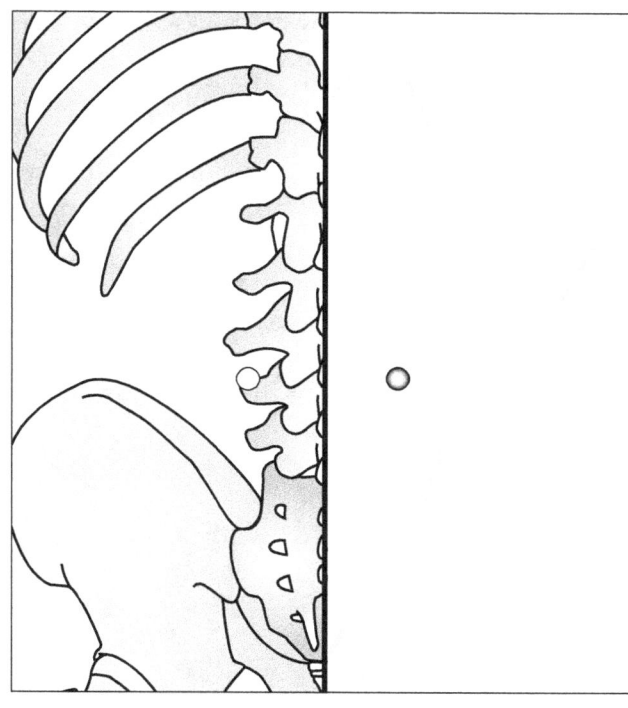

Location: On the lower back, below the spinous process of the 3rd lumbar vertebra, 1.5 cun lateral to the posterior midline.

Functions: Removes obstructions from the channel, strengthens the low back.
Indications: Lumbar pain, dysmenorrhea, abdominal distention, borborygmus, anal fistula.
Attributes: Sea of Qi point.

Notes

Point Combinations

UB 25
DACHANGSHU

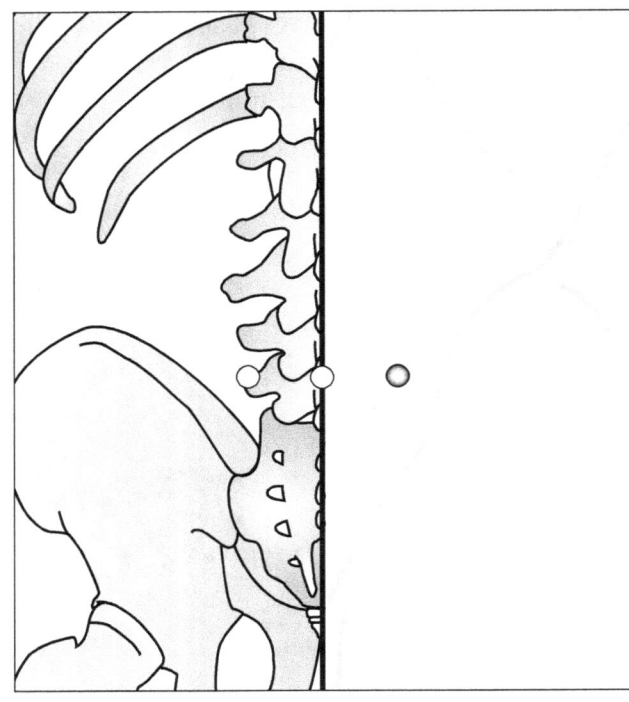

Location: On the lower back, below the spinous process of the 4th lumbar vertebra, 1.5 cun lateral to the posterior midline.

Functions: Regulates the Large Intestine, removes obstructions from the channel, strengthens the low back.

Indications: Lumbar pain, abdominal distention, diarrhea, constipation, urticaria, bleeding hemorrhoids.

Attributes: Back Shu of the Large Intestine.

Notes
_____
_____
_____
_____
_____
_____
_____
_____
_____

Point Combinations
_____
_____
_____
_____
_____
_____
_____

UB 26
GUANYUANSHU

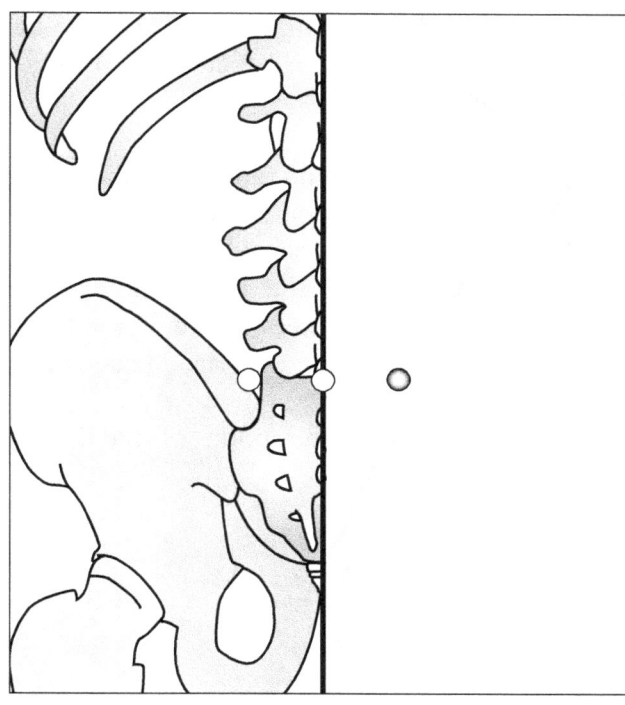

Location: On the lower back, below the spinous process of the 5th lumbar vertebra, 1.5 cun lateral to the posterior midline.

Functions: Removes obstructions from the channel, strengthens the lower back.

Indications: Pain in the lumbar and sacral region, abdominal distention, enuresis, diarrhea, frequent urination, dysuria.

Attributes: Source point.

Notes

_____
_____
_____
_____
_____
_____
_____
_____
_____

Point Combinations

_____
_____
_____
_____
_____
_____
_____

UB 27
XIAOCHANGSHU

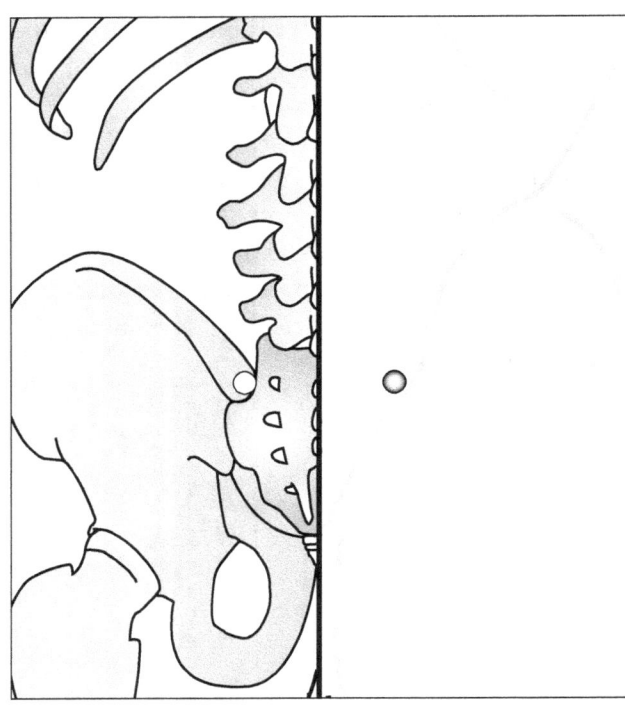

Location: On the sacrum, at the level of the 1st posterior sacral foramen, 1.5 cun lateral to the median sacral crest.

Functions: Promotes the function of the Small Intestine, resolves damp, resolves damp-heat, benefits urination.

Indications: Pain in the lumbar and sacral region, pain in the knees, lower abdominal pain and distention, dysuria, leukorrhea, spermatorrhea.

Attributes: Back Shu point of the Small Intestine.

Notes
_____
_____
_____
_____
_____
_____
_____
_____

Point Combinations
_____
_____
_____
_____
_____
_____
_____

UB 28
PANGUANGSHU

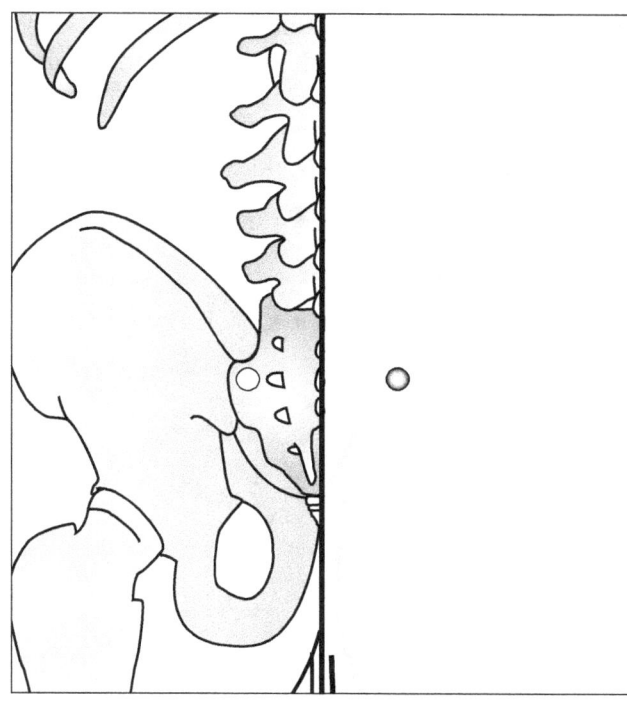

Location: On the sacrum, at the level of the 2nd posterior sacral foramen, 1.5 cun lateral to the median sacral crest.

Functions: Regulates the Bladder, resolves damp, clears damp-heat, open water passages, removes stagnation in the channel.

Indications: Enuresis, dysuria, stiffness and pain of the lower back, knee pain, leg pain, diarrhea, constipation.

Attributes: Back Shu point of the Urinary Bladder.

Notes

_____
_____
_____
_____
_____
_____
_____
_____

Point Combinations

_____
_____
_____
_____
_____
_____
_____

UB 29
ZHONGLUSHU

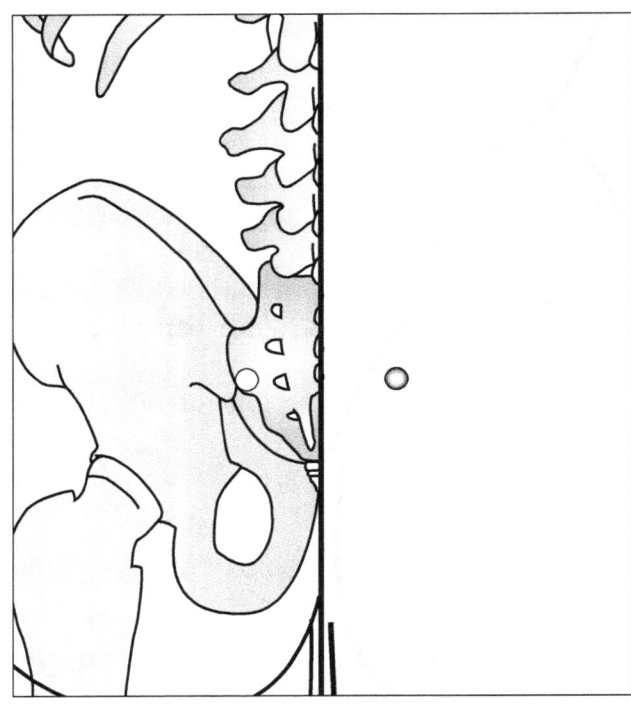

Location: On the sacrum, at the level of the 3rd posterior sacral foramen, 1.5 cun lateral to the median sacral crest.

Functions: Strengthens the low back, warms the channel and region, relieves diarrhea.
Indications: Hernia, low back pain, stiffness in the lumbar region, diarrhea.
Attributes: Center back muscles point.

Notes

Point Combinations

UB 30
BAIHUANSHU

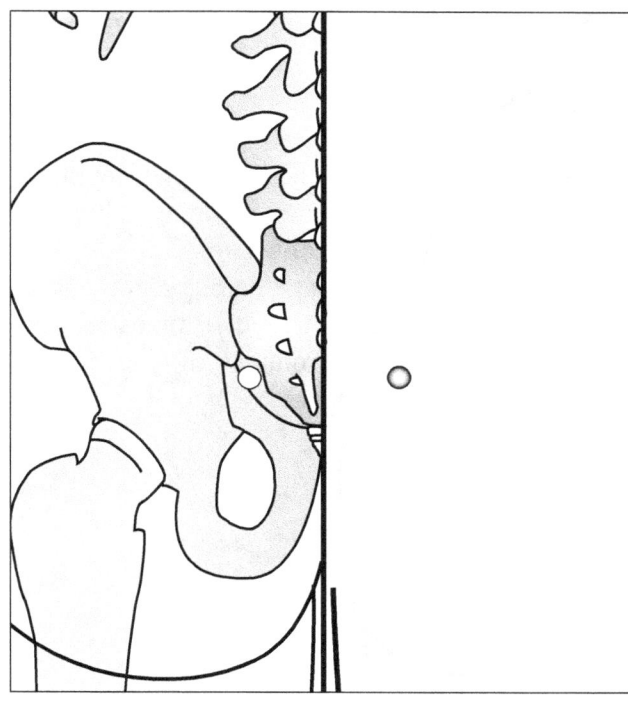

Location: On the sacrum, at the level of the 4th posterior sacral foramen, 1.5 cun lateral to the median sacral crest.

Functions: Benefits the lower back, regulates menstruation.

Indications: Irregular menstruation, enuresis, spermatorrhea, leukorrhea, lumbosacral pain, hernia.

Notes

_____
_____
_____
_____
_____
_____
_____
_____

Point Combinations

_____
_____
_____
_____
_____
_____
_____

UB 31
SHANGLIAO

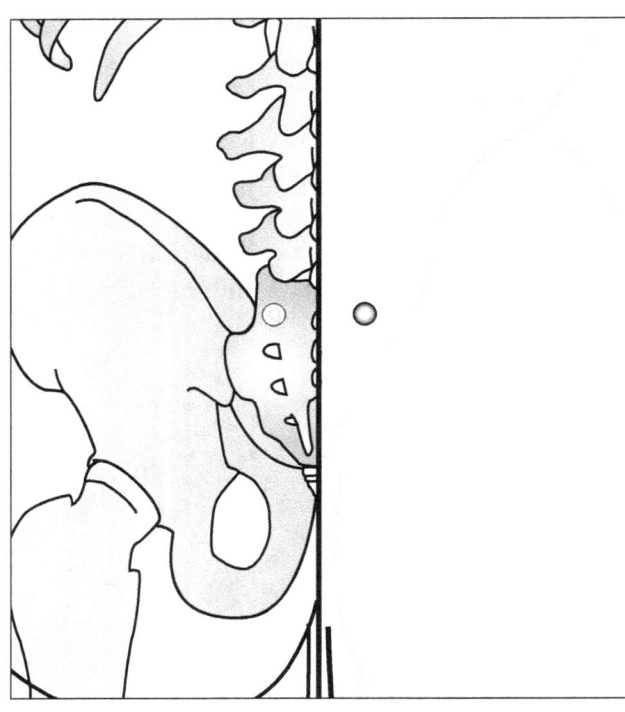

Location: On the sacrum, medial and inferior to the posterosuperior iliac spine, at the 1st posterior sacral foramen.

Functions: Regulates the lower jiao, regulates menstruation, benefits the lumbar area, benefits the knees, benefits urination.

Indications: Lumbar pain, sacral pain, constipation, dysuria, irregular menstruation, bloody leukorrhea, prolapse of the uterus, impotence, spermatorrhea.

Notes

_____
_____
_____
_____
_____
_____
_____
_____

Point Combinations

_____
_____
_____
_____
_____
_____

UB 32
CILIAO

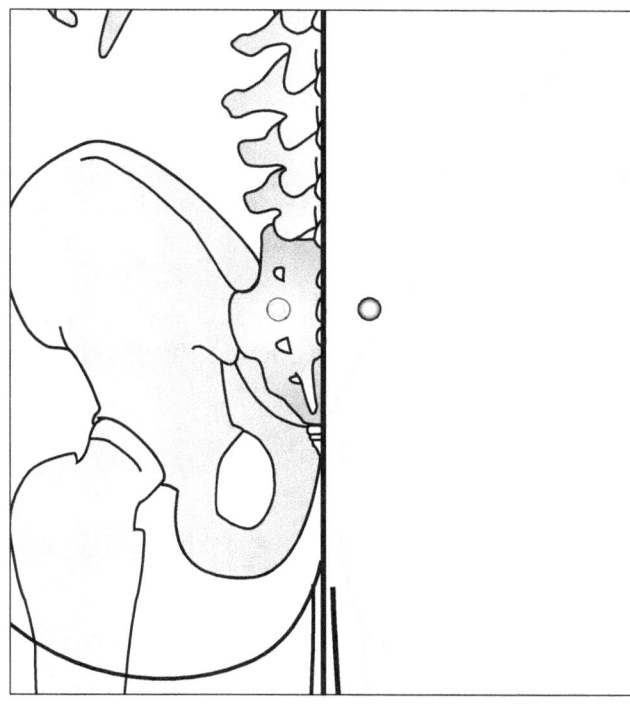

Location: On the sacrum, medial and inferior to the posterosuperior iliac spine, at the 2nd posterior sacral foramen.

Functions: Regulates the lower jiao, regulates menstruation, benefits the lumbar area, benefits the knees, benefits urination.

Indications: Lumbar pain, sacral pain, weakness and numbness of the lower extremities, spermatorrhea, impotence, irregular menstruation, bloody leukorrhea.

Notes

_____

_____

_____

_____

_____

_____

_____

_____

Point Combinations

_____

_____

_____

_____

_____

_____

UB 33
ZHONGLIAO

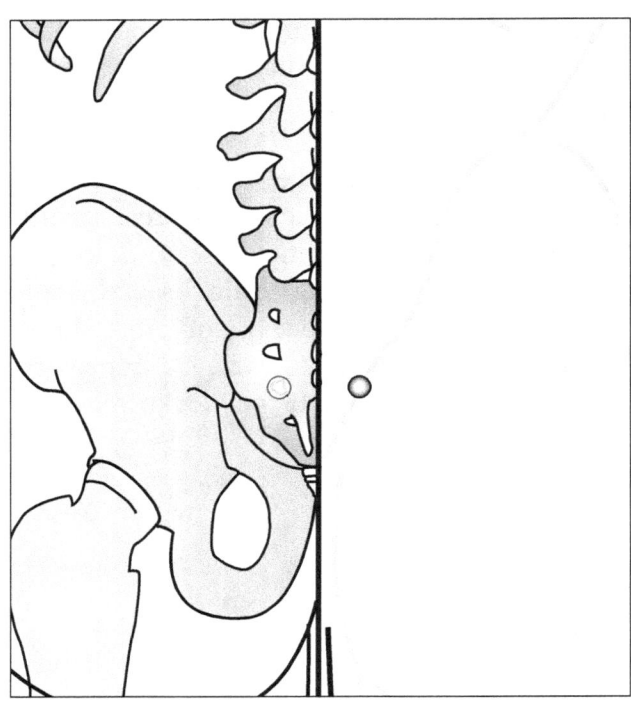

Location: On the sacrum, medial and inferior to the posterosuperior iliac spine, at the 3rd posterior sacral foramen.

Functions: Regulates the lower jiao, regulates menstruation, benefits the lumbar area, benefits the knees, benefits the knees, benefits urination.

Indications: Lumbar pain, sacral pain, irregular menstruation, leukorrhea, dysuria, constipation, diarrhea.

Notes

_____
_____
_____
_____
_____
_____
_____
_____

Point Combinations

_____
_____
_____
_____
_____
_____
_____

UB 34
XIALIAO

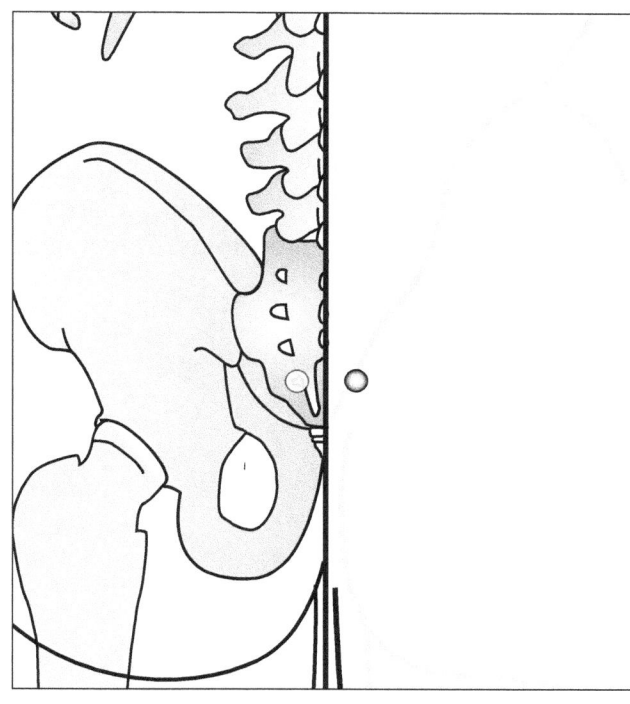

Location: On the sacrum, medial and inferior to the posterosuperior iliac spine, at the 4th posterior sacral foramen.

Functions: Regulates the lower jiao, regulates menstruation, benefits the lumbar area, benefits the knees, benefits the legs, benefits urination.
Indications: Lumbar pain, sacral pain, lower abdominal pain, dysuria, bloody leukorrhea.

Notes

_____

_____

_____

_____

_____

_____

_____

_____

_____

Point Combinations

_____

_____

_____

_____

_____

_____

_____

UB 35
HUIYANG

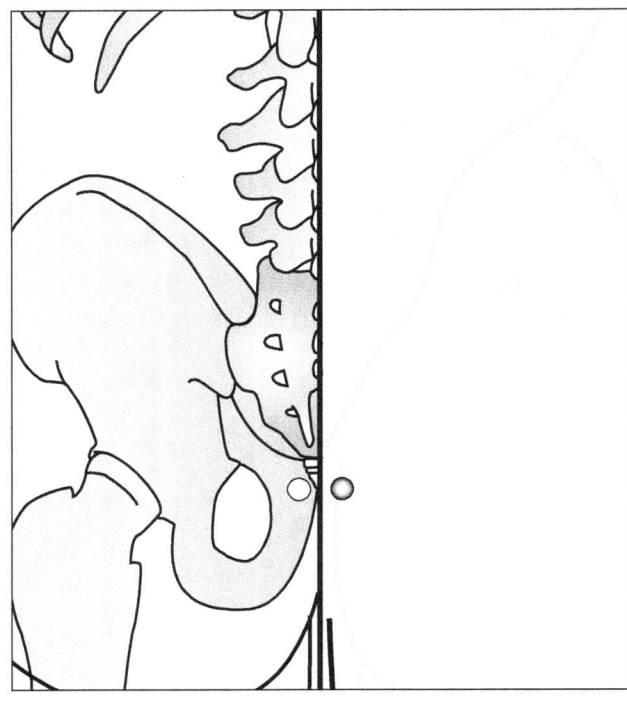

Location: In the region of the sacrum, 0.5 cun lateral to the tip of the coccyx.

Functions: Resolves damp-heat, treats trauma of the coccyx, treats hemorrhoids.

Indications: Bowel incontinence, diarrhea, blood in the stool, hemorrhoids, impotence, bloody leukorrhea.

Notes

Point Combinations

UB 36
CHENGFU

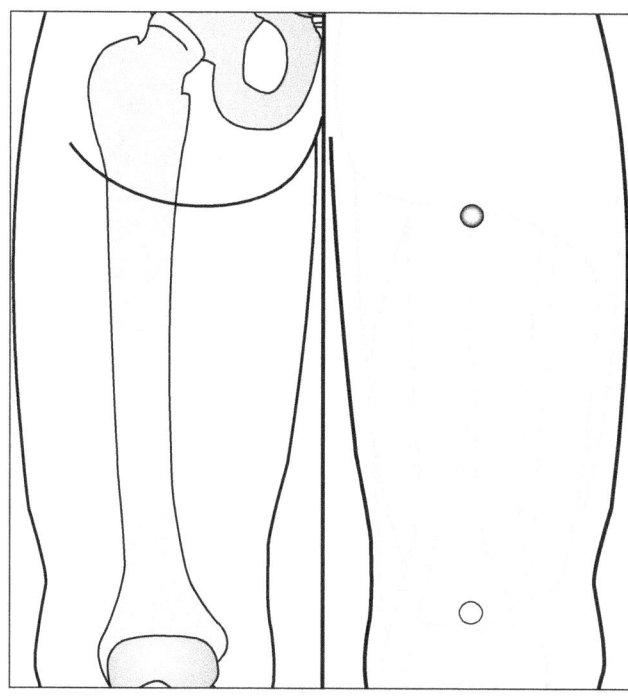

Location: On the posterior aspect of the leg, at the midpoint of the transverse gluteal crease.

Functions: Extinguishes wind, remove blockages from the channel, relaxes the connecting vessels, tendons and ligaments, relieves pain.

Indications: Motor impairment, pain, numbness and paralysis of the lower extremity, lower back and gluteal region, pain in the genitals, muscular atrophy, retention of urine, swelling of the coccyx, constipation, hemorrhoids.

Attributes: Local point for sciatic pain and pain in lower back radiating down posterior thigh.

Notes
_____
_____
_____
_____
_____
_____
_____
_____
_____

Point Combinations
_____
_____
_____
_____
_____
_____
_____

UB 37
YINMEN

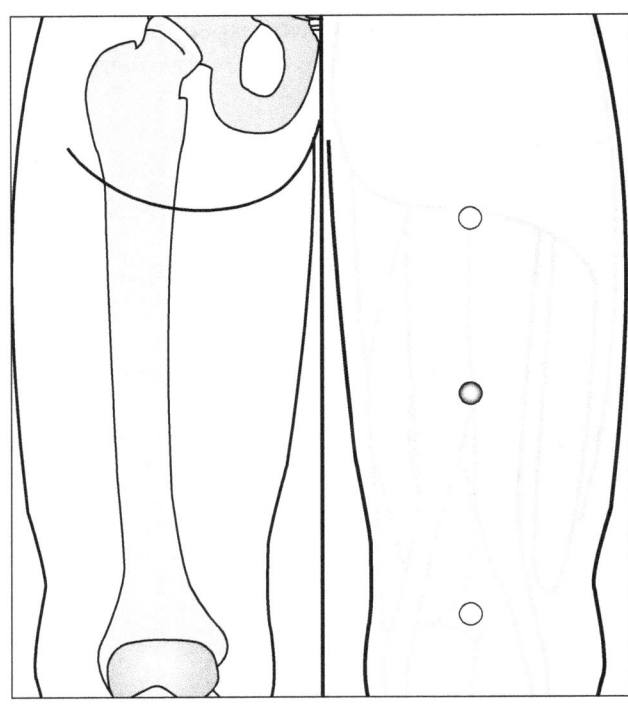

Location: On the posterior aspect of the leg, 6 cun below BL-36 Chengfu on the line joining BL-36 Chengfu and BL-40 Weizhong.

Functions: Removes blockages from the channel, nourishes the lumbar spine, relaxes the connecting vessels, tendons and ligaments, relieves pain.

Indications: Motor impairment, pain, numbness and paralysis of the lower extremity, lower back and thigh, herniated disk, occipital headache.

Attributes: Local point for sciatic pain.

Notes
_____
_____
_____
_____
_____
_____
_____
_____

Point Combinations
_____
_____
_____
_____
_____
_____

UB 38
FUXI

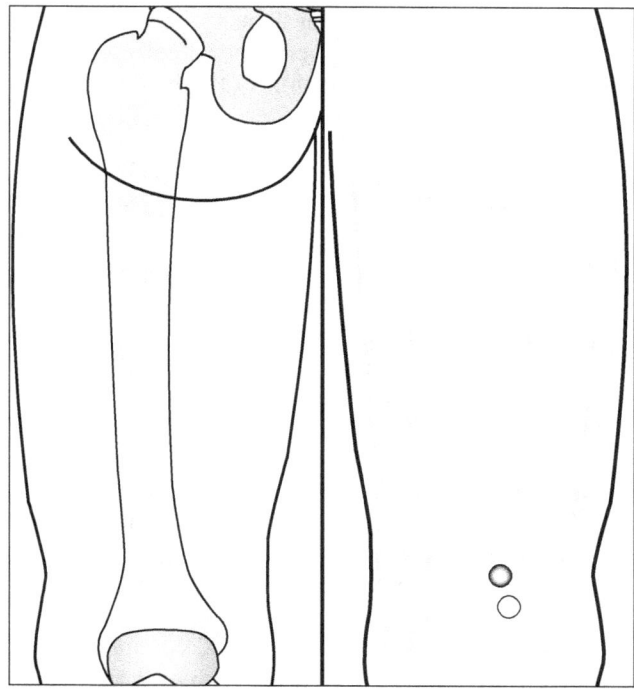

Location: On the posterior aspect of the leg, at the lateral end of the transverse popliteal crease, on the medial side of the tendon of the biceps femoris muscle, 1 cun above BL-39 Weiyang.

Functions: Clears heat, moves blood, relaxes the connecting vessels, tendons and ligaments, remove blockages from the channel and relieves pain, nourishes the lumbar spine.

Indications: Constipation, vomiting and diarrhea with muscle spasms (acute gastroenteritis), numbness of the femoral and gluteal regions, paralysis of lateral aspect of leg and thigh, cystitis, contraction and motor impairment of the popliteal fossa.

Notes

_____

_____

_____

_____

_____

_____

_____

_____

Point Combinations

_____

_____

_____

_____

_____

_____

UB 39
WEIYANG

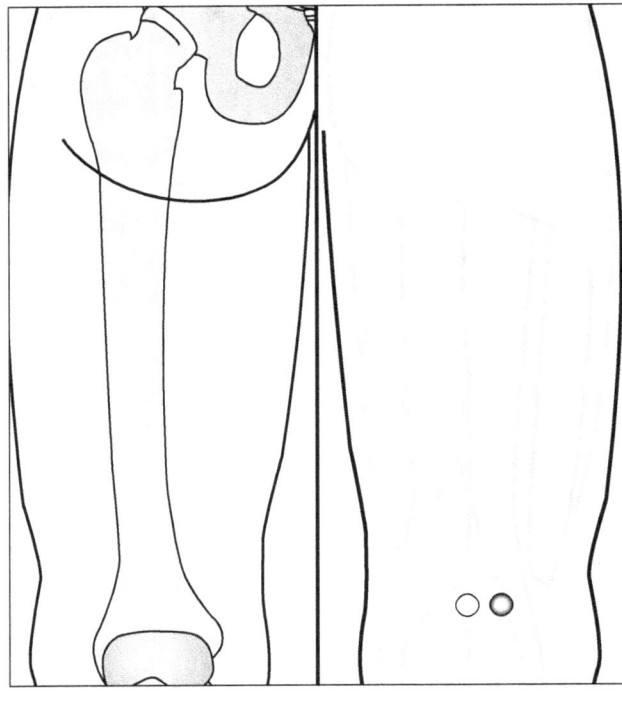

Location: On the posterior aspect of the leg, at the lateral end of the transverse popliteal crease, on the medial side of the tendon of the biceps femoris muscle.

Functions: Benefits the Urinary Bladder, opens the three jiao's, remove blockages from the channel and courses the water pathways, relaxes the connecting vessels, tendons and ligaments, nourishes the lower jiao, promotes urination, transformation and transportation of fluids and transformation of damp-heat, relieves pain.

Indications: Constipation, edema of the ankles, edema causing urinary retention, incontinence, burning, discomfort or difficulty, pain in lower back and/or extending to the abdomen, spasm of leg and/or foot, cystitis, nephritis, chyluria, fullness in chest or abdomen.

Attributes: Lower He-Sea point of San Jiao channel.

*Main point for any urinary issues, edema, or fluid issues in the body.

Notes
_____
_____
_____
_____
_____
_____
_____
_____

Point Combinations
_____
_____
_____
_____
_____
_____
_____

UB 40
WEIZHONG

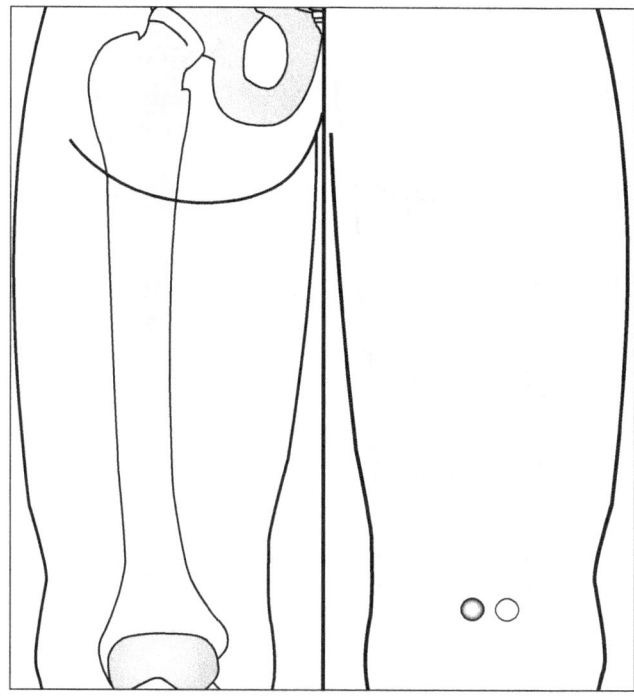

Location: On the posterior aspect of the leg, at the midpoint of the transverse popliteal crease of the popliteal fossa, between the tendons of the biceps femoris muscle and the semitendinosus muscle.

Functions: Remove blockages from the channel, relaxes the connecting vessels, muscles, tendons and ligaments, resolves damp, cools and moves blood and clears damp and heat, expels wind-damp, benefits the lower back, hips and knees, nourishes the Spleen, calms the fetus, relieves pain.

Indications: Arthritis, pain and stiffness of lumbar spine, low back, hip and knee, sciatica, paralysis of the lower limb, spasm of gastrocnemius muscle, hemiplegia, carbuncles and skin problems due to heat, heat exhaustion, seizures, coma from stroke, tidal fevers, abdominal pain, diarrhea and vomiting, muscular atrophy.

Attributes: Earth point, He-Sea point and Lower He-Sea point of Urinary Bladder, Command point for upper and lower back.

* Major point for sciatica.

** Good point for Heat and/or toxins in blood.

Notes

Point Combinations

UB 41
FUFEN

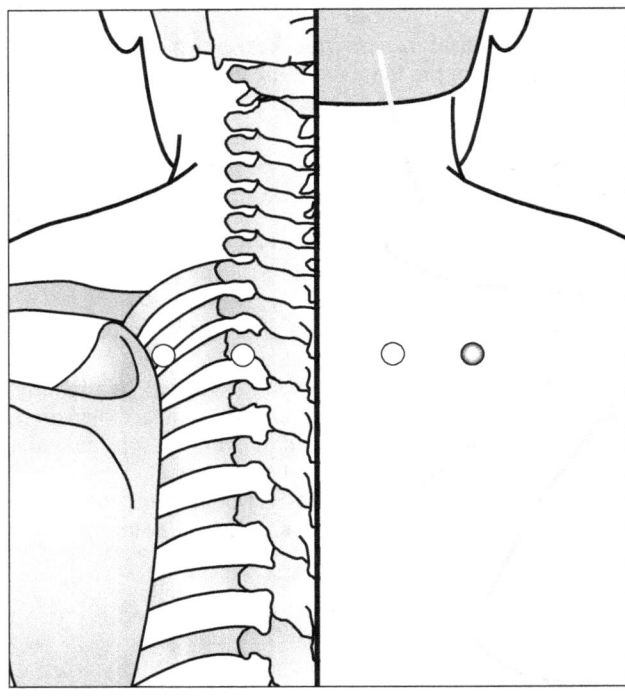

Location: On the back, below the spinous process of the 2nd thoracic vertebra, 3 cun lateral to the posterior midline.

Functions: Remove blockages from the channel, relaxes and nourishes the connecting vessels, tendons and bones, supports the lumbar spine and knee, clears summer-heat and cools blood, relieves pain and expels wind and cold.

Indications: Soreness, pain and stiffness of the neck, shoulder and back, numbness of the arm and elbow.

Notes

Point Combinations

UB 42
POHU

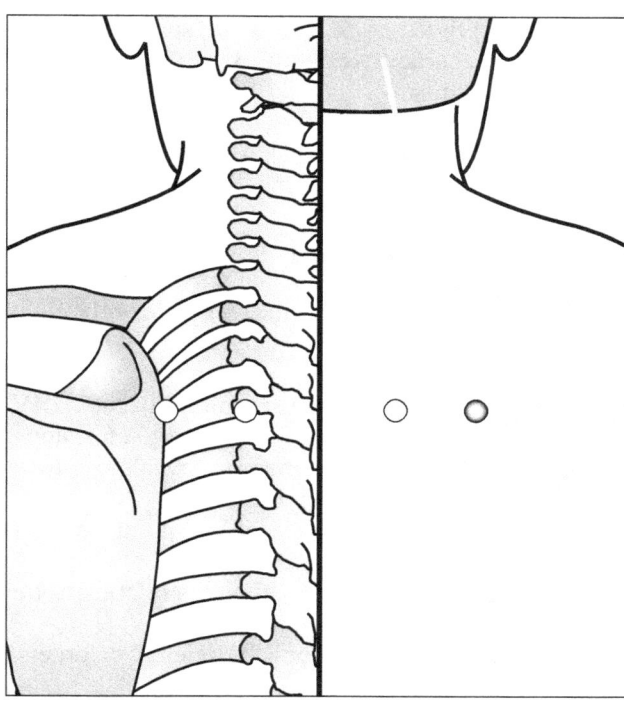

Location: On the back, below the spinous process of the 3rd thoracic vertebra, 3 cun lateral to the posterior midline.

Functions: Benefits and opens the Lung, stops cough and asthma, supports descending function of Lung Qi, corrects rebellious and regulates Lung Qi, clears heat.

Indications: Asthma, cough, bronchitis, pulmonary tuberculosis, pleurisy, stiff neck, pain in the shoulder and back, hemoptysis.

Attributes: Outer Back Shu point of the Lung.
*Point used to treat emotional issues relating to the Lung.

Notes
_____
_____
_____
_____
_____
_____
_____
_____
_____

Point Combinations
_____
_____
_____
_____
_____
_____

UB 43
GAOHUANGSHU

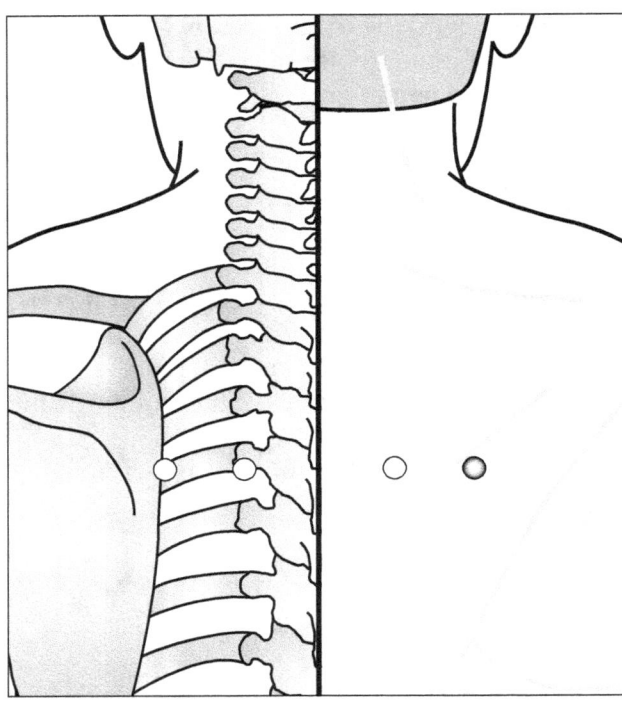

Location: On the back, below the spinous process of the 4th thoracic vertebra, 3 cun lateral to the posterior midline.

Functions: Stops cough and asthma, opens the chest and benefits the Lung, tonifies Qi, blood, Heart yin, Kidney, Spleen, Lung yin, moistens dryness, transforms phlegm, nourishes deficiencies and essence, supports and calms the Heart and spirit and stimulates the mind, regulates rebellious Stomach Qi.

Indications: Cough, asthma, bronchitis, hiccups, pleurisy, hemoptysis, night sweats, HIV, pulmonary tuberculosis, nocturnal emissions, absent mindedness, poor memory, weakness from prolonged illness, spinal pain.

Attributes: Outer Back Shu point of the Pericardium.

*Point used to treat emotional issues relating to the Pericardium.

**Point for late stage chronic deficiency disorders.

Notes
_____
_____
_____
_____
_____
_____
_____
_____

Point Combinations
_____
_____
_____
_____
_____
_____

UB 44
SHENTANG

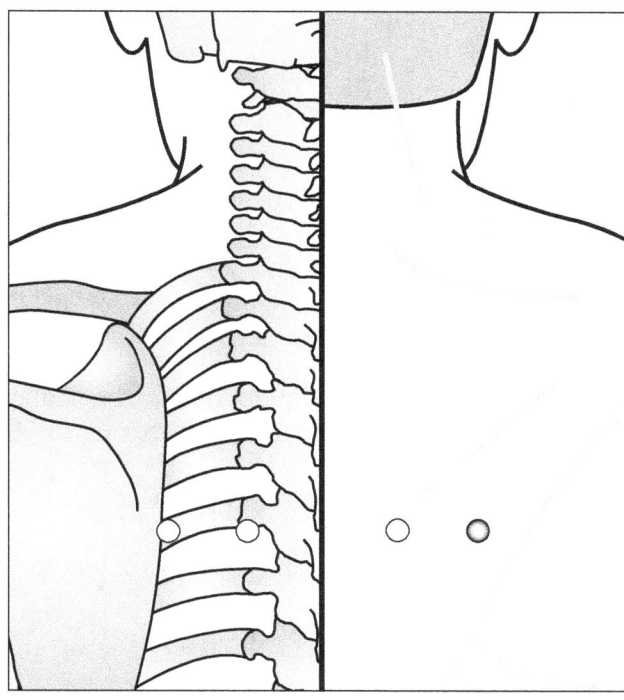

Location: On the back, below the spinous process of the 5th thoracic vertebra, 3 cun lateral to the posterior midline.

Functions: Remove blockages from the channel, relaxes and nourishes the connecting vessels, clears heat, manages Heart Qi, soothes the chest, calms shen, courses Qi, stops cough and dyspnea.

Indications: Asthma, cough, bronchitis, cardiac pain and palpitations, insomnia, anxiety, depression, Heart disease, chest congestion, pain and stiffness of the back and intercostal neuralgia.

Attributes: Outer Back Shu point of the Heart.

*Point used to treat emotional issues relating to the Heart.

**Good point for shen disturbances.

Notes

Point Combinations

UB 45
YIXI

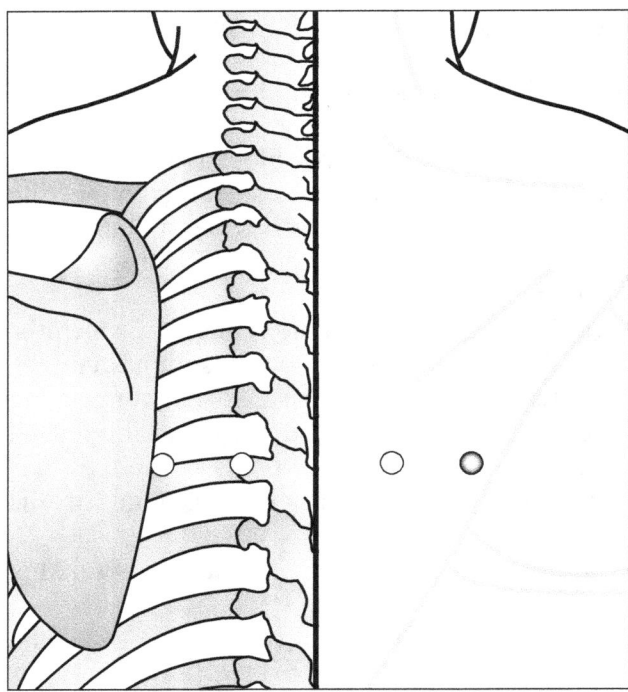

Location: On the back, below the spinous process of the 6th thoracic vertebra, 3 cun lateral to the posterior midline.

Functions: Remove blockages from the channel, benefits the Lung, extinguishes wind and relieves pain, calms the Stomach, releases the exterior, clears heat and induces sweat, moves Qi and blood, directs Lung Qi downward, relaxes the connecting vessels, tendons and ligaments.

Indications: Asthma, cough, hiccup, back and shoulder pain, intercostal neuralgia, pericarditis, malaria.

Attributes: Outer Back Shu point of the DU Channel.

*Also used to treat eye and vision problems.

Notes _____
_____
_____
_____
_____
_____
_____
_____
_____

Point Combinations _____
_____
_____
_____
_____
_____
_____

UB 46
GEGUAN

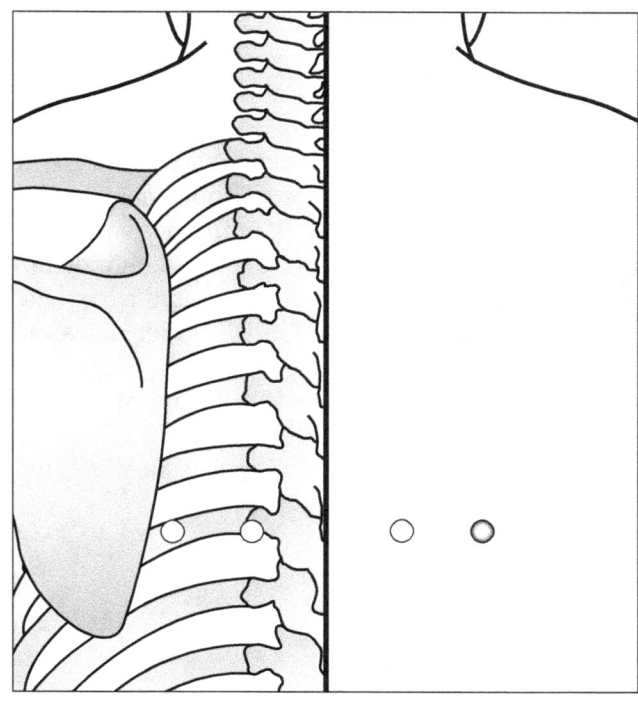

Location: On the back, below the spinous process of the 7th thoracic vertebra, 3 cun lateral to the posterior midline.

Functions: Remove blockages from the channel, relaxes the connecting vessels, muscles, tendons and ligaments, benefits the middle jiao, regulates the stomach and strengthens the Spleen, resolves damp, regulates the diaphragm, moves Qi and blood, relieves pain.

Indications: Hiccups, belching, vomiting, spasm of the esophagus, dysphasia, gastric hemorrhage, stiffness and pain of the back, intercostal neuralgia.

Notes

Point Combinations

UB 47
HUNMEN

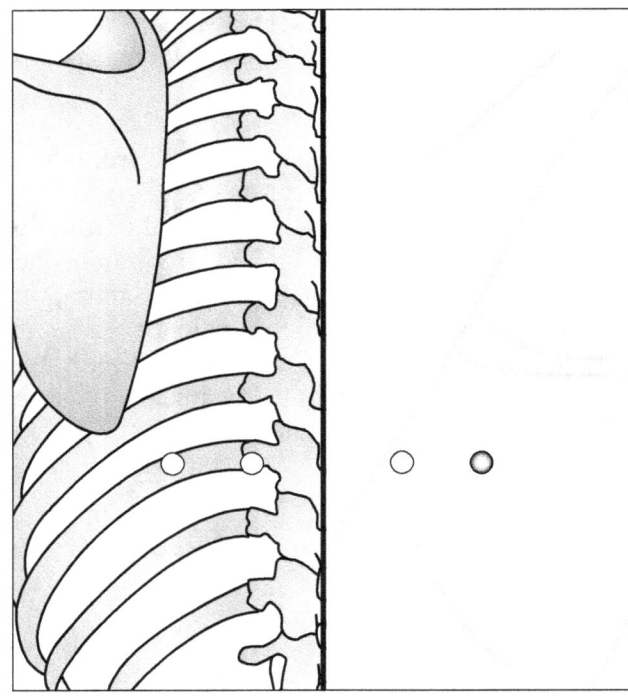

Location: On the back, below the spinous process of the 9th thoracic vertebra, 3 cun lateral to the posterior midline.

Functions: Remove blockages from the Liver channel, secures the ethereal soul, manages Qi of Fu organs and Stomach, nourishes Spleen.

Indications: Back, chest, and hypochondrium pain, stomach pain, vomiting and diarrhea, neurasthenia, Liver and Gall Bladder diseases, pleurisy.

Attributes: Outer Back Shu point of the Liver.

*Point used to treat emotional issues relating to the Liver.

Notes
_____
_____
_____
_____
_____
_____
_____
_____

Point Combinations
_____
_____
_____
_____
_____
_____
_____

UB 48
YANGGANG

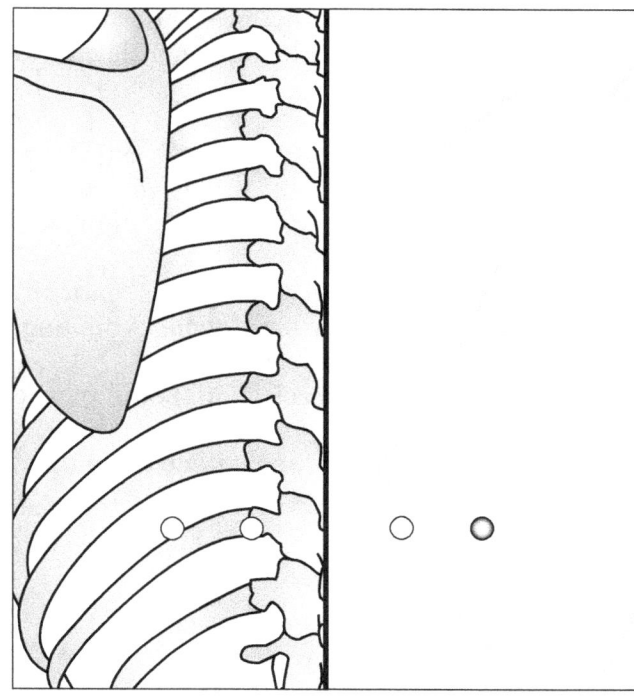

Location: On the back, below spinous process of the 10th thoracic vertebra, 3 cun lateral to the posterior midline.

Functions: Manages Gall Bladder and Stomach, clears damp-heat from Gall Bladder, balances the middle jiao and nourishes Spleen.

Indications: Hepatitis, jaundice, cholecystitis, gastritis, borborygmus, pain in abdominal and hypochondrium regions, diarrhea.

Attributes: Outer Back Shu point of the Gall Bladder.

*Point used to treat emotional issues relating to the Gall Bladder.

Notes

_____

_____

_____

_____

_____

_____

_____

_____

Point Combinations

_____

_____

_____

_____

_____

_____

UB 49
YISHE

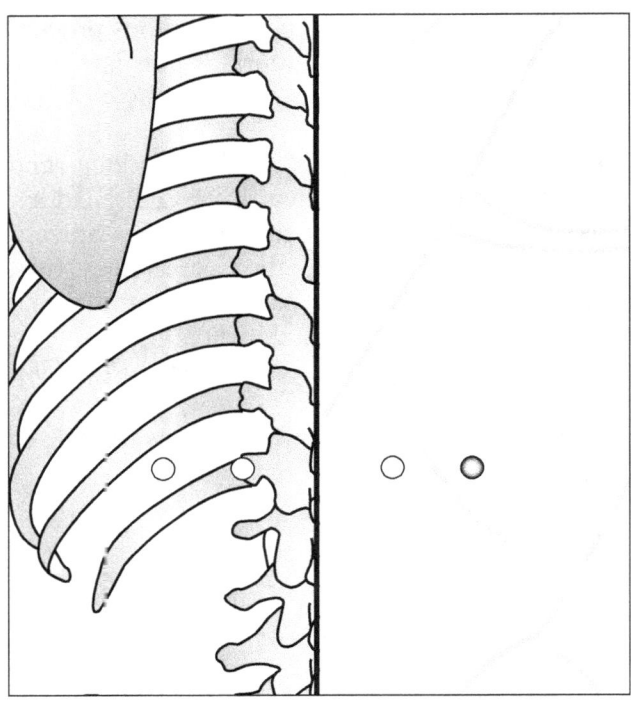

Location: On the back, below spinous process of the 11th thoracic vertebra, 3 cun lateral to the posterior midline.

Functions: Nourishes Spleen Qi and yang, manages Qi of Stomach and Liver, soothe rebellious Qi, clears damp-heat, stimulates memory and concentration.
Indications: Hepatitis, cholecystitis, gastritis, borborygmus, difficulty swallowing, vomiting, diarrhea, abdominal distention.
Attributes: Outer Back Shu point of the Spleen.
*Point used to treat emotional issues relating to the Spleen.

Notes
_____
_____
_____
_____
_____
_____
_____
_____

Point Combinations
_____
_____
_____
_____
_____
_____

UB 50
WEICANG

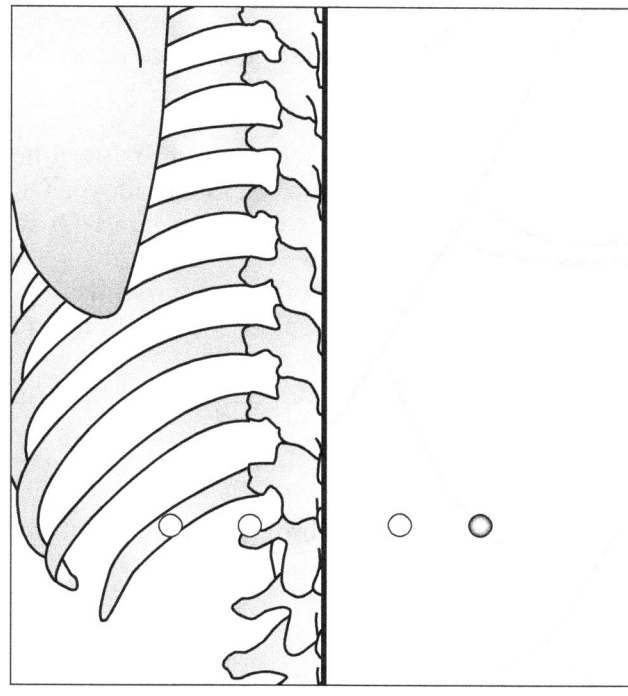

Location: On the back, below spinous process of the 12th thoracic vertebra, 3 cun lateral to the posterior midline.

Functions: Unblocks and manages the middle jiao, courses Qi, resolves damp, balances the Stomach and nourishes the Spleen.

Indications: Abdominal distention, Stomach ache, back pain, abdominal pain and pain in the epigastric region, infantile indigestion, gastritis.

Attributes: Outer Back Shu point of the Stomach.

*Point used to treat emotional issues relating to the Stomach.

Notes
_____
_____
_____
_____
_____
_____
_____
_____
_____

Point Combinations
_____
_____
_____
_____
_____
_____
_____

UB 51
HUANGMEN

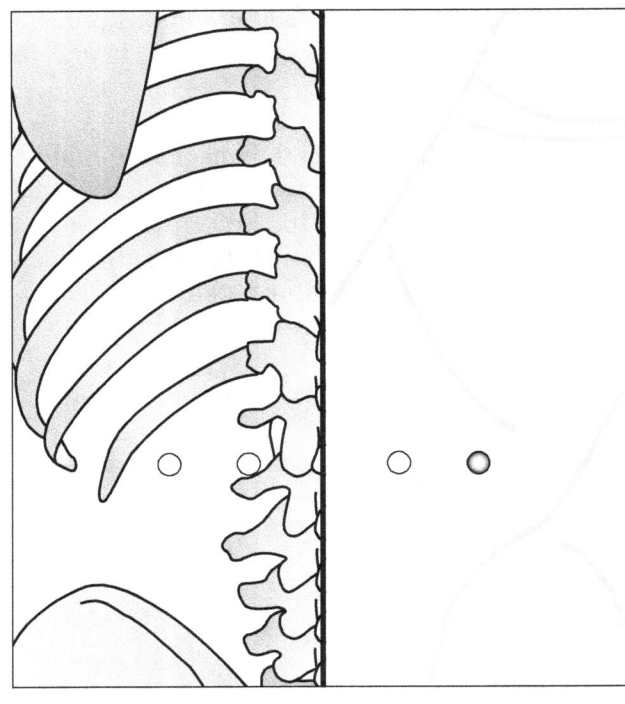

Location: On the back, below spinous process of the 1st lumbar vertebra, 3 cun lateral to the posterior midline.

Functions: Sedates heat in Large Intestine and encourage the digestive system, moves Qi, manages the three jiaos and distributes Qi in upper jiao, abate masses.

Indications: Paralysis of lower extremity, low back and abdominal pain, constipation and abdominal masses.

Attributes: Outer Back Shu point of the San Jiao.

*Point used to treat emotional issues relating to the San Jiao.

**Useful for treating chronic stagnation of Qi, blood or phlegm.

Notes

_____

_____

_____

_____

_____

_____

_____

_____

Point Combinations

_____

_____

_____

_____

_____

_____

UB 52
ZHISHI

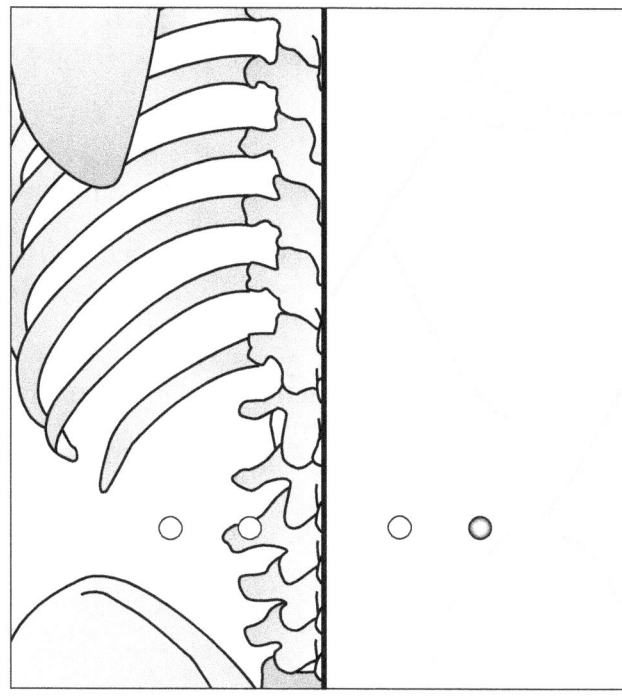

Location: On the low back, below the spinous process of the 2nd lumbar vertebra, 3 cun lateral to the posterior midline.

Functions: Nourishes the Kidneys and essence, supports and reinforces the lower back, manages urination and resolves damp, strengthens will power.

Indications: Dermatitis, edema, sexual function and impotence, prostatitis, eczema of the scrotum, spermatorrhea, nephritis, swelling and pain of the genitals, incontinence, nocturnal emissions, irregular menstruation, depression, disorientation, vomiting, low back pain, paralysis of the lower extremity.

Attributes: Outer Back Shu point of the Kidney.

*Point used to treat emotional issues relating to the Kidney.

**Major point to increase will power to set and accomplish goals as well as the will to live.

***Good for Kidney yang, better for Kidney yin and Qi.

Notes

Point Combinations

UB 53
BAOHUANG

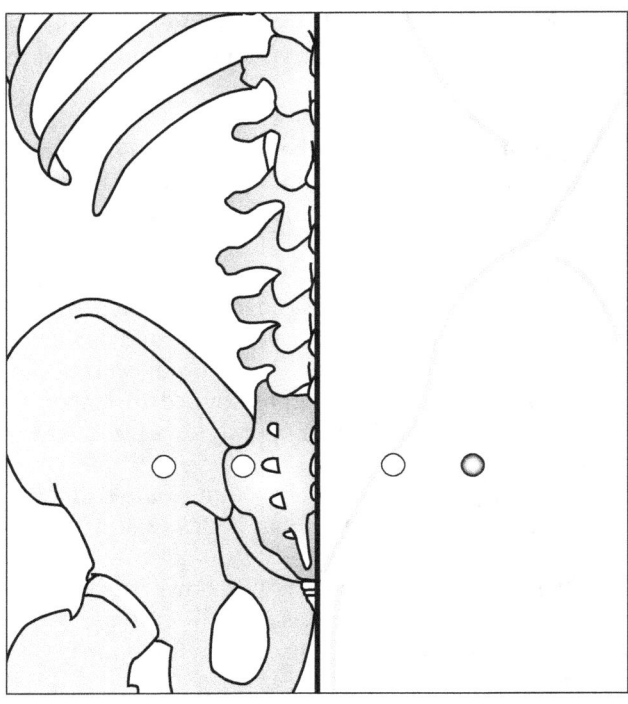

Location: On the buttock and at the level of the 2nd posterior sacral foramen, 3 cun lateral to the median sacral crest.

Functions: Opens waterways and bowels, manages and disperses Qi in lower jiao, manages Qi in Fu organs and nourishes Spleen Qi, nourishes and supports the lumbar spine, encourages the transformation of fluids and elimination of waste.

Indications: Borborygmus, low back and abdominal pain and distention, sciatica, urinary retention or difficulty, edema.

Attributes: Outer Back Shu point of the Large Intestine.

*Point used to treat emotional issues relating to the Large Intestine.

Notes
_____
_____
_____
_____
_____
_____
_____
_____

Point Combinations
_____
_____
_____
_____
_____
_____

UB 54
ZHIBIAN

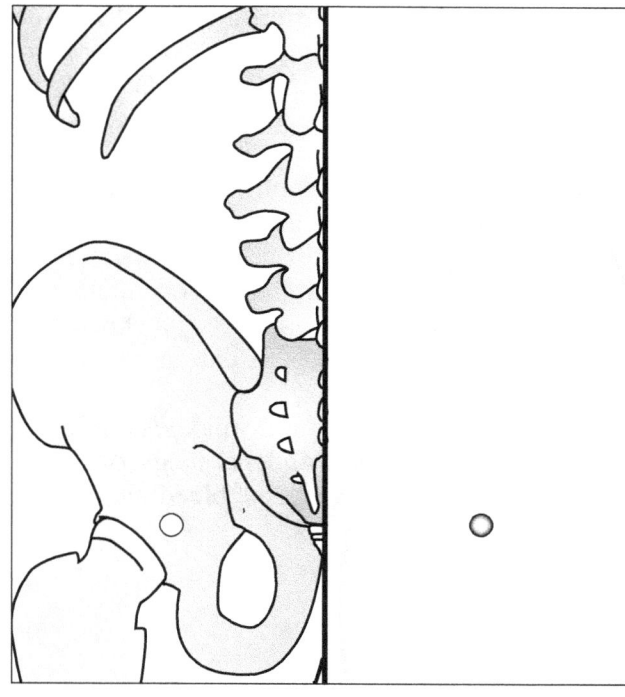

Location: On the buttock and at the level of the 4th posterior sacral foramen, 3 cun lateral to the median sacral crest.

Functions: Remove blockages from the channel, relaxes the connecting vessels, muscles, tendons and ligaments, resolves damp and clears heat, nourishes and supports the knee and lumbar spine.

Indications: Sciatica and lumbosacral pain with pain radiating down buttock and posterior leg, motor impairment of the lower extremities, muscular atrophy, hemorrhoids, constipation, dysuria, swelling and diseases of reproductive organs and anus.

Attributes: Outer Back Shu point of the Small Intestine.
*Point used to treat emotional issues relating to the Small Intestine.

Notes
_____
_____
_____
_____
_____
_____
_____
_____
_____

Point Combinations
_____
_____
_____
_____
_____
_____
_____

UB 55
HEYANG

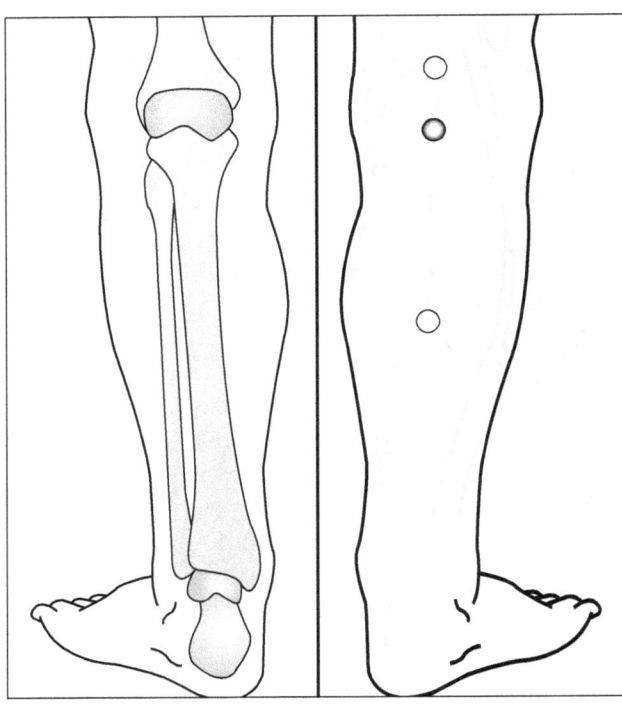

Location: On the posterior aspect of the lower leg, 2 cun below BL-40 Weizhong on the line joining BL-40 Weizhong and BL-57 Chengshan.

Functions: Remove blockages from the channel, relaxes and nourishes the connecting vessels, benefits the back and lower extremities, manages Penetrating and Ren channels and supports the Kidneys, supports the knee and lumbar spine, relieves pain and stops uterine bleeding.

Indications: Soreness and weakness in lower back and knees, pain and paralysis of lower extremities, abnormal uterine bleeding.

Notes

Point Combinations

UB 56
CHENGJIN

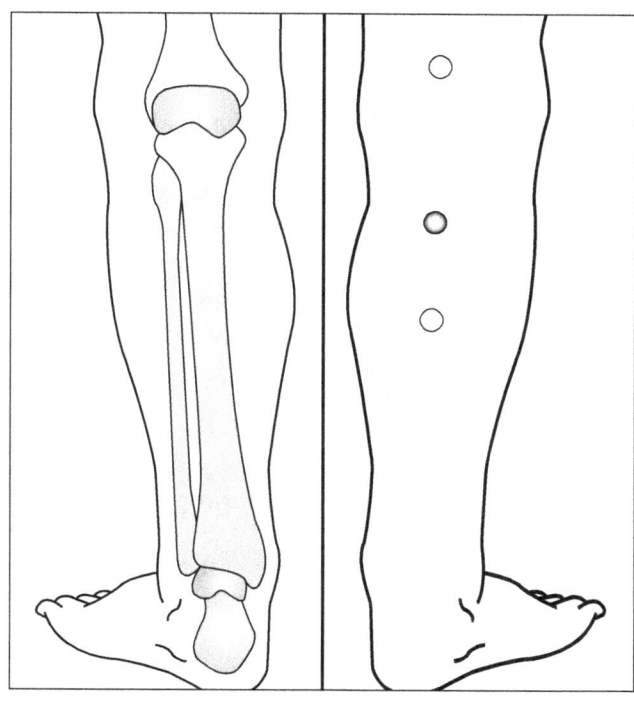

Location: On the posterior aspect of the lower leg, 5 cun below BL-40 Weizhong on the line joining BL-40 Weizhong and BL-57 Chengshan, in the center of the belly of the gastrocnemius muscle.

Functions: Remove blockages from the channel, relaxes and nourishes the connecting vessels, benefits the back, arms, legs, foot and heel.

Indications: Calf spasms, acute low back pain, sciatica, pain and spasm in gastrocnemius muscle, paralysis of lower extremity, hemorrhoids, headache.

Notes

Point Combinations

UB 57
CHENGSHAN

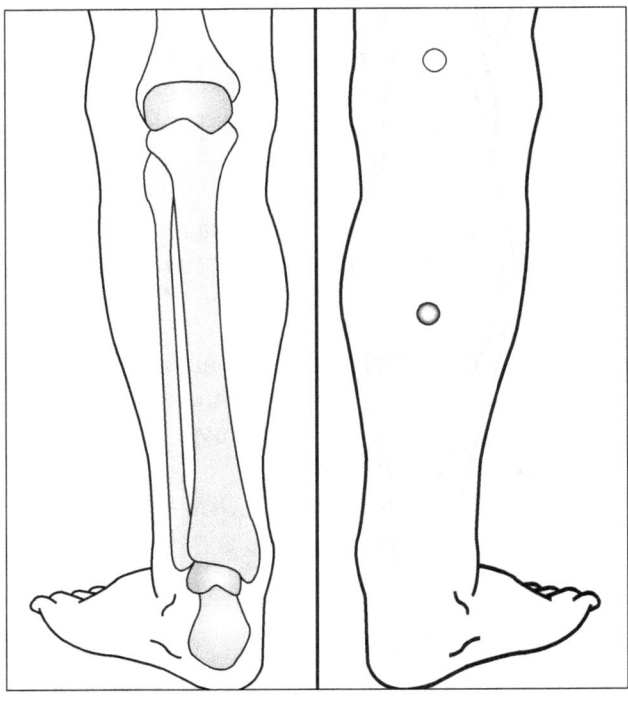

Location: On the posterior midline of the lower leg, 8 cun below BL-40 Weizhong in the depression below the gastrocnemius muscle, when the leg is extended or the heel is lifted.

Functions: Remove blockages from the channel, relaxes and nourishes the connecting vessels and muscles, benefits the Large Intestine courses and cools blood, clears heat and resolves damp, manages Qi of yang organs.

Indications: Sciatica, rheumatoid arthritis, hemorrhoids, vomiting, sore throat, diarrhea, anal prolapse, digestive issues, soreness, weakness and pain of the lower back and mgastrocnemius muscle, paralysis of lower limb.

Attributes: Main point for hemorrhoids.

Notes
_____
_____
_____
_____
_____
_____
_____
_____

Point Combinations
_____
_____
_____
_____
_____
_____

UB 58
FEIYANG

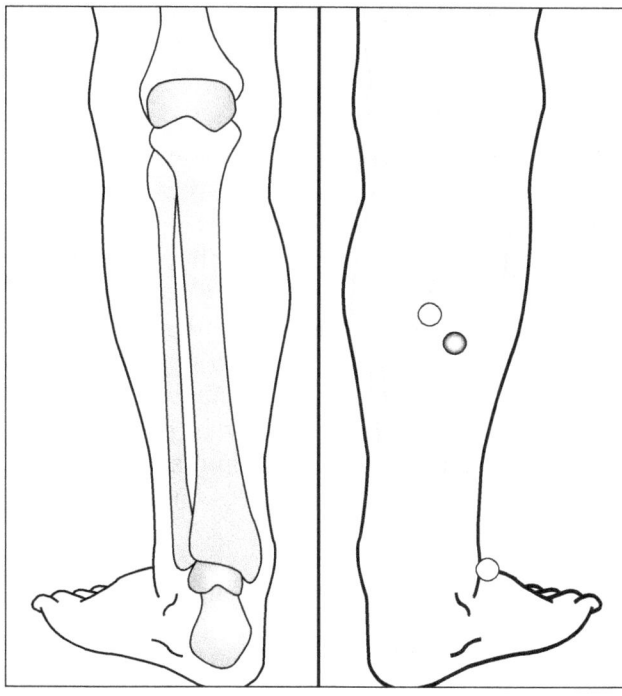

Location: On the posterior aspect of the lower leg, 7 cun above BL-60 Kunlun, 1 cun lateral and inferior to BL-57 Chengshan.

Functions: Remove blockages from the channel, relaxes and nourishes the connecting vessels, nourishes the Kidneys, expels wind-damp, and pathogens in Tai Yang channel, courses Qi, relieves pain.

Indications: Vertigo, seizures, insanity, nasal congestion or obstruction, blurred vision, epistaxis, pain in the head, back, lower back, legs and calf muscle and joints, cystitis, rheumatoid arthritis, nephritis, hemorrhoids.

Attributes: Luo-Connecting point of Urinary Bladder channel.

*Main point for chronic low back pain.

**No.1 point for rheumatoid arthritis.

Notes

Point Combinations

UB 59
FUYANG

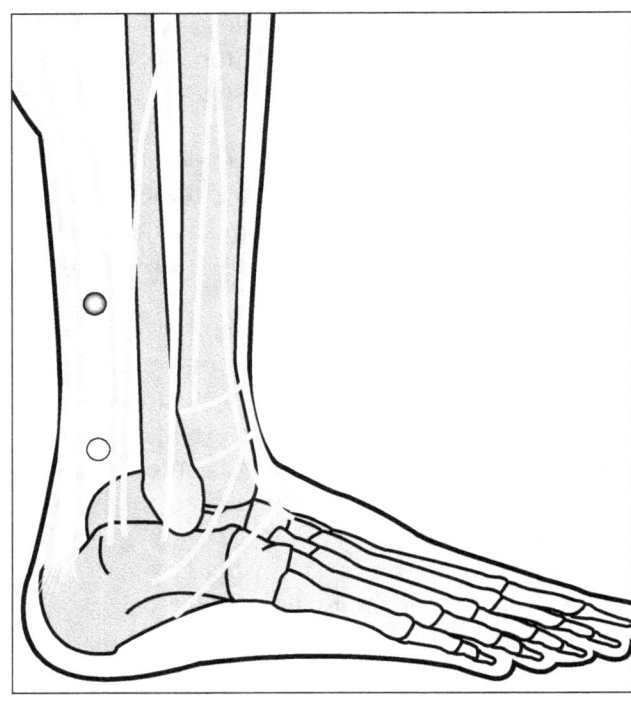

Location: On the posterior / lateral aspect of the lower leg, 3 cun above BL-60 Kunlun, behind the lateral malleolus.

Functions: Remove blockages from the channel, supports and reinforces the back, extinguishes wind, clears heat, wind-damp, and pathogens in Tai Yang channel and damp-heat in the Bladder, encourages Yang Qiao Mai Vessel, courses Qi, encourages agility, relaxes pain.

Indications: Headache or heaviness of the head, low back pain, paralysis of the lower limb, inflammation at external malleolus.

Attributes: Xi-cleft point of the Yang Qiao Mai Vessel.

Notes
_____
_____
_____
_____
_____
_____
_____
_____

Point Combinations
_____
_____
_____
_____
_____
_____
_____

UB 60
KUNLUN

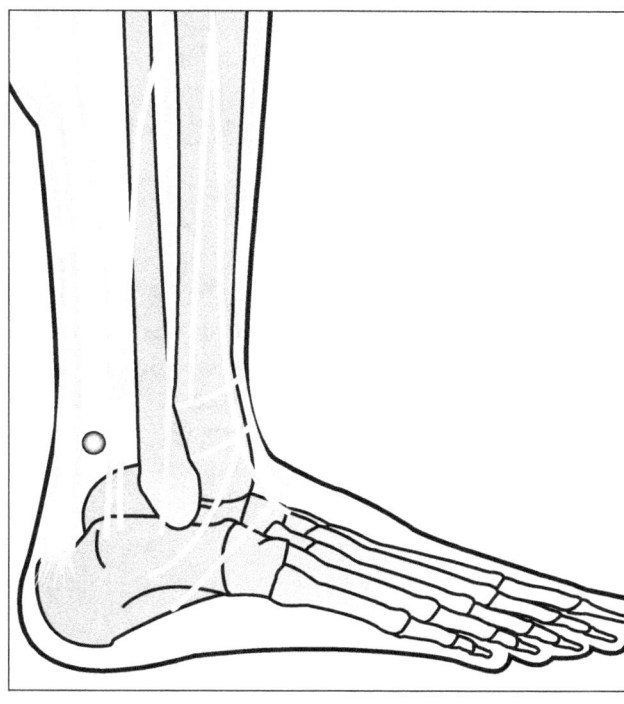

Location: On the posterior / lateral aspect of the lower leg, posterior to the lateral malleolus, in the depression between the tip of the external malleolus and Achilles tendon.

Functions: Remove blockages from the channel, relaxes and nourishes the connecting vessels and muscles, extinguishes wind, resolves damp, clears heat, extinguishes wind-cold, courses Qi and blood, supports the Kidneys, low back, legs and heels, manages Shao Yang Qi, expels Tai Yang pathogens.

Indications: Headache, stiff neck, blurred vision, epistaxis, pain in the lower arm, shoulder, lower back, and heel, plantar fasciitis, sciatica, paralysis of lower extremity, delayed, painful or dark clotted menses, difficult labor, retained placenta, infantile fright, tidal fever.

Attributes: Fire point and Jing River point of the Urinary Bladder channel.

*Main point back and neck pain and occipital headaches.

**CONTRAINDICATED IN PREGNANCY.

Notes

_____
_____
_____
_____
_____
_____
_____
_____

Point Combinations

_____
_____
_____
_____
_____
_____

UB 61
PUCAN

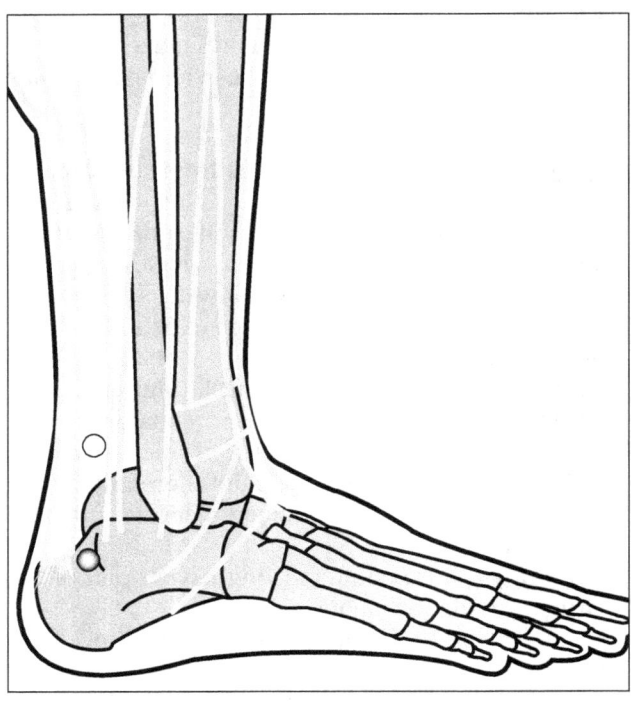

Location: On the lateral side of the foot, posterior and inferior to the lateral malleolus, inferior to BL-60 Kunlun, lateral to the calcaneum at the junction of the red and white skin.

Functions: Remove blockages from the channel, relaxes and nourishes the connecting vessels, nourishes the Kidneys, supports bones, relieves pain, reduces swelling, extinguishes wind, resolves damp, calms shen and spirit.

Indications: Meniere's disease, headache, mania, psychosis, epilepsy, seizures, hemiplegia, low back pain, pain in the ankle, foot and heel, muscular atrophy.

Notes

Point Combinations

UB 62
SHENMAI

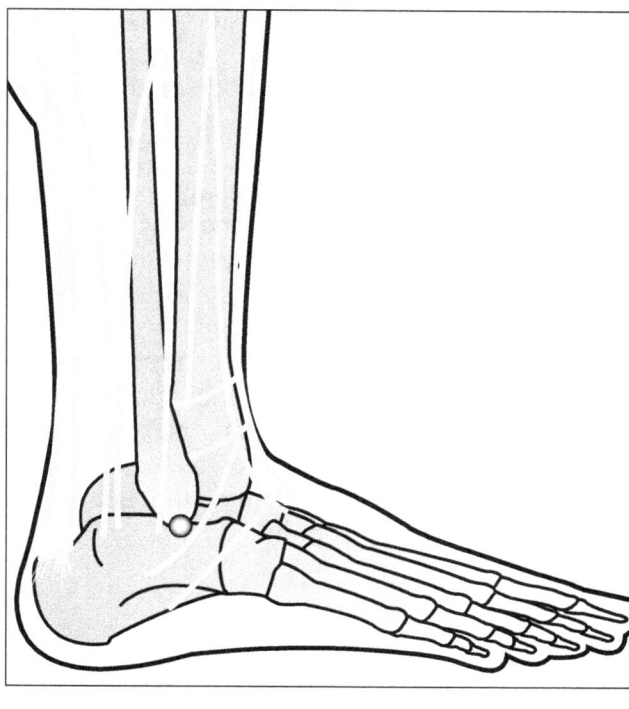

Location: On the lateral side of the foot, in the depression 0.5 cun below the external malleolus.

Functions: Remove blockages from the channel, relaxes the connecting vessels, muscles, tendons and ligaments, expels exterior pathogens, interior wind, heat and releases the exterior, calms shen, opens Yang Qiao Mai channel, benefits the eyes.

Indications: Meniere's disease, headache, palpitations, mania, psychosis, insanity, epilepsy, seizures, hemiplegia, insomnia, dizziness, meningitis, low back pain, pain in the ankle, foot and heel, hemiplegia, aphasia, tinnitus.

Attributes: Confluent point of Yang Qiao channel and Ghost point.
*Main point for epilepsy.

Notes

Point Combinations

UB 63
JINMEN

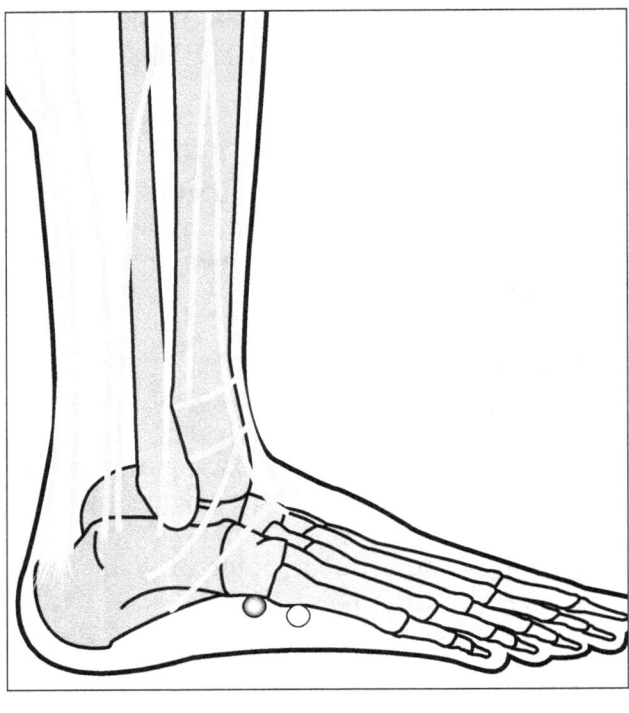

Location: On the lateral side of the foot, directly below the anterior border of the lateral malleolus, on the lower border of the cuboid bone.

Functions: Remove blockages from the channel, relaxes the connecting vessels, extinguishes wind-heat, extinguishes wind-damp, relieves pain, calms shen, restores consciousness.

Indications: Epilepsy, seizures, mania, infantile convulsions, insomnia, palpitations, abdominal inflammation or spasm, motor impairment or pain of lower back, legs, and bottom of the foot, bladder incontinence.

Attributes: Xi-Cleft point.

Notes _____

_____

_____

_____

_____

_____

_____

_____

_____

Point Combinations _____

_____

_____

_____

_____

_____

_____

UB 64
JINGGU

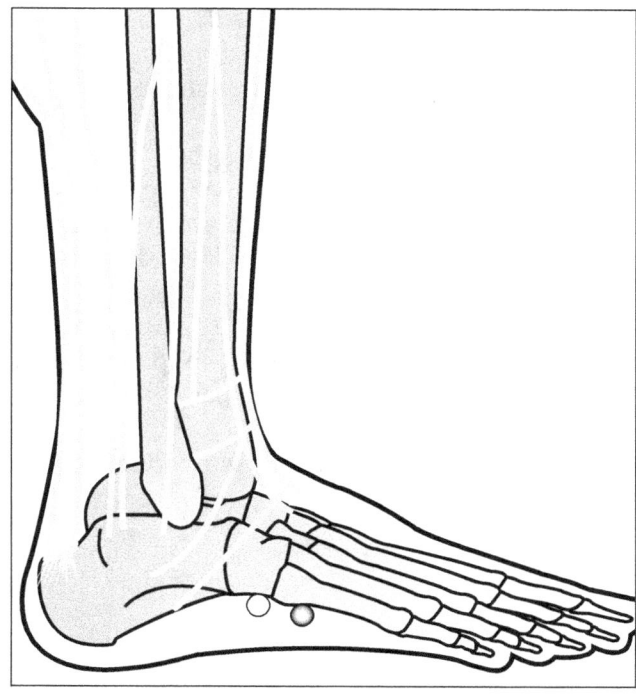

Location: On the lateral side of the foot, below the tuberosity of the 5th metatarsal bone at the junction of the red and white skin.

Functions: Remove blockages from the channel, relaxes the connecting vessels, extinguishes wind-heat, extinguishes wind-damp, calms shen and mind.

Indications: Headache or heaviness in the head, seizure, insanity, blurred vision, stiff neck, meningitis, palpitations, myocarditis, pain in lower back and leg, cold in legs, painful urination, tidal fever.

Attributes: Yuan Source point.

Notes

Point Combinations

UB 65
SHUGU

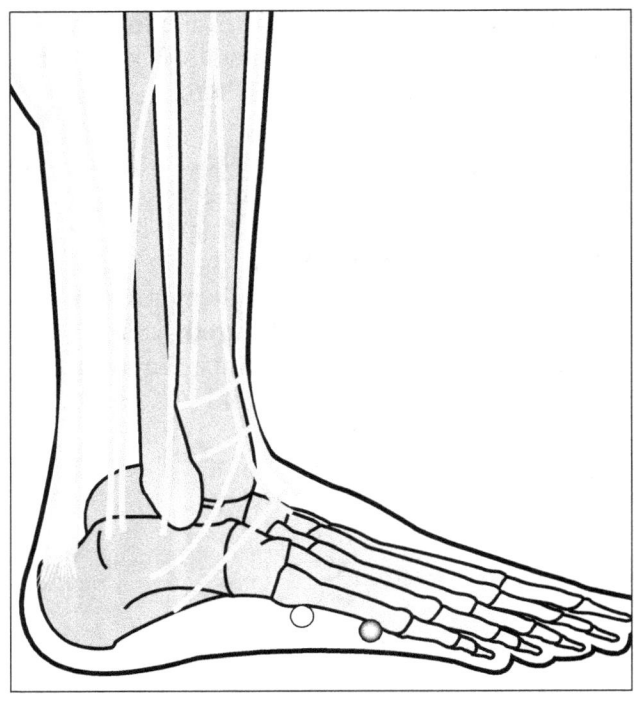

Location: On the lateral side of the foot, posterior to the 5th metatarsalphalangeal joint at the junction of the red and white skin.

Functions: Remove blockages from the channel, relaxes the connecting vessels, supports the back, bones, head, shen and vision, extinguishes wind-heat, clears Heart fire, toxins and pathogens.

Indications: Mental illness, seizures, mania, malaria, headache, blurred vision, pannus, stiff neck, diarrhea, hemorrhoids, paralysis, broken bones.

Attributes: Wood point, Shu Stream point, Sedation point.

Notes

_____
_____
_____
_____
_____
_____
_____
_____

Point Combinations

_____
_____
_____
_____
_____
_____
_____

UB 66
ZUTONGGU

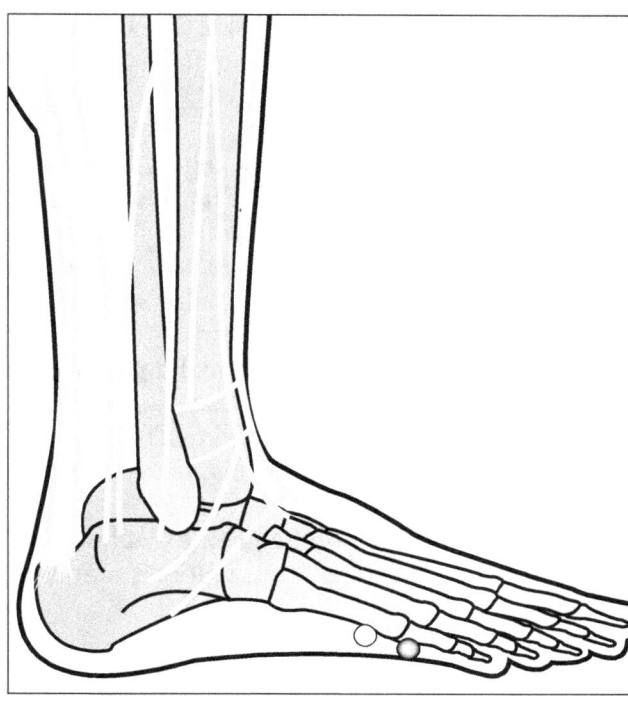

Location: On the lateral side of the foot, anterior to the 5th metatarsalphalangeal joint at the junction of the red and white skin.

Functions: Remove blockages from the channel, extinguishes wind-heat, calms shen, subdues fright.

Indications: Mental illness, mania, headache, blurred vision, stiff neck, asthma, epistaxis, vertigo, indigestion.

Attributes: Water point, Ying Spring point and Horary point.

Notes
_____
_____
_____
_____
_____
_____
_____
_____

Point Combinations
_____
_____
_____
_____
_____
_____

UB 67
ZHIYIN

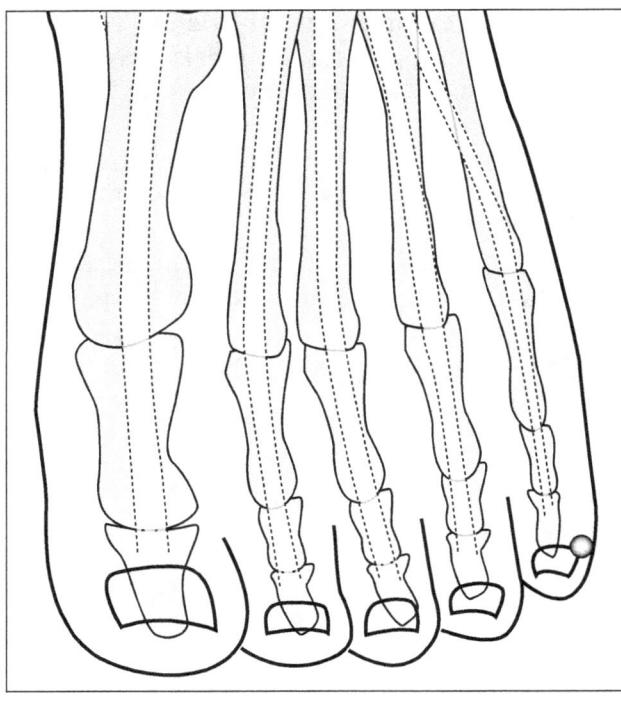

Location: On the lateral side of the distal segment of the little toe, 0.1 cun from the corner of the toenail.

Functions: Remove blockages from the channel, extinguishes wind-heat, extinguishes damp-heat, interior and exterior wind, courses and manages Qi and blood, loosens the nasal passageways, relieves pain, calms shen and calms the fetus, improves vision.

Indications: Headache opthalmalgia, epistaxis, nasal obstruction, clear nasal discharge, difficult labor, malposition of fetus, retention of placenta, infantile convulsions, heat sensation in the sole, stroke.

Attributes: Metal point and Jing Well point of the Urinary Bladder, Tonification point and Exit point.

*Main point for turning a breech baby.

Notes

_____
_____
_____
_____
_____
_____
_____
_____

Point Combinations

_____
_____
_____
_____
_____
_____

KD 1
YONGQUAN

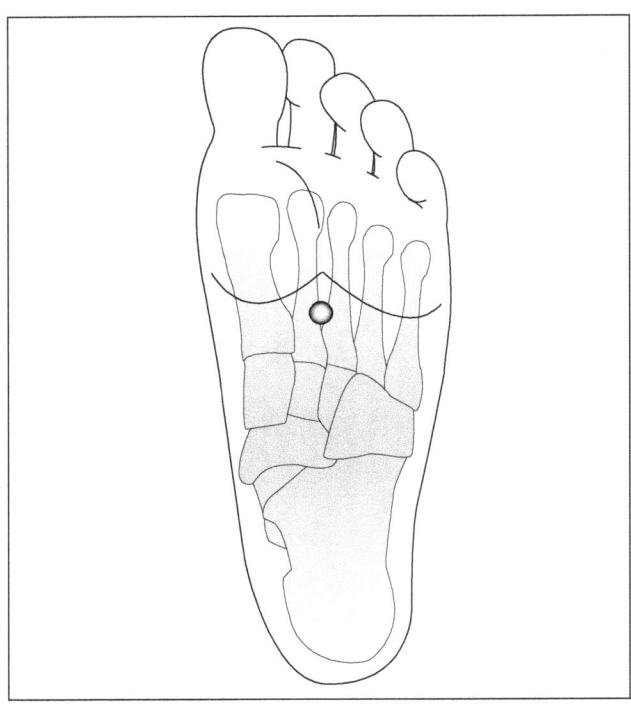

Location: On the sole, in the depression appearing on the anterior part of the sole when the foot is in plantar flexion, approximately at the junction of the anterior third and posterior two-thirds of the line connecting the base of the 2nd and 3rd toes and the heel.

Functions: Descends Qi, calms shen, revives consciousness and relieves yang collapse.

Indications: Anxiety, palpitations, dizziness, cloudy vision, hypertension, poor memory, benefits the throat and tongue.

Attributes: Wood point, Jing Well point.

Notes

_____

_____

_____

_____

_____

_____

_____

Point Combinations

_____

_____

_____

_____

_____

KD 2
RANGGU

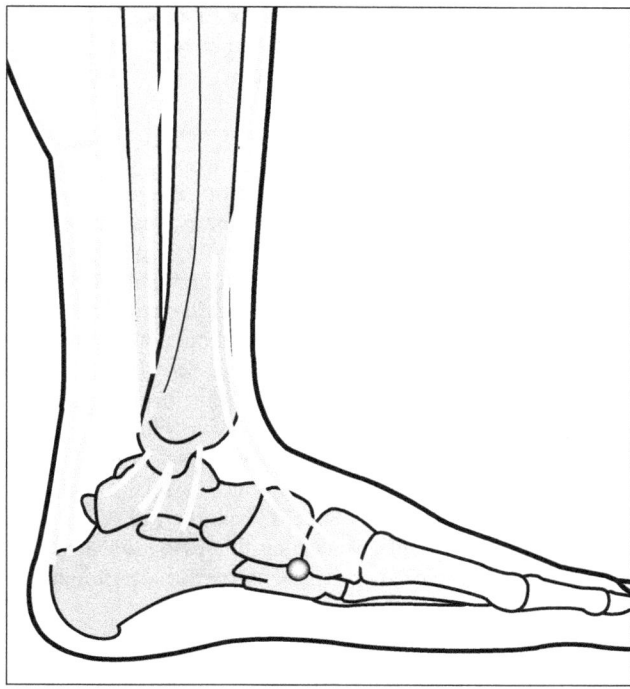

Location: On the medial side of the foot, in the depression below the tuberosity of the navicular bone at the junction of the red and white skin.

Functions: Clears deficient heat, regulates the Kidneys, tonifies Kidney yang.

Indications: Sore throat, obstruction of the throat, night sweats, irritability, local foot pain, emotional imbalances (fright), irregular menstruation, infertility, genital itching, seminal emissions.

Attributes: Fire point, Ying Spring point.

Notes
_____
_____
_____
_____
_____
_____
_____
_____

Point Combinations
_____
_____
_____
_____
_____
_____
_____

KD 3
TAIXI

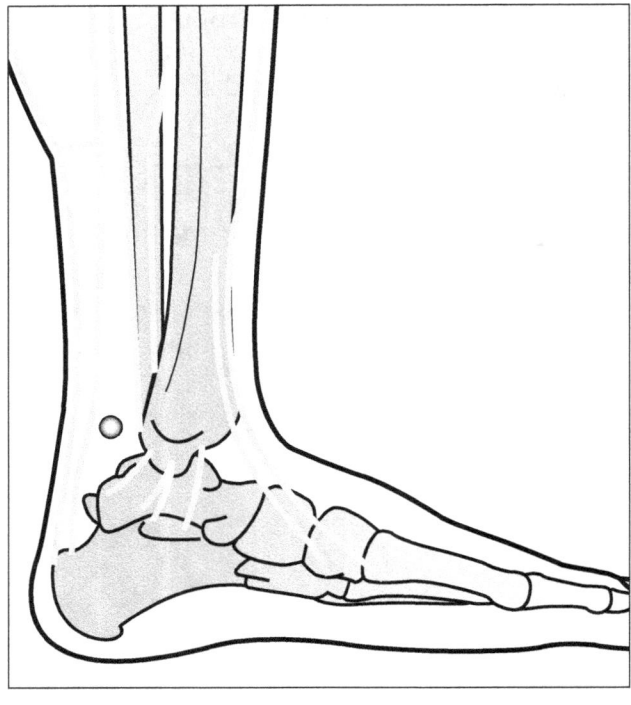

Location: On the medial side of the foot, posterior to the medial malleolus, in the depression between the tip of the medial malleolus and Achilles tendon.

Functions: Tonify the Kidneys, strengthens the lower back, relieves ankle/heel pain.

Indications: Sore throat, hemoptysis, irregular menses, impotence, toothache, deafness/tinnitus, asthma/cough, diabetes, insomnia, seminal emission, spermatorrhea, urinary frequency, pain in low back, paralysis of lower limb, headache, constipation, breast abscess, dark yellow urine, cardiac pain, cold limbs, thirst/sticky mouth, neuraesthenia, uterine diseases, cold shan, nephritis, cystitis, enuresis, alopecia, pain in the sole of foot, dizziness, spasms of diaphragm, infantile convulsions, chronic malaria, Kidney disease, heat disease with copious sweating, severe emaciation; dyspnoea and coughing fits, severe jaundice, vomiting abundant glairy mucus, vomiting, diarrhea, pain in abdomen and flanks, branching fullness in the chest and lateral costal region, pulmonary empyema, damp itch and sores on the inside of the thigh, pruritus.

Attributes: Earth point, Yuan Source point, Shu Stream point.

Notes
_____
_____
_____
_____
_____
_____
_____
_____

Point Combinations
_____
_____
_____
_____
_____
_____

KD 4
DAZHONG

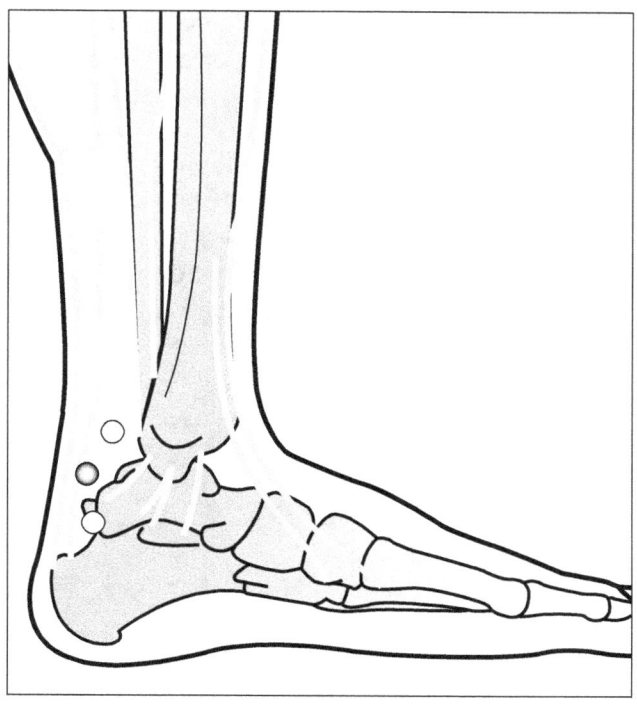

Location: On the medial side of the foot, posterior and inferior to the medial malleolus, in the depression anterior to the medial attachment of the Achilles tendon.

Functions: Benefits the Kidneys, strengthens the will, local point for ankle/heel pain.

Indications: Hemoptysis, asthma, pain in the lower back, dysuria, enuresis, constipation, pain in the heel, dementia.

Attributes: Luo-Connecting point.

Notes

Point Combinations

KD 5
SHUIQUAN

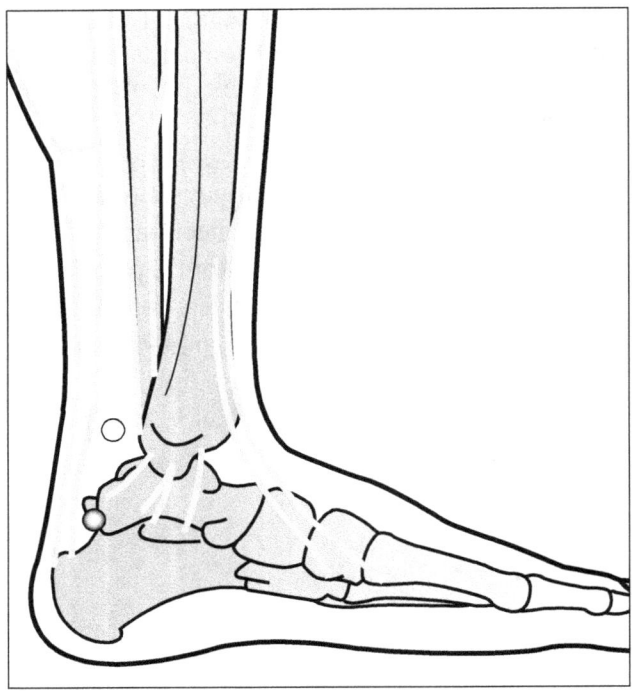

Location: On the medial side of the foot, 1 cun below KI-3 Taixi, posterior and inferior to the medial malleolus in the depression on the medial side of the tuberosity of the calcaneum.

Functions: Regulates menstruation, benefits urination.

Indication: Irregular menstruation, dysmenorrhea, amenorrhea, uterine prolapse, blurred vision.

Attributes: Xi-Cleft point.

Notes

Point Combinations

KD 6
ZHAOHAI

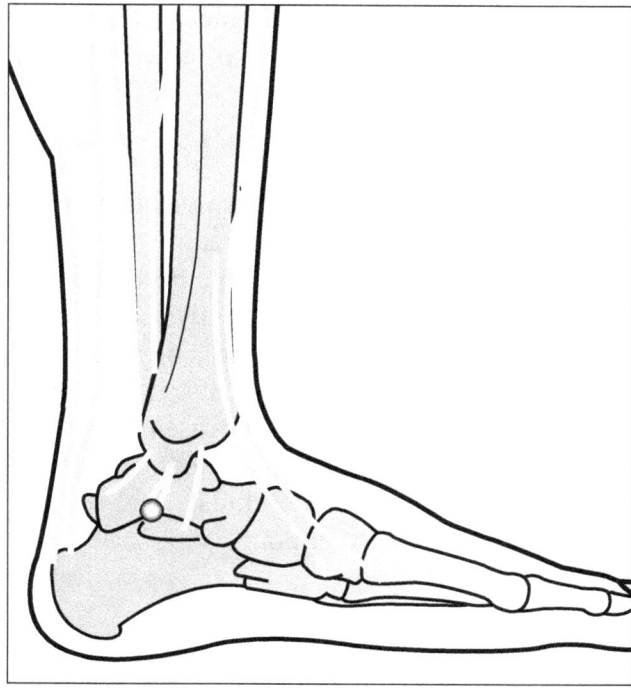

Location: On the medial side of the foot, in the depression below the tip of the medial malleolus.

Functions: Nourishes the Kidneys, clears deficient heat, benefits the throat, benefits the eyes, calms shen, regulates the Yin Qiao channel.

Indications: Sore throat, dry throat, irregular menses, uterine prolapse, vaginal discharge, bloody leukorrhea, pruritis vulvae, urinary frequency, urinary retention, constipation, difficult labor, foot swelling/limb swelling, epilepsy, psychosis, neuraesthenia, insomnia/hypersomnia, hernia, edema, hemiplegia, excessive erection, intestinal tuberculosis, eye pain, visual problems, eye disorders, unilateral lower abdominal pain in women, retention of placenta, chronic malaria, fever, asthma, thoracic oppression, no desire to eat, nocturnal enuresis, yellow urine, heat in the lower abdomen, pain and weakness of the limbs, running piglet syndrome, postpartum abdominal pain, persistent flow of lochia, female lassitude due to Qi and blood vacuity, heat vexation in the five Hearts, cramp in the hands and feet preventing movement, cholera with vomiting and diarrhea, headache.

Attributes: Master point of the Yin Qiao channel, (coupled with LU7).

Notes

Point Combinations

KD 7
FULIU

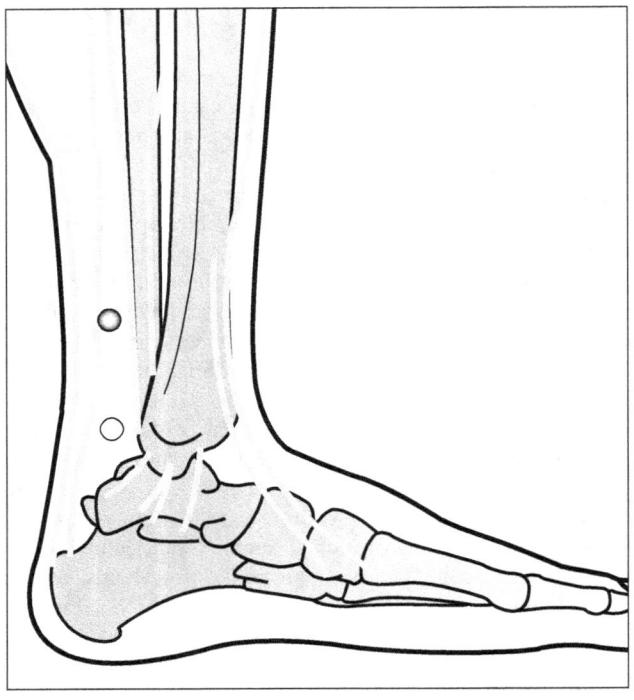

Location: On the medial side of the leg, 2 cun directly above KI-3 Taixi, anterior to the Achilles tendon.

Functions: Strengthens the Kidneys, strengthens the low back, resolves dampness, regulates sweating, treats edema.

Indications: Low back pain, borborygmus, diarrhea/dysentry, edema, paralysis of lower limb swelling (wei syndrome), night sweats, minute pulse, abdominal distension, foot swelling/limb swelling, febrile diseases without sweating, spontaneous sweating/absence of sweating, lin syndrome, orchitis.

Attributes: Jing River point.

Notes

Point Combinations

KD 8
JIAOXIN

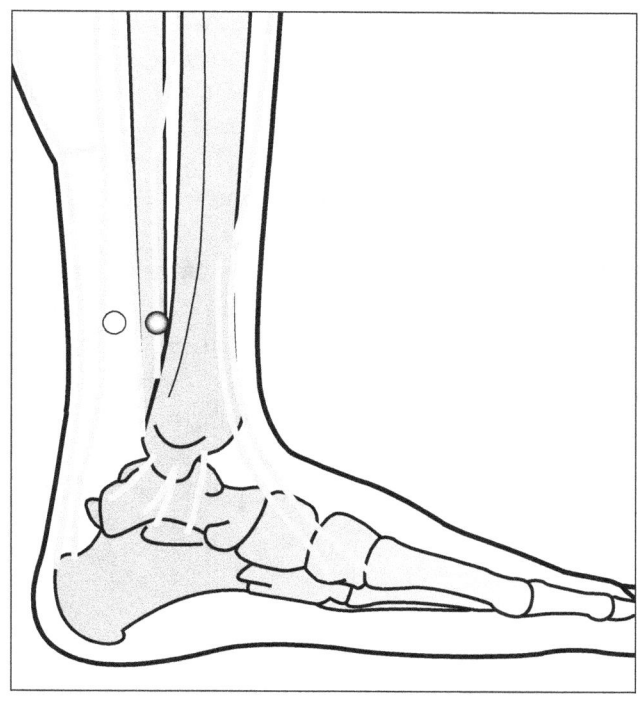

Location: On the medial side of the leg, .5 cun anterior to KI-7 Fuliu, 2 cun directly above KI-3 Taixi, posterior to the tibia.

Functions: Regulates the Ren channel and Penetrating Vessel, regulates menstruation.

Indications: Irregular menstruation, dysmenorrhea, metorrhagia, metrostaxis, prolapse of the uterus, diarrhea, constipation, pain and swelling of testis.

Attributes: Xi-Cleft point of the Yin Qiao Vessel.

Notes

Point Combinations

KD 9
ZHUBIN

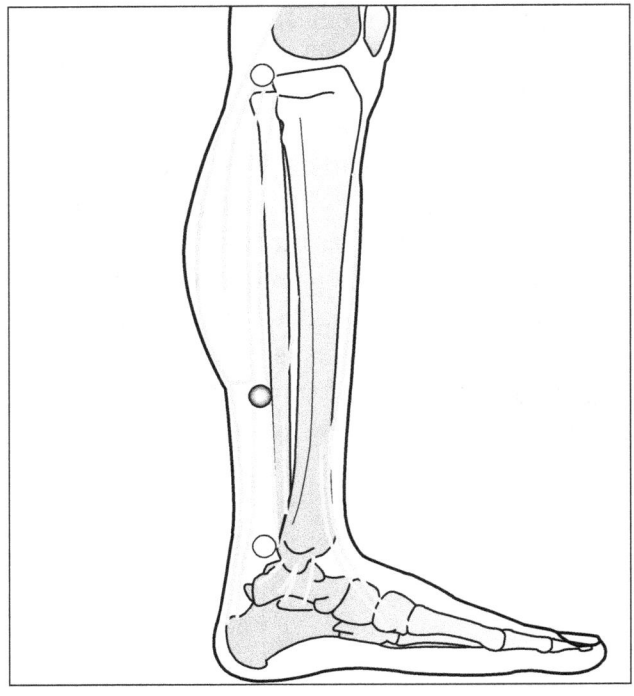

Location: On the medial side of the leg, 5 cun above KI-3 Taixi, on the line joining KI-3 Taixi and KI-10 Yingu, at the medial and inferior end of the belly of the gastrocnemius muscle.

Functions: Calms shen, clears heat, relieves pain.

Indications: Pain in the lower limb, manic psychosis, hernia, orchitis, drug detoxification, epilepsy, abnormal menstruation, vomiting saliva, absence of milk, colic, pelvic inflammatory disease, nephritis, cystitis, swollen tongue, muscle spasms.

Attributes: Xi-Cleft point of the Yin Wei Vessel.

Notes _____

_____

_____

_____

_____

_____

_____

_____

Point Combinations _____

_____

_____

_____

_____

_____

_____

KD 10
YINGU

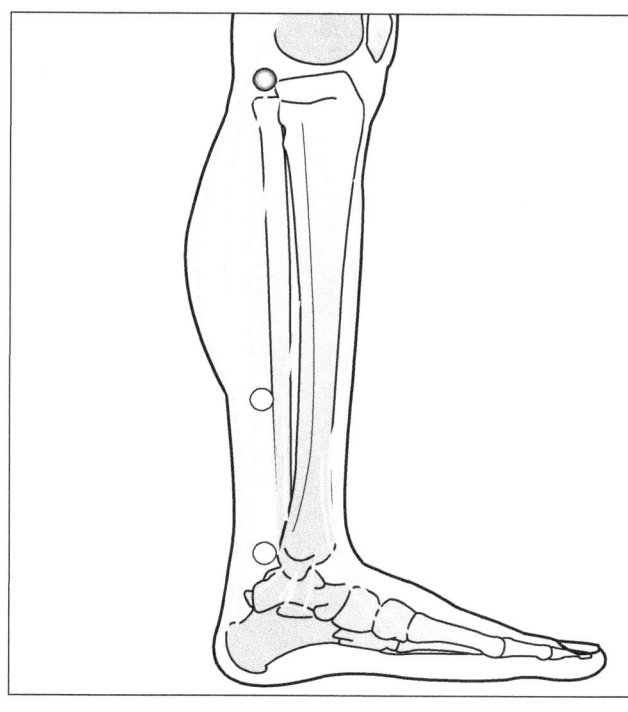

Location: On posterior side of the leg, on the medial side of the popliteal fossa, between the tendons of the semitendinosus muscle and semimembranosus muscle.

Functions: Resolves damp, resolves damp-heat from the lower jiao, benefits the Kidneys, relieves pain.

Indications: Impotence, uterine bleeding, pain in the medial aspect of the thigh and knee, hernia, dysuria, pain in the knee, pain in the popliteal fossa, male genital disorders, tongue protrusion without drooling, abdominal distension, psychosis, vaginal discharge, intestinal tuberculosis with knots in the abdomen, abdominal pain radiating to the navel, addictions, cholera.

Attributes: He-Sea point.

Notes

Point Combinations

KD 11
HENGGU

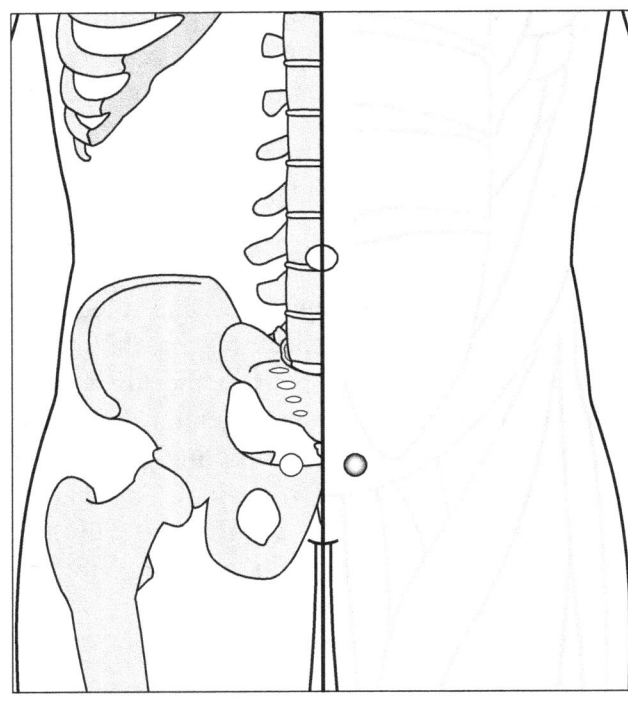

Location: On the abdomen, 5 cun below the center of the umbilicus at the upper border of the pubic symphysis, 0.5 cun lateral to the anterior midline.

Functions: Resolves damp, regulates the lower jiao.

Indications: Fullness and pain in the lower abdomen, enuresis, dysuria, nocturnal emission, impotence, pain in the genitals, hernia, spermatorrhea.

Attributes: Meeting point of the Kidney channel and Penetrating Vessel.

Notes

Point Combinations

KD 12
DAHE

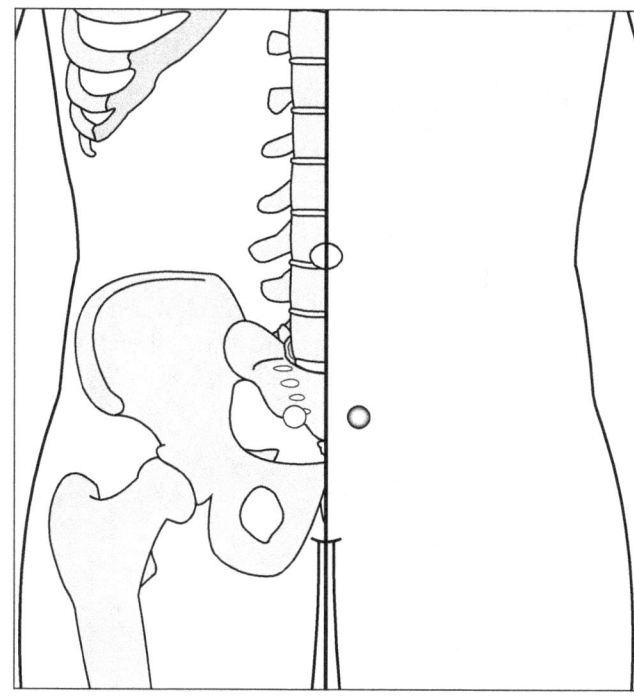

Location: On the abdomen, 4 cun below the center of the umbilicus, 0.5 cun lateral to the anterior midline.

Functions: Tonifies Kidney Qi, binds essence, regulates the Ren channel and Penetrating Vessel.

Indications: Spermatorrhea, nocturnal emission, impotence, prolapse uterus, morbid leukorrhea, pain in the external genitalia.

Attributes: Meeting point of the Kidney channel and Penetrating Vessel.

Notes

Point Combinations

KD 13
QIXUE

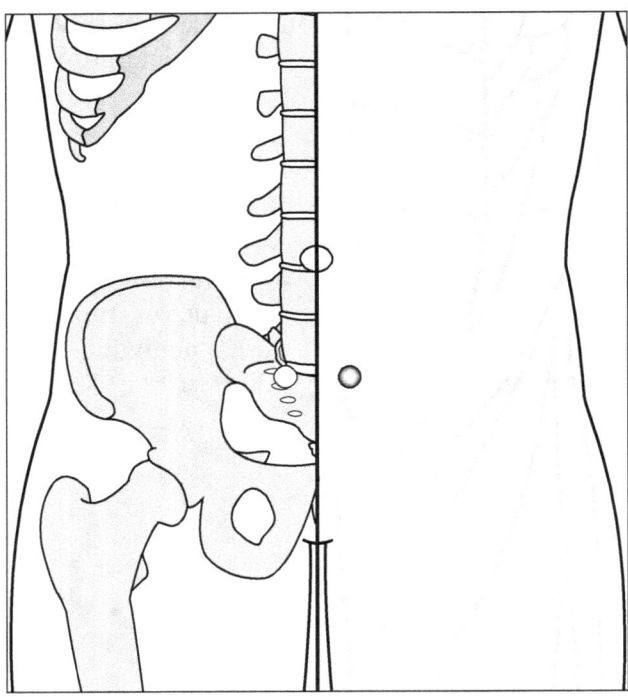

Location: On the abdomen, 3 cun below the center of the umbilicus, 0.5 cun lateral to the anterior midline.

Functions: Tonifies Kidney Qi, regulates the lower jiao, regulates the Ren channel and Penetrating Vessel.

Indications: Irregular menstruation, dysuria, dysmenorrhea, diarrhea, morbid leukorrhea.

Attributes: Meeting point of the Kidney channel and Penetrating Vessel.

Notes

Point Combinations

KD 14
SIMAN

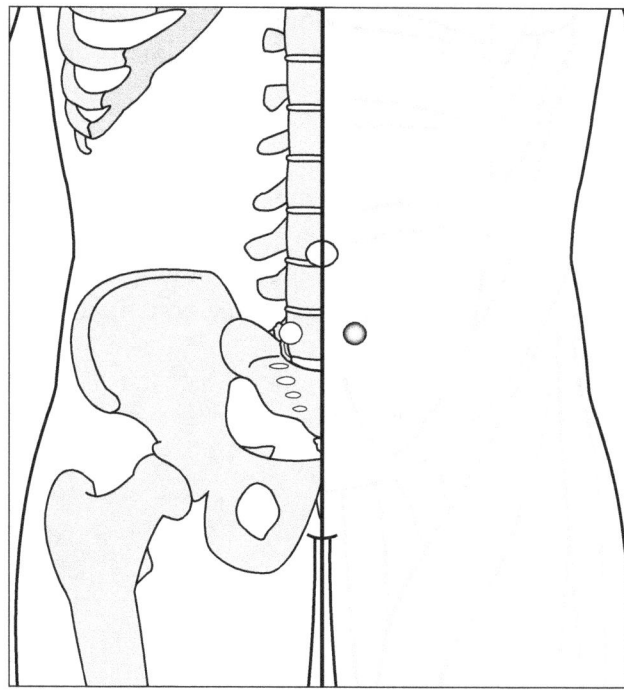

Location: On the abdomen, 2 cun below the center of the umbilicus, 0.5 cun lateral to the anterior midline.

Functions: Tonifies Kidney Qi, regulates the water passage ways, regulates the lower jiao, moves blood stagnation, regulates the Ren channel and Penetrating Vessel.

Indications: Abdominal pain and distention, diarrhea, nocturnal emission, irregular menstruation, dysmenorrhea, postpartum abdominal pain.

Attributes: Meeting point of the Kidney channel and Penetrating Vessel.

Notes

_____
_____
_____
_____
_____
_____
_____
_____

Point Combinations

_____
_____
_____
_____
_____
_____

KD 15
ZHONGZHU

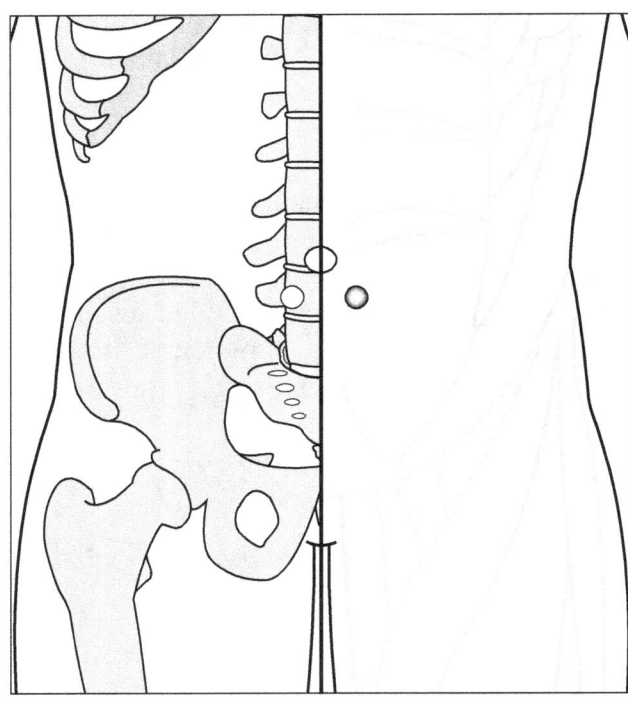

Location: On the abdomen, 1 cun below the center of the umbilicus, 0.5 cun lateral to the anterior midline.

Functions: Regulates the lower jiao and intestines, regulates the Ren channel and Penetrating Vessel.

Indications: Irregular menstruation, dysmenorrhea, abdominal pain, constipation, diarrhea.

Attributes: Meeting point of the Kidney channel and Penetrating Vessel.

Notes

Point Combinations

KD 16
HUANGSHU

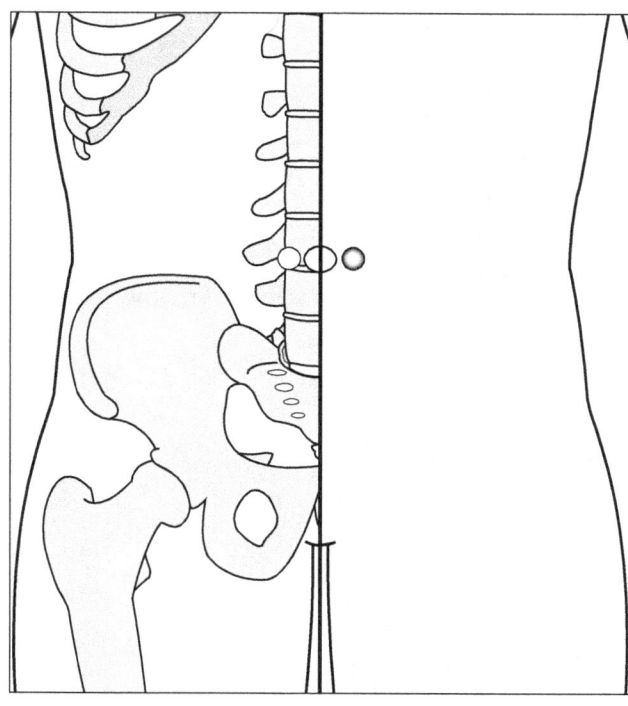

Location: On the abdomen, 0.5 cun lateral to the center of the umbilicus, 0.5 cun lateral to the anterior midline.

Functions: Regulates Qi, removes channel obstructions, regulates the Intestines.

Indications: Abdominal pain and distention, diarrhea, constipation, vomiting.

Attributes: Meeting point of the Kidney channel and Penetrating Vessel.

Notes

Point Combinations

KD 17
SHANGQU

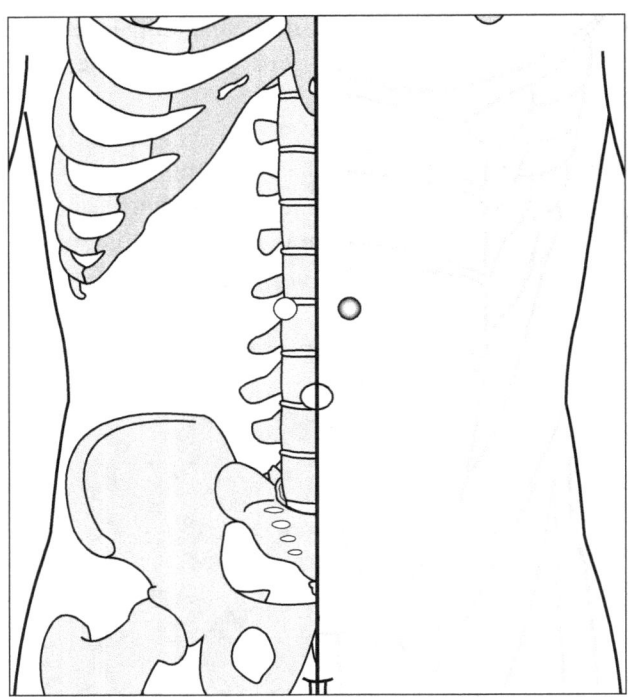

Location: On the abdomen, 2 cun above the center of the umbilicus, 0.5 cun lateral to the anterior midline.

Functions: Removes accumulation in the channel and relieves pain.

Indications: Abdominal pain and distention, vomiting, constipation and diarrhea.

Attributes: Meeting point of the Kidney channel and Penetrating Vessel.

Notes
_____
_____
_____
_____
_____
_____
_____
_____

Point Combinations
_____
_____
_____
_____
_____
_____

KD 18
SHIGUAN

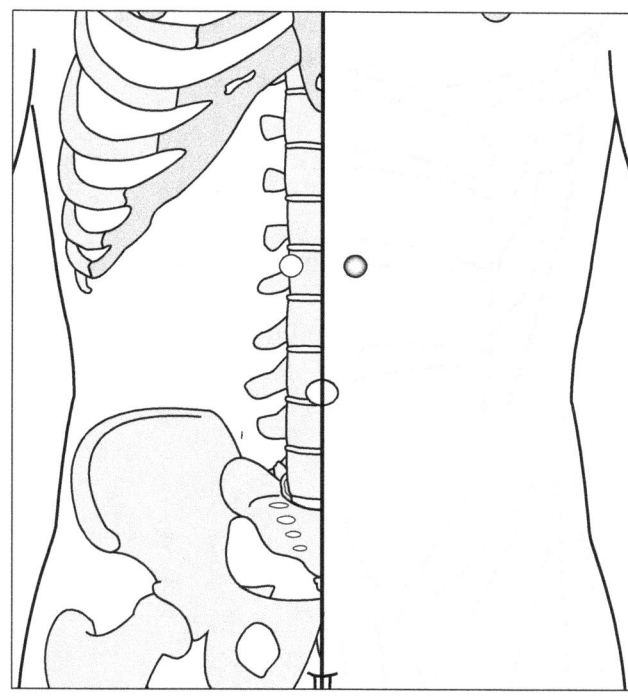

Location: On the abdomen, 3 cun above the center of the umbilicus, 0.5 cun lateral to the anterior midline.

Functions: Harmonizes Stomach, regulates lower jiao, relieves pain, regulates Penetrating Vessel and Ren channel.

Indications: Abdominal pain and distention, postpartum abdominal pain, nausea and vomiting, constipation and infertility.

Attributes: Meeting point of the Kidney channel and Penetrating Vessel.

Notes

_____
_____
_____
_____
_____
_____
_____
_____
_____

Point Combinations

_____
_____
_____
_____
_____
_____
_____
_____

KD 19
YINDU

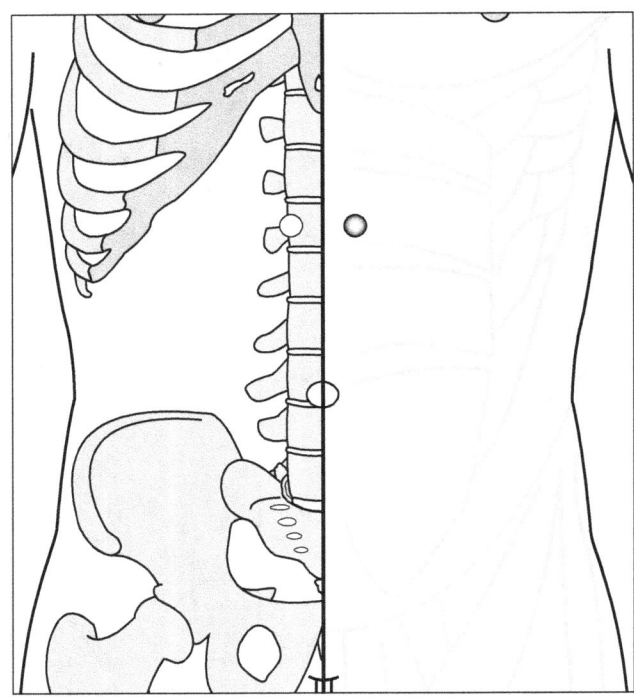

Location: On the abdomen, 4 cun above the center of the umbilicus, 0.5 cun lateral to the anterior midline.

Functions: Harmonizes Stomach, descends rebellious Qi, regulates Penetrating Vessel and Ren channel.

Indications: Abdominal pain and distention, epigastric pain, borborygmus, constipation, nausea and vomiting and infertility.

Attributes: Meeting point of the Kidney channel and Penetrating Vessel.

Notes

_____

_____

_____

_____

_____

_____

_____

_____

Point Combinations

_____

_____

_____

_____

_____

_____

KD 20
FUTONGGU

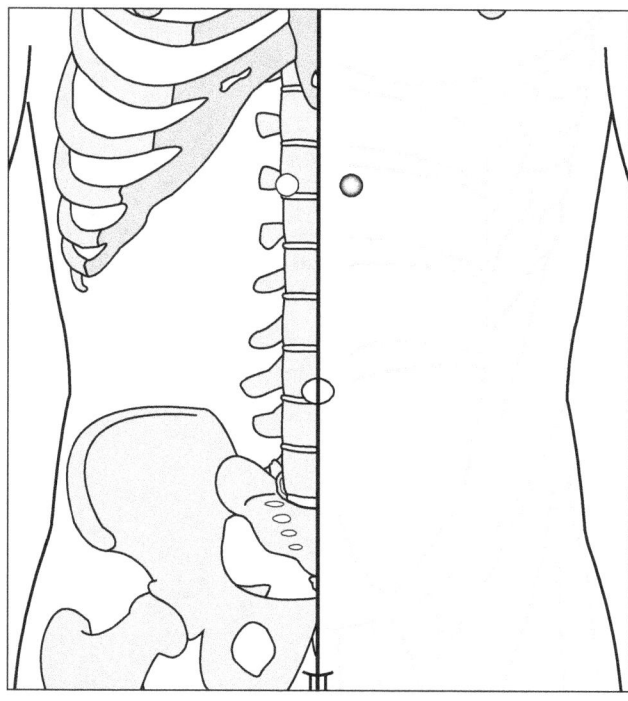

Location: On the abdomen, 5 cun above the center of the umbilicus, 0.5 cun lateral to the anterior midline.

Functions: Harmonizes middle jiao, opens the chest and transforms phlegm.

Indications: Abdominal pain and distention, chest pain and distention, vomiting, indigestion and diarrhea.

Attributes: Meeting point of the Kidney channel and Penetrating Vessel.

Notes

Point Combinations

KD 21
YOUMEN

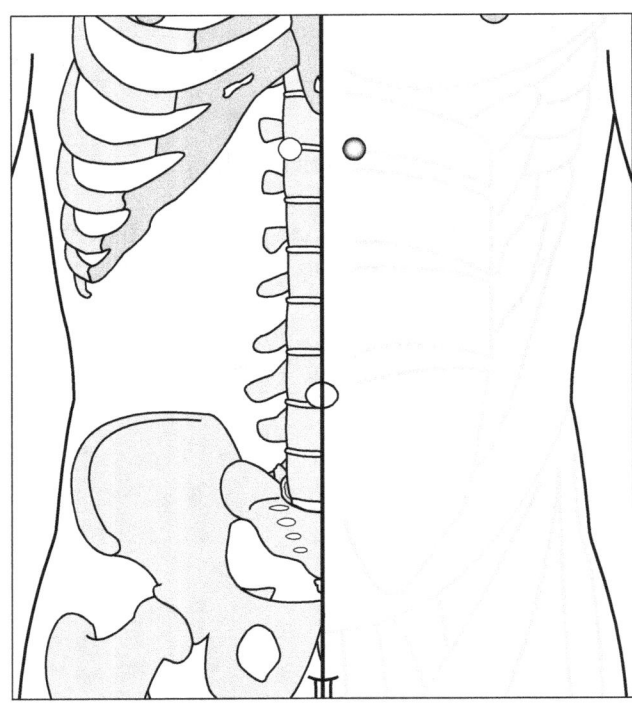

Location: On the abdomen, 6 cun above the center of the umbilicus, 0.5 cun lateral to the anterior midline.

Functions: Harmonizes middle jiao, descends rebellious Qi, soothes Liver Qi.

Indications: Abdominal pain and distention, chest pain and distention, nausea and vomiting, morning sickness, indigestion and diarrhea.

Attributes: Meeting point of the Kidney channel and Penetrating Vessel.

Notes

_____
_____
_____
_____
_____
_____
_____
_____
_____

Point Combinations

_____
_____
_____
_____
_____
_____
_____
_____

KD 22
BULANG

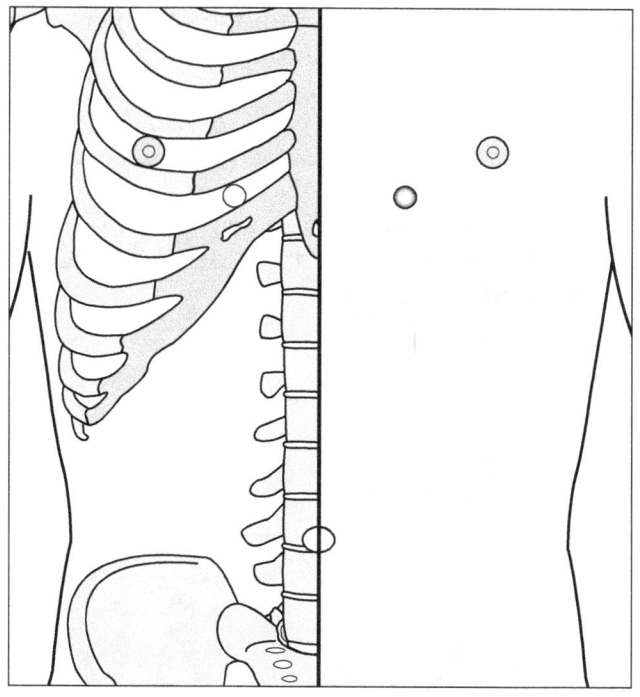

Location: On the chest, in the 5th intercostal space, 2 cun lateral to the anterior midline.

Functions: Opens the chest, descends rebellious Lung and Stomach Qi.

Indications: Cough, asthma, vomiting, chest pain and fullness, shortness of breath, breast abscess or nodules.

Notes

Point Combinations

KD 23
SHENFENG

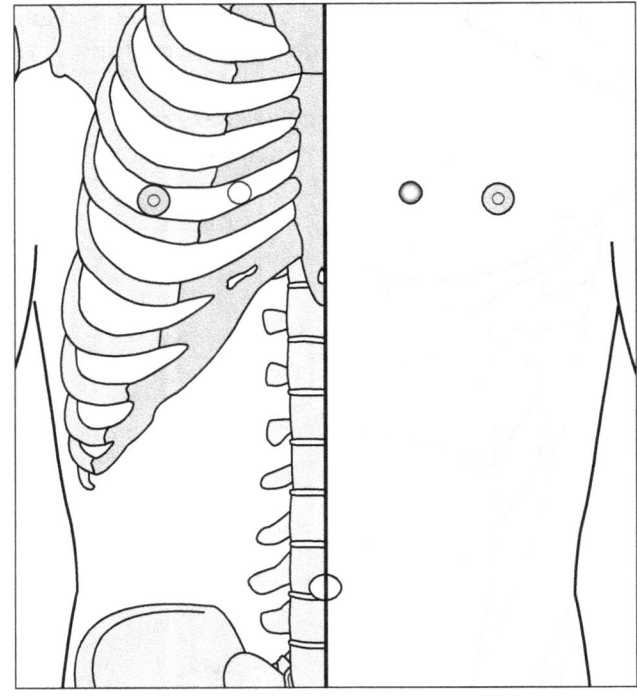

Location: On the chest, in the 4th intercostal space, 2 cun lateral to the anterior midline.

Functions: Opens the chest, descends rebellious Lung and Stomach Qi and benefits the breasts.

Indications: Cough, asthma, vomiting, chest pain and fullness, shortness of breath, breast abscess or nodules.

Notes

Point Combinations

KD 24
LINGXU

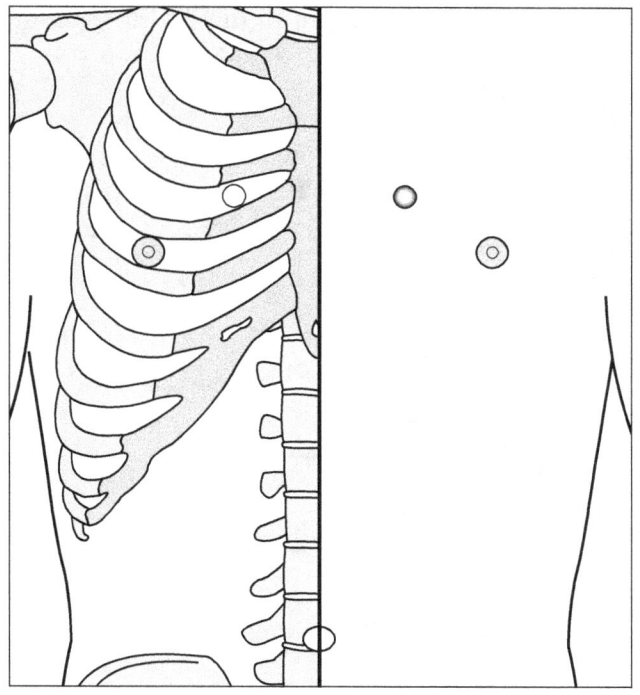

Location: On the chest, in the 3rd intercostal space, 2 cun lateral to the anterior midline.

Functions: Opens the chest, descends rebellious Lung and Stomach Qi and benefits the breasts.

Indications: Cough, asthma, vomiting, chest pain and fullness, shortness of breath, breast abscess or nodules.

Notes

Point Combinations

KD 25
SHENCANG

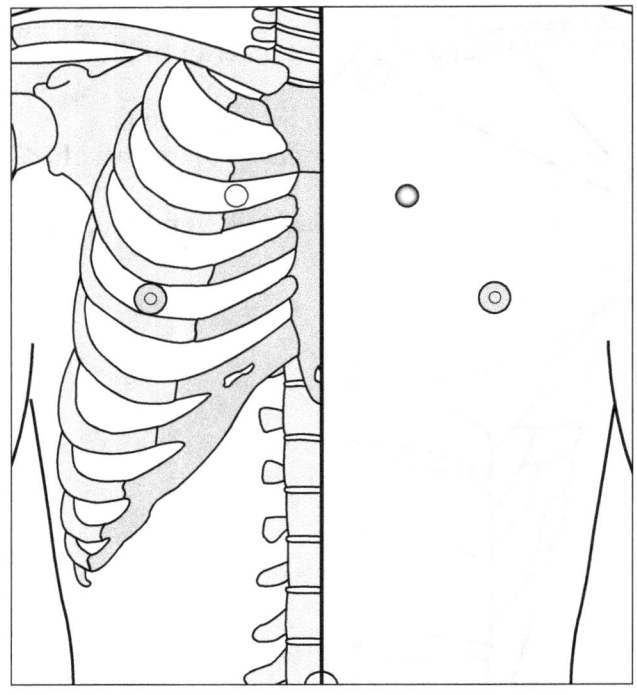

Location: On the chest, in the 2nd intercostal space, 2 cun lateral to the anterior midline.

Functions: Opens the chest, descends rebellious Lung and Stomach Qi.

Indications: Cough, asthma, chest pain and fullness and vomiting.

Notes

Point Combinations

KD 26
YUZHONG

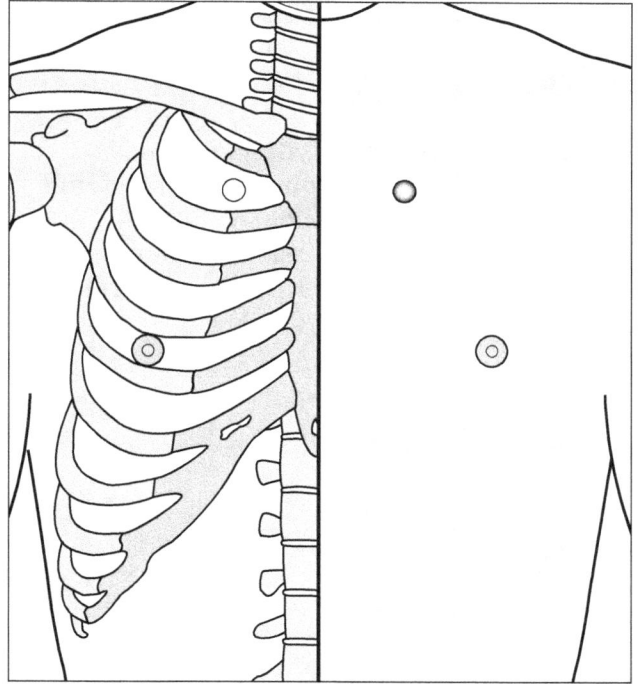

Location: On the chest, in the 1st intercostal space, 2 cun lateral to the anterior midline.

Functions: Opens the chest, descends rebellious Lung and Stomach Qi and relieves cough.

Indications: Cough, asthma, chest pain and fullness.

Notes

_____
_____
_____
_____
_____
_____
_____
_____

Point Combinations

_____
_____
_____
_____
_____
_____

KD 27
SHUFU

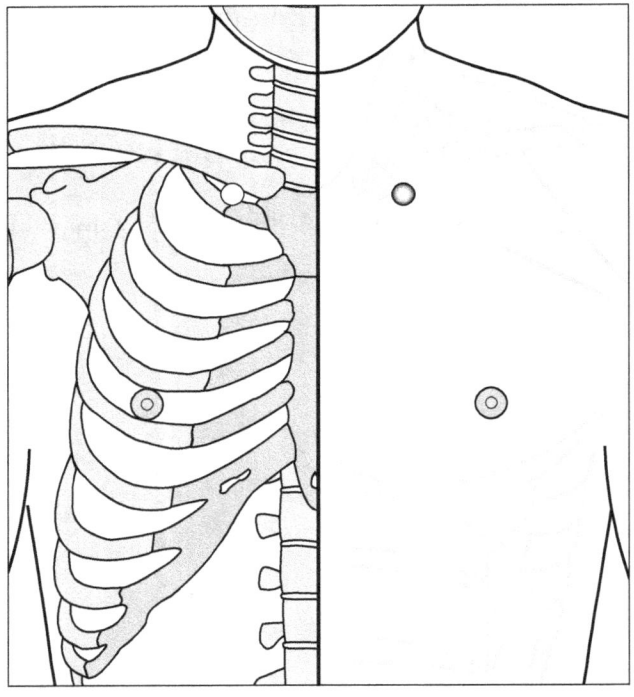

Location: On the chest, on the lower border of the clavicle, 2 cun lateral to the anterior midline.

Functions: Opens the chest, descends rebellious Lung and Stomach Qi, transforms phlegm and relieves cough.

Indications: Cough, asthma, vomiting with phlegm, chest pain and fullness, shortness of breath.

Notes

Point Combinations

PC 1
TIANCHI

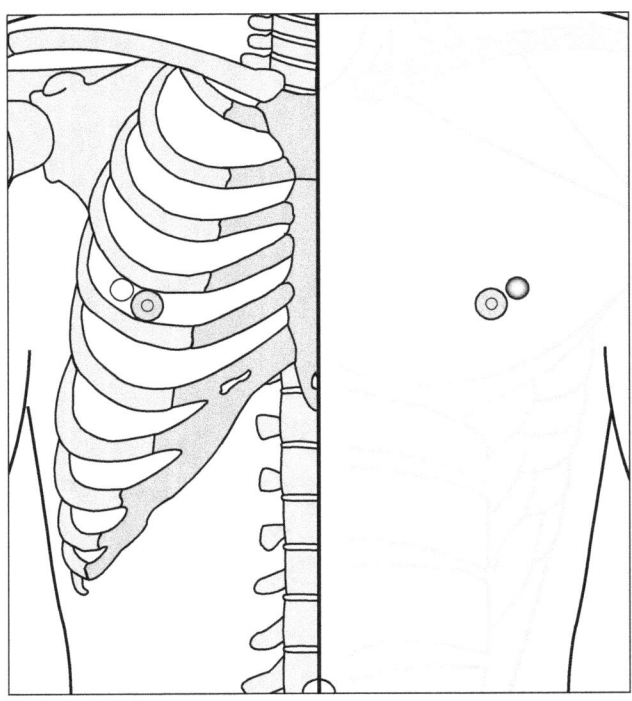

Location: On the chest, in the 4th intercostal space, 1 cun lateral to the center of the nipple, 5 cun lateral to the anterior midline.

Functions: Unblocks the chest, opens the lung, courses Liver Qi, clears heat, reduces shortness of breath, wheezing, and coughing.

Indications: Angina pectoris, swelling, pain, and tenderness of axilla area, intercostal neuralgia, pain or distention at breast, axillary or hypochondrium region.

Attributes: Point of intersection for Pericardium, San Jiao, Gall Bladder and Liver.
*Major point for insufficient lactation.
**Caution when needling to avoid breast tissue and puncturing the Lung.

Notes

Point Combinations

PC 2
TIANQUAN

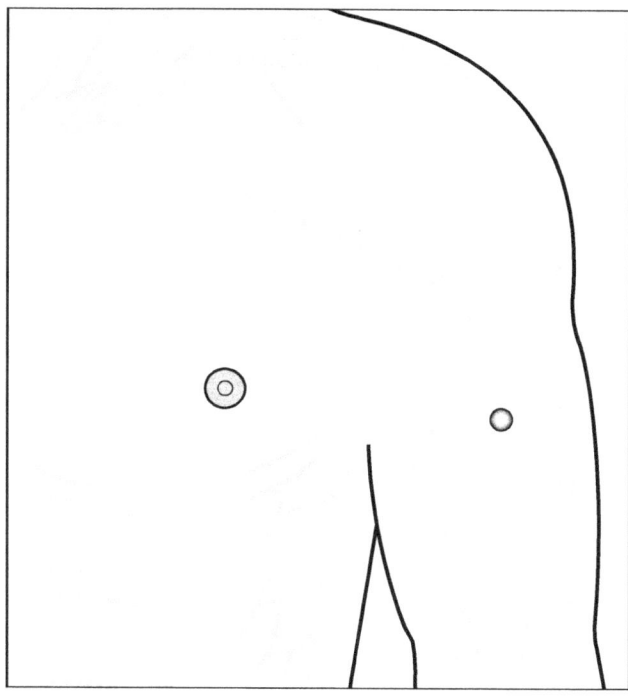

Location: On the medial upper arm, between the heads of the biceps brachii longus muscle and the biceps brachii brevis muscle, 2 cun below the axillary fossa.

Functions: Unblocks the chest and assists the Lung, nourishes Heart Qi and yang, courses Liver Qi, moves blood, calms shen, manages and supports the Heart, expands the chest, removes blockages, relieves pain.

Indications: Angina pectoris, cardiac pain, pain or distention in the chest, hypochondrium, or lateral lumbar regions and medial aspect of arm, palpitations and cough.

Notes

_____
_____
_____
_____
_____
_____
_____
_____

Point Combinations

_____
_____
_____
_____
_____
_____

PC 3
QUZE

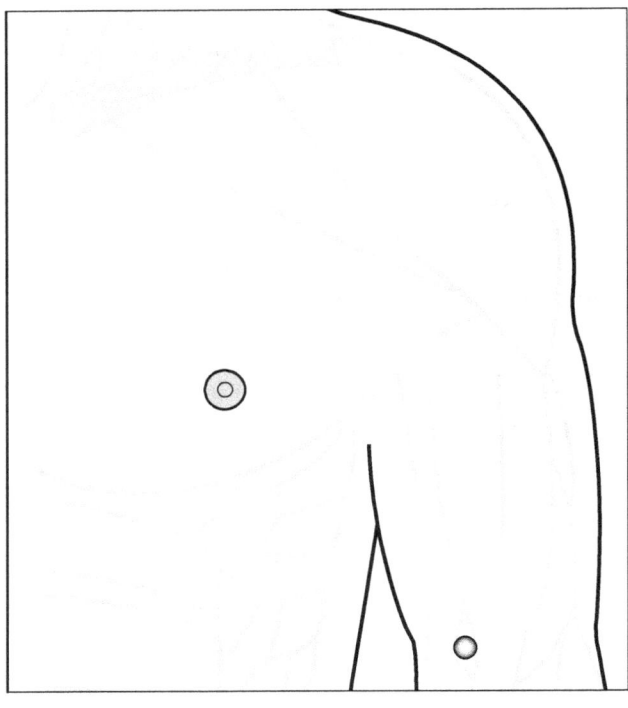

Location: On the cubital crease of the arm, on the ulnar side of the biceps brachii tendon.

Functions: Regulates Intestines and calms the Stomach, clears toxic heat, extinguishes internal wind, unblocks Heart Qi, cools and moves blood, calms shen, stops spasms and vomiting.

Indications: Myocarditis, rheumatic Heart disease, chest pain, bronchitis, pain in arm and elbow, heat exhaustion, irritability and easily startled, enteritis, acute gastritis and gastroenteritis, diarrhea and vomiting.

Attributes: Water point, He-Sea point.

* Good point for heat rash.

** Frequently bled for blood level pathogens.

Notes

_____
_____
_____
_____
_____
_____
_____
_____

Point Combinations

_____
_____
_____
_____
_____
_____

PC 4
XIMEN

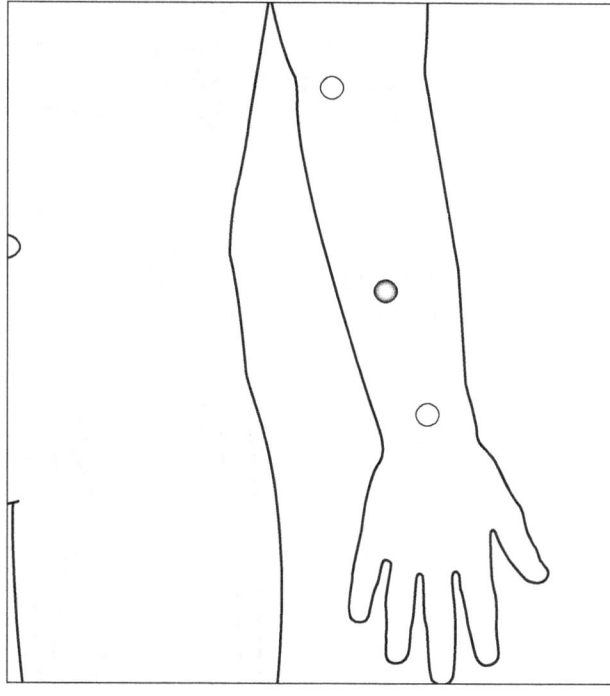

Location: On the palmar side of the forearm and on the line connecting PC-3 Quze and PC-7 Daling, 5 cun above the crease of the wrist, between the tendons of the palmaris longus muscle and radial flexor muscle of the wrist.

Functions: Remove blockages from the channel, clears heat and cools blood, regulates Qi and blood, courses Qi and manages Heart Qi, calms the Heart and calms shen, nourishes the mind, expands the chest and diaphragm, relieves pain.

Indications: Angina pectoris, palpitations, irritability, cardiac pain and vomiting, rheumatic Heart disease, myocarditis, spasm of the diaphragm, pleurisy, mastitis, epistaxis, hematemesis, hemorrhoids, epilepsy, hysteria, depression, irritability, fear of strangers.

Attributes: Xi-Cleft point.
*Most important point for angina.
**Very effective for palpitations.

Notes
_____
_____
_____
_____
_____
_____
_____
_____
_____

Point Combinations
_____
_____
_____
_____
_____
_____
_____

PC 5
JIANSHI

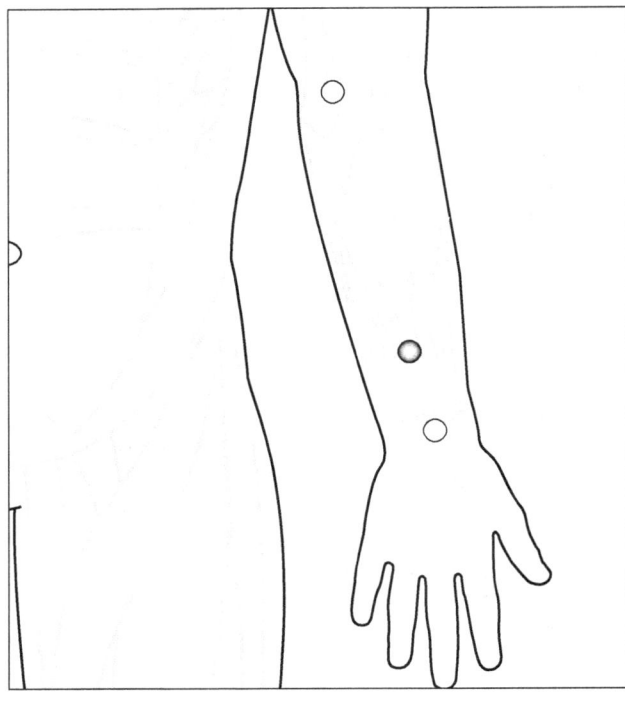

Location: On the palmar side of the forearm and on the line connecting PC-3 Quze and PC-7 Daling, 3 cun above the crease of the wrist, between the tendons of the palmaris longus muscle and radial flexor muscle of the wrist.

Functions: Remove blockages from the channel, stimulates the connecting vessel, tendons and ligaments, transforms phlegm, clears heat and Heart fire, manages and supports the Heart and Heart yang, expands the chest, manages Stomach, calms shen.

Indications: Cardiac pain, rheumatic Heart disease, palpitations, malaria, tidal fever, Stomach ache and vomiting, menstrual irregularities, irritability, hysteria, psychosis, insanity, seizures/epilepsy, nightmares, pain, tenderness or swelling of the axilla, contracture of the elbow and arm, scabies.

Attributes: Metal point, Jing River point and Meeting point for three arm yin channels.

*Good point for motion or morning sickness.

Notes
_____
_____
_____
_____
_____
_____
_____
_____

Point Combinations
_____
_____
_____
_____
_____
_____

PC 6
NEIGUAN

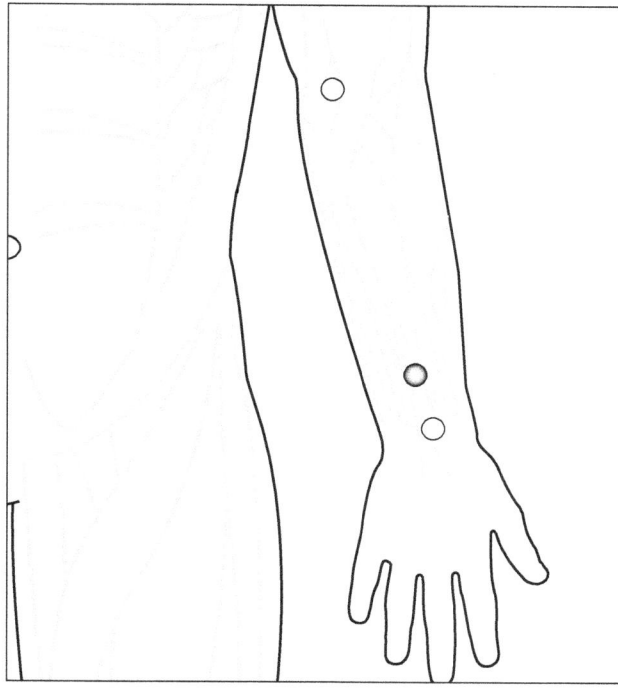

Location: On the palmar side of the forearm and on the line connecting PC-3 Quze and PC-7 Daling, 2 cun above the crease of the wrist, between the tendons of the palmaris longus muscle and radial flexor muscle of the wrist.

Functions: Manages the Qi of the Heart, Liver, and Stomach, calms the Heart, calms shen, expands the chest and supports the diaphragm, nourishes the Heart, balances the Stomach and middle jiao, courses San Jiao channel, resolves damp, summer-heat and phlegm, manages blood, relieves pain, supports the occiput.

Indications: Angina pectoris, cardiac and abdominal pain, rheumatic Heart disease, palpitations, swollen and painful throat, hyperthyroidism, spasm of the diaphragm/hiccup, cough, chest oppression, asthma, pain in hypochondrium region, Stomach ache, nausea, vomiting, febrile disease, malaria, irritability, mental disorders, nervousness, insomnia, migraines, hysteria, seizures/epilepsy, shock, jaundice, contracture and pain in elbow and arm, jaundice, gall stones, painful menses, rectal prolapse.

Attributes: Luo-Connecting point, Master point of Yin Wei Mai channel.

*Main point for nausea and very effective for asthma.

Notes

_____
_____
_____
_____
_____
_____
_____
_____

Point Combinations

_____
_____
_____
_____
_____
_____

PC 7
DALING

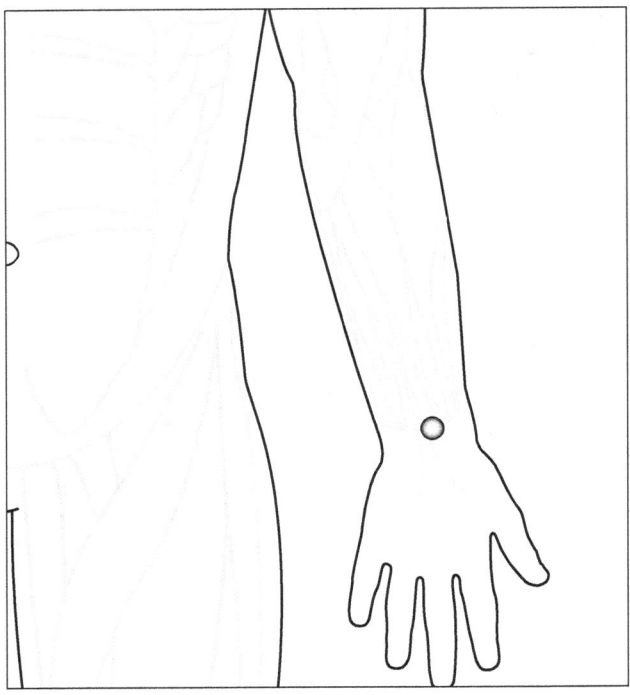

Location: At the midpoint of the crease of the wrist, between the tendons of the palmaris longus muscle and radial flexor muscle of the wrist.

Functions: Clears heat and calms shen, clears Heart fire, moves and cools blood, manages Heart Qi, harmonizes the Stomach, loosens the chest.

Indications: Cardiac and hypochondrium region pain, palpitation, chest oppression, hemoptysis, throat blockage or pain at root of the tongue, tonsillitis, foul breath, myocarditis, intercostal neuralgia, Stomach ache, gastritis, vomiting, mental disorders, panic, insomnia, seizures/epilepsy, convulsions, wrist pain and issues of the wrist, damp skin diseases.

Attributes: Earth point, Shu Stream point and Yuan Source point, Sedation and Ghost point.
*Main point for carpal tunnel syndrome and very effective for insomnia.

Notes _____

_____

_____

_____

_____

_____

_____

_____

Point Combinations _____

_____

_____

_____

_____

_____

_____

PC 8
LAOGONG

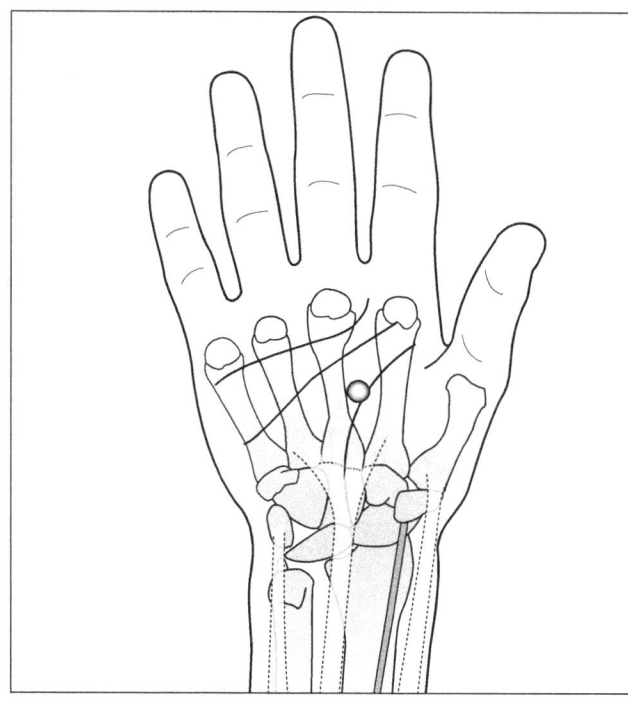

Location: At the center of the palm, between the 2nd and 3rd metacarpal bones, but close to the latter, and in the part touching the tip of the middle finger when a fist is made.

Functions: Manages Heart Qi, supports Heart Yin, clears heat and Heart fire, resolves damp-heat, extinguishes wind and resolves damp and transforms phlegm, balances Stomach.

Indications: Angina pectoris, foul breath, mouth ulcers, difficulty in swallowing food, stomatitis, gastritis, jaundice, post stroke coma, hyperhidrosis, numbness of the fingers, athletes foot, mental illness, hysteria, madness, nausea and vomiting.

Attributes: Fire point, Ying Spring point. Horary point, Exit point and Ghost point.
*Main point for issues in the oral cavity.

Notes

_____
_____
_____
_____
_____
_____
_____
_____

Point Combinations

_____
_____
_____
_____
_____
_____

PC 9
ZHONGCHONG

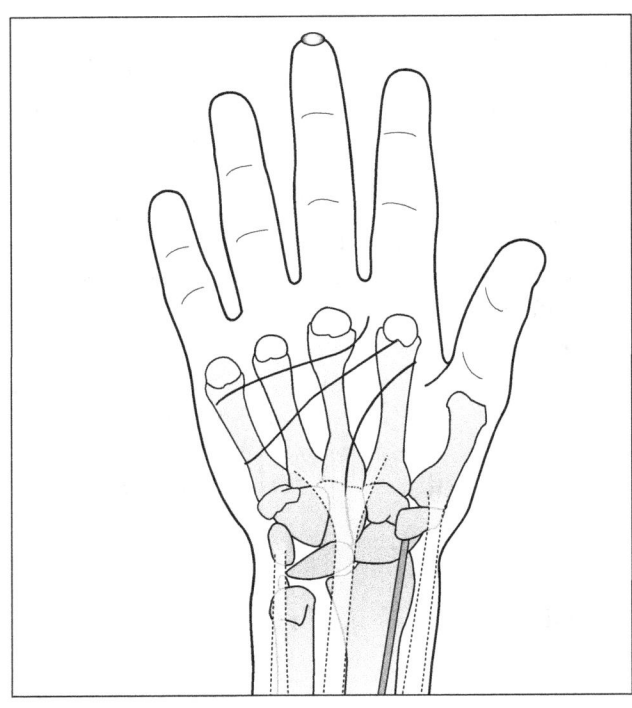

Location: In the center of the tip of the distal segment of the middle finger.

Functions: Clears heat, extinguishes wind, manages the Heart, moves Qi, resuscitates collapsed yang, restores consciousness.

Indications: Angina pectoris, apoplectic loss of consciousness, palpitations, aphasia, heat exhaustion, hot palms, high fever, convulsions, shock.

Attributes: Wood point and Jing Well point, tonification point and resuscitation point.
*Main Jing Well point for resuscitation.

Notes

Point Combinations

SJ 1
GUANCHONG

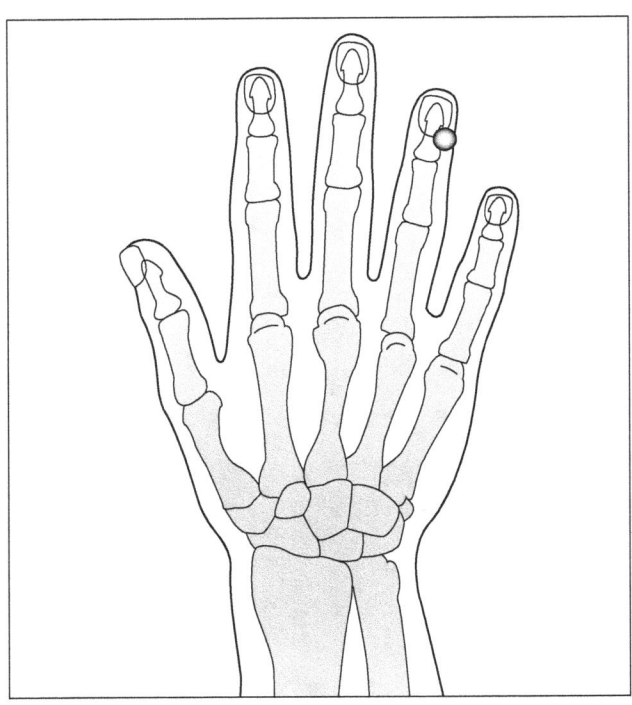

Location: On the ulnar side of the distal segment of the ring finger, 0.1 cun from the corner of the fingernail.

Functions: Activates the channel, clears heat in the upper jiao, clears heat, fire, extinguishes wind and expels toxins, removes blockages in the channel, relieves pain, benefits the tongue and ears.

Indications: Headache, dizziness, conjunctivitis, earache, tinnitus, deafness, sore throat, dry mouth, stiff tongue, laryngitis, fever.

Attributes: Metal point, Jing Well point.
*Resuscitation point for loss of consciousness.

Notes _____

_____

_____

_____

_____

_____

_____

_____

_____

Point Combinations _____

_____

_____

_____

_____

_____

_____

SJ 2
YEMEN

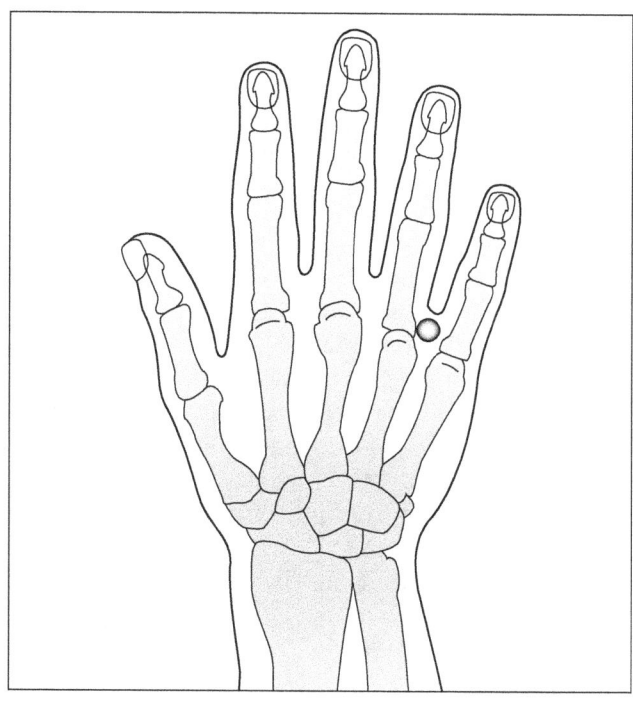

Location: On the dorsum of the hand, between the 4th and 5th fingers, at the junction of the red and white skin, 0.5 cun proximal to the margin of the web.

Functions: Activates the channel, clears heat in the upper jiao, removes blockages in the channel, extinguishes wind, generates fluid, stimulates the connecting vessel, moves Qi and unblocks stagnation, relieves pain and swelling, supports the ears, calms shen.

Indications: Headache, earache, deafness, tinnitus, toothache in lower jaw, palpitations from fear, epilepsy, mania, laryngitis, laryngopharyngitis, pain of hands and arm and painful swelling of the fingers, malaria

Attributes: Water point, Ying Spring point.

Notes

Point Combinations

SJ 3
ZHONGZHU

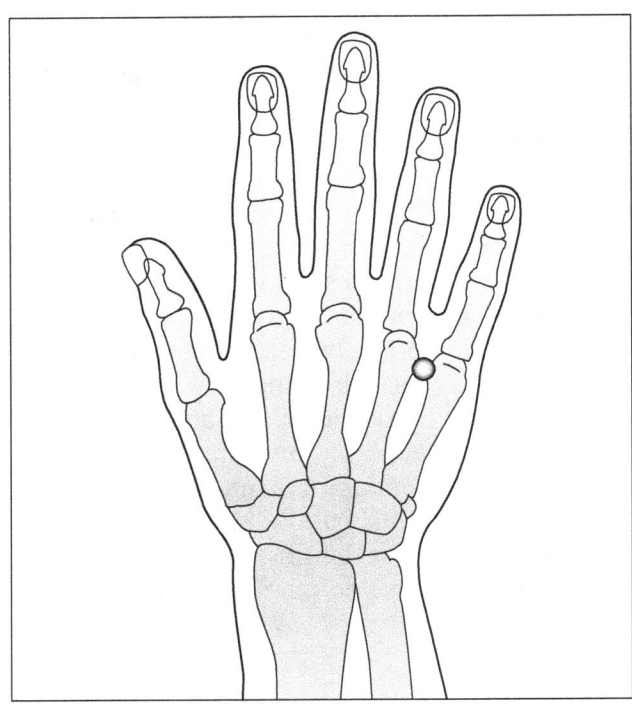

Location: On the dorsum of the hand, proximal to the 4th metacarpophalangeal joint, in the depression between the 4th and 5th metacarpal bones.

Functions: Activates the channel and moves Qi and blood, extinguishes wind, clears heat ,relieves pain, generates fluid for the throat, supports the ears, head and eyes.

Indications: Headache, earache, deafness, deaf-mutism, tinnitus, blurred vision, temporal pain, itchiness of the face and body, intercostal neuralgia, pain of the back, shoulder, elbow and arm, stiff fingers, malaria, fever.

Attributes: Wood point, Shu Stream point and Tonification point.

*Main distal point for issues of the ear and temporal headaches.

Notes

Point Combinations

SJ 4
YANGCHI

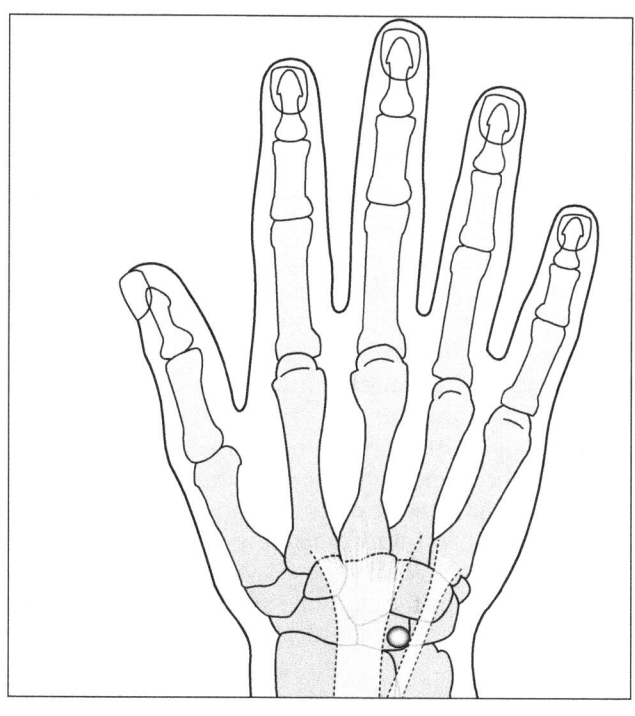

Location: On the ulnar side of the tranverse wrist crease, in the depression on the ulnar side of the extensor digitorum communis tendon.

Functions: Removes blockages and calms the channel, tendons and ligaments, clears heat, extinguishes wind, clears fire, relieves pain, resolves damp, lubricates dryness, benefits the ears and stomach.

Indications: Deafness, swollen, red eyes, dry mouth and throat, tonsillitis, chest pain and fullness, swelling and pain in the neck and upper extremity, common cold (from heat), malaria, fever.

Attributes: Yuan-Source point.

Notes

Point Combinations

SJ 5
WAIGUAN

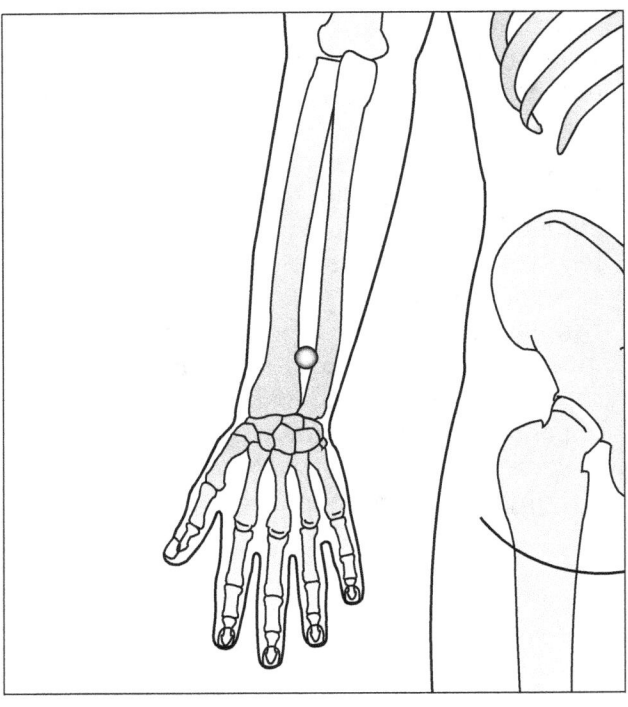

Location: On the dorsal side of the forearm and on the line connecting SJ-4 Yangchi and the tip of the olecranon, 2 cun proximal to the dorsal crease of the wrist, between the radius and ulna.

Functions: Removes blockages in the channel and stimulates the connecting vessel, moves Qi, extinguishes wind, induces sweat and releases the exterior for hot and cold pathogens, expels toxins, relieves pain and reduces swelling, opens Yang Wei Vessel, benefits the head and ears.

Indications: Headache/migraine, earache, tinnitus, deafness, nose bleed, stiff neck, swollen throat, aphasia, pain of the ribs, stomach ache, constipation, scrofula, common cold, fever, weak fingers, pain in joints of the upper extremity, paralysis.

Attributes: Luo-Connecting point, Confluent point of Yang Wei Vessel.

*Main point of the Immune system and good point for migraines. Paired with confluent point GB-41.

Notes _____

_____

_____

_____

_____

_____

_____

_____

Point Combinations _____

_____

_____

_____

_____

_____

SJ 6
ZHIGOU

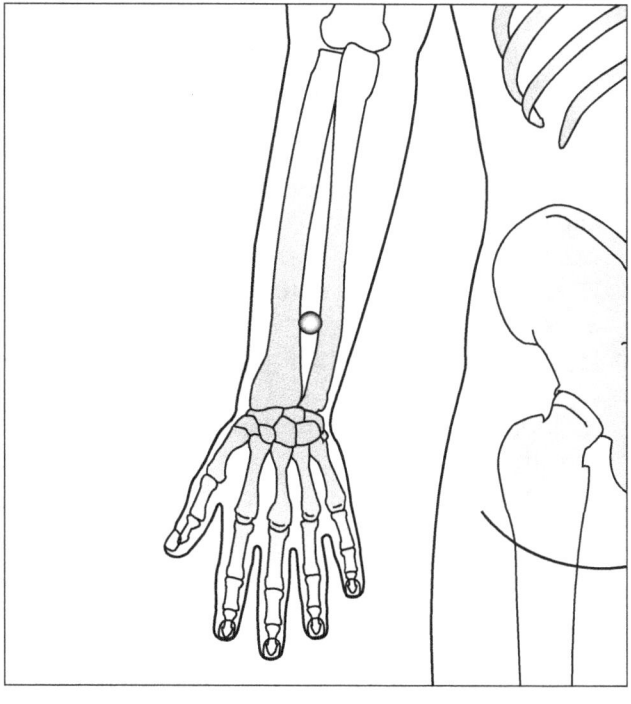

Location: On the dorsal side of the forearm and on the line connecting SJ-4 Yangchi and the tip of the olecranon, 3 cun proximal to the dorsal crease of the wrist, between the radius and ulna.

Functions: Removes blockages from the channel, activates the channel and relieves pain, manages Qi and clears heat and fire in the three jiaos, generates fluid, extinguishes wind -cold, manages the Zang Fu organs, corrects Qi counter flow, restores consciousness, transforms phlegm, supports the chest and lateral costal regions, promotes lactation, moves bowels, assists the voice.

Indications: Sore or swollen throat, pleurisy, intercostal neuralgia, chest pain, angina pectoris, belching, pain in the shoulder, axilla, ribs or arm, hand tremor, insufficient lactation, constipation, vomiting, diarrhea.

Attributes: Fire point, Jing River point.

*Main point for constipation.

Notes

_____
_____
_____
_____
_____
_____
_____
_____

Point Combinations

_____
_____
_____
_____
_____
_____

SJ 7
HUIZONG

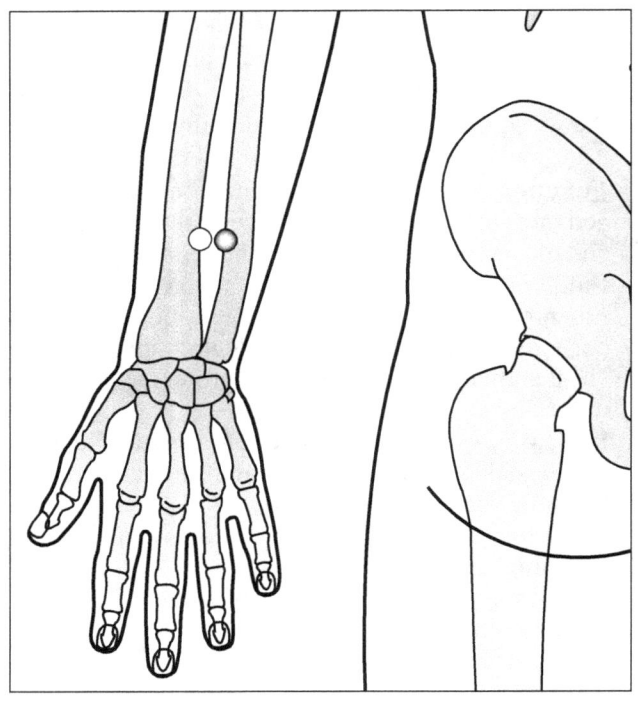

Location: On the dorsal side of the forearm, one finger breadth lateral to SJ-6 Zhigou, 3 cun proximal to the dorsal crease of the wrist, on the radial border of the ulna.

Functions: Removes blockages in the channel and clears heat, converts internal wind damp and extinguishes wind-heat, moves Qi, courses Liver Qi and relieves pain, benefits the ears and eyes.

Indications: Tinnitus, deafness, superficial pain of skin, pain in the arm, trembling, parkinson's, seizures, epilepsy, confusion and senility in the elderly.

Attributes: Xi-Cleft point.

Notes

_____

_____

_____

_____

_____

_____

_____

_____

_____

Point Combinations

_____

_____

_____

_____

_____

_____

_____

SJ 8
SANYANGLUO

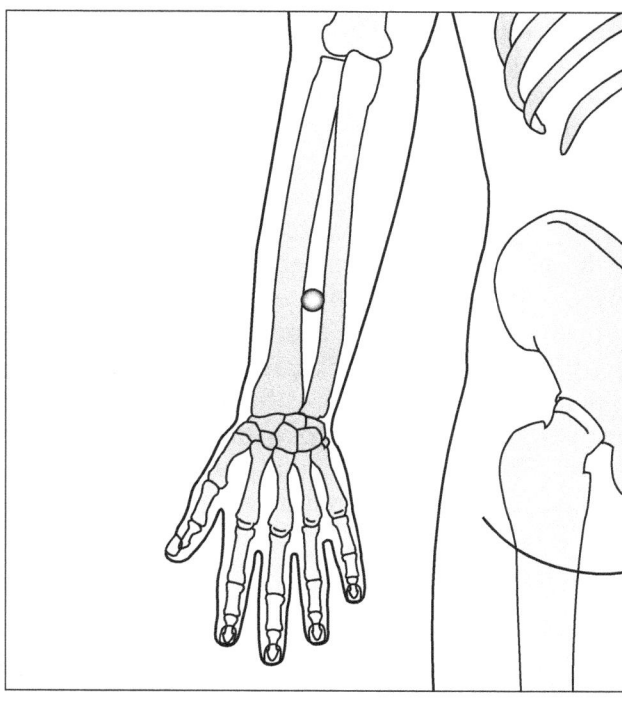

Location: On the dorsal side of the forearm and on the line connecting SJ-4 Yangchi and the tip of the olecranon, 4 cun proximal to the dorsal crease of the wrist, between the radius and ulna.

Functions: Removes blockages and activates the channel and connecting vessels, relieves pain, clears heat, clears fire, resolves damp, extinguishes wind, clears heat, restores consciousness.

Indications: Deafness, loss of voice, aphasia, pain and motor impairment of the upper extremity, low back pain caused by injury.

Notes
_____
_____
_____
_____
_____
_____
_____
_____

Point Combinations
_____
_____
_____
_____
_____
_____

SJ 9
SIDU

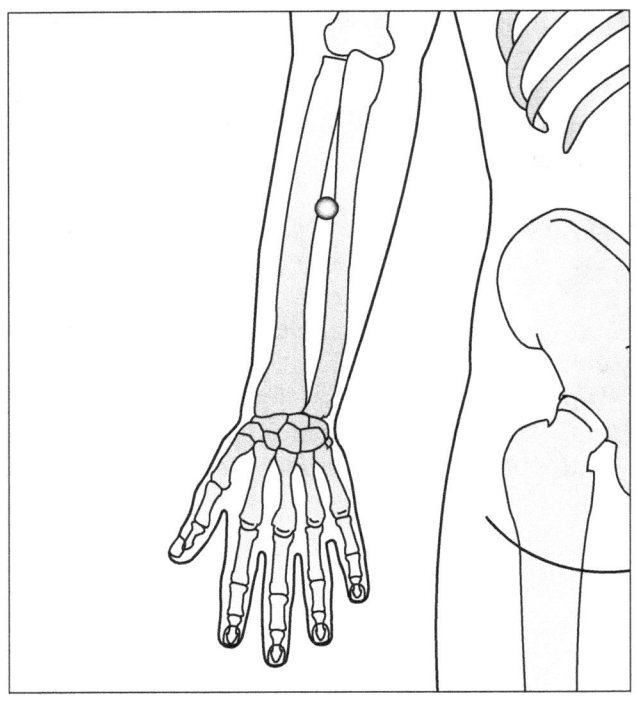

Location: On the dorsal side of the forearm and on the line connecting SJ-4 Yangchi and the tip of the olecranon, 5 cun proximal to the dorsal crease of the wrist, between the radius and ulna.

Functions: Removes blockages and activates the channel and connecting vessels, manages the waterways and courses Qi, calms the chest, opens and assists the ears and throat.

Indications: Headache, neurasthenia, vertigo, deafness, tinnitus, sore throat, loss of voice, obstruction of the throat, toothache in lower jaw, shortness of breath, paralysis of upper extremity, pain in forearm, nephritis.

Notes

Point Combinations

SJ 10
TIANJING

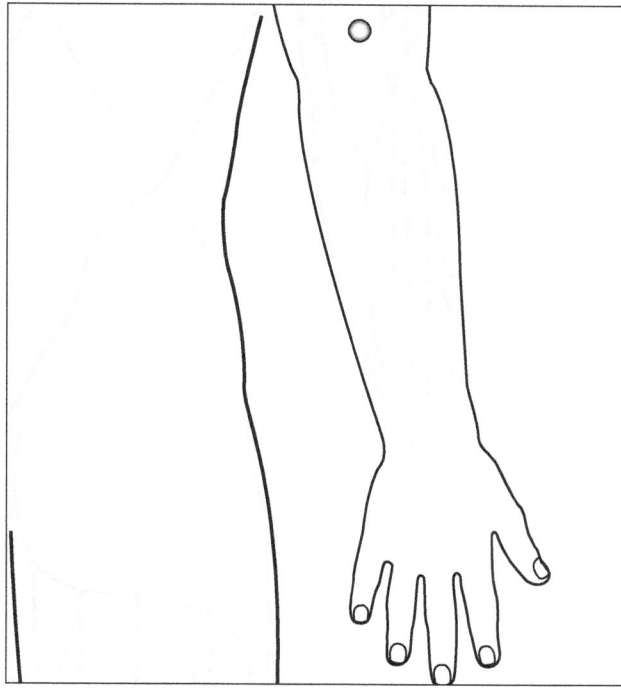

Location: On the dorsal side of the arm, 1 cun above the tip of the olecranon process in the depression when the arm is flexed.

Functions: Clears fire, calms the Heart, calms shen, removes blockages and activates the channel and connecting vessels, loosens the muscles and tendons, courses Qi, transforms phlegm, calms the chest coughing, manages Ying and Wei channels.

Indications: Headache, migraine, deafness, pain in the eyes, neck, shoulder and back, pain or numbness of the arm, tonsillitis, blockage of the throat, hemoptysis, coughing/vomiting blood and puss, pain in the chest, Heart, and lateral costal region, abdominal distention, spastic colon, scrofula, hives, epilepsy, mania, insanity, fright, sadness.

Attributes: Earth point, He-Sea point, sedation point for San Jiao channel.

*Main point for swollen lymph nodes of the neck.

Notes

_____
_____
_____
_____
_____
_____
_____
_____

Point Combinations

_____
_____
_____
_____
_____
_____

SJ 11
QINGLENGYUAN

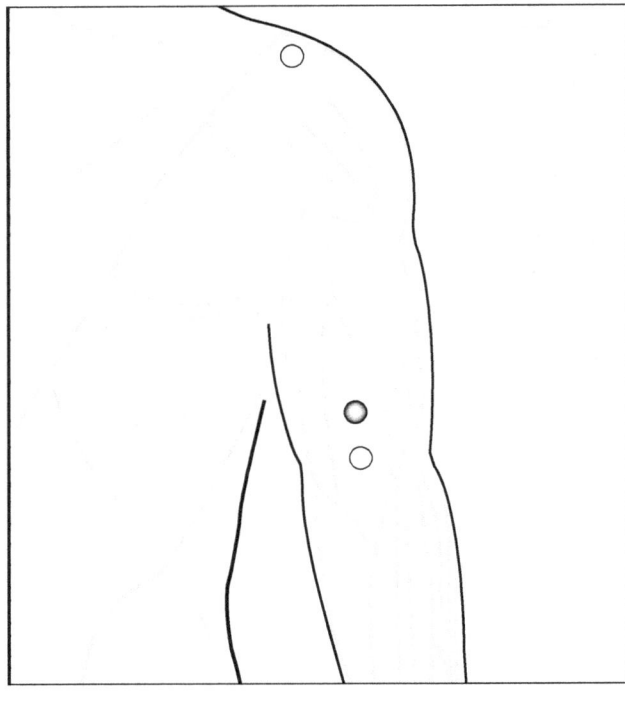

Location: On the dorsal side of the arm, 2 cun above the tip of the olecranon process in the depression when the arm is flexed, 1 cun above SJ-10 Tianjing.

Functions: Activates the channel, extinguishes wind-damp, resolves damp-heat.

Indications: Headache, yellowness of the eyes, pain of the shoulder and arm.

Notes

Point Combinations

SJ 12
XIAOLUO

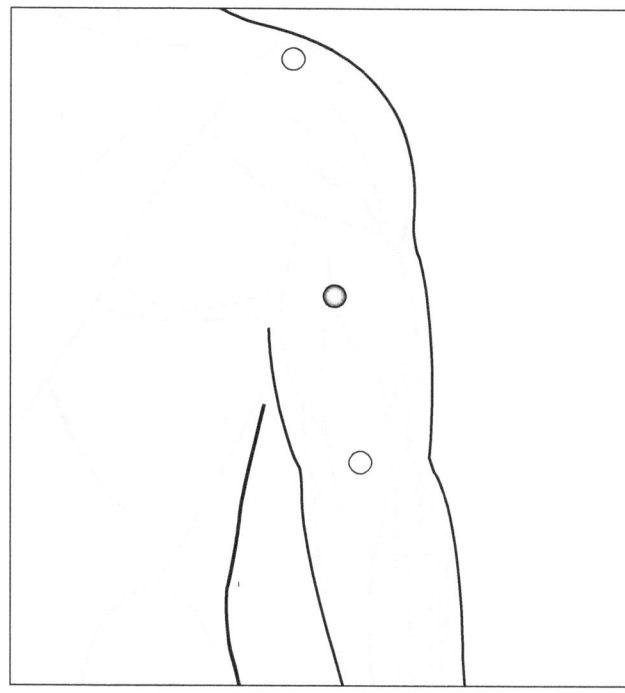

Location: On the dorsal side of the arm, at the midpoint on the line connecting SJ-11 Qinglengyuan and SJ-13 Naohui.

Functions: Activates the channel, relieves pain.

Indications: Headache, stiffness of the neck, pain in the shoulder, arm and back.

Notes

_____
_____
_____
_____
_____
_____
_____
_____
_____

Point Combinations

_____
_____
_____
_____
_____
_____
_____

SJ 13
NAOHUI

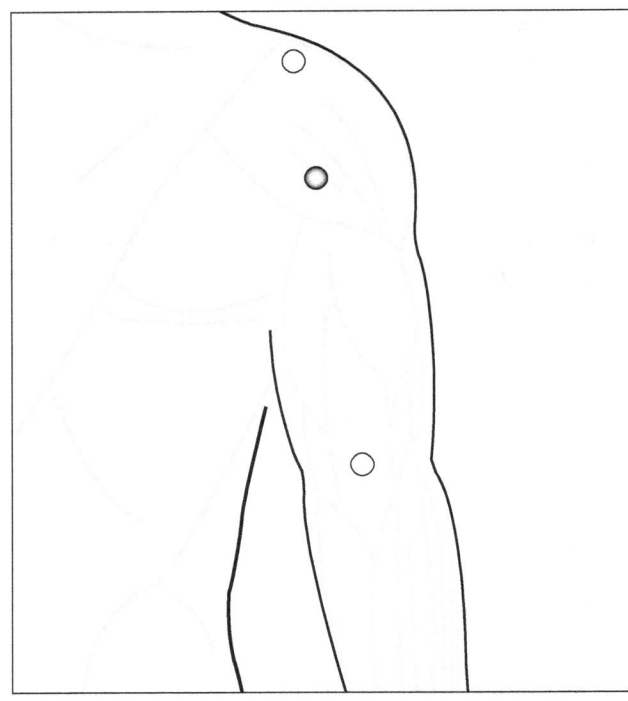

Location: On the dorsal side of the arm, on the posterior border of the deltoid muscle and on the line connecting SJ-14 Jianliao and the olecranon process, 3 cun below SJ-14 Jianliao

Functions: Activates the channel, relieves pain, transforms phlegm.

Indications: Pain in the shoulder and upper arm, goiter, scrofula.

Notes
_____
_____
_____
_____
_____
_____
_____
_____

Point Combinations
_____
_____
_____
_____
_____
_____
_____

SJ 14
JIANLIAO

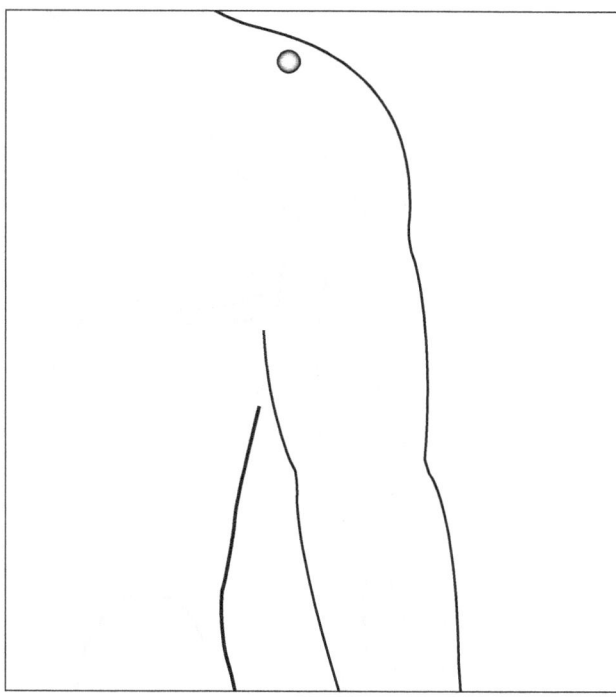

Location: On the shoulder, posterior to LI-15 Jianyu in the depression posterior and inferior to the acromion when the arm is abducted or raised to the level of the shoulder.

Functions: Activates the channel, relieves pain in the shoulder, extinguishes wind-damp.
Indications: Pain in the shoulder.
Attributes: *Typically combined with LI-15 for shoulder pain.

Notes

_____
_____
_____
_____
_____
_____
_____
_____
_____

Point Combinations

_____
_____
_____
_____
_____
_____

SJ 15
TIANLIAO

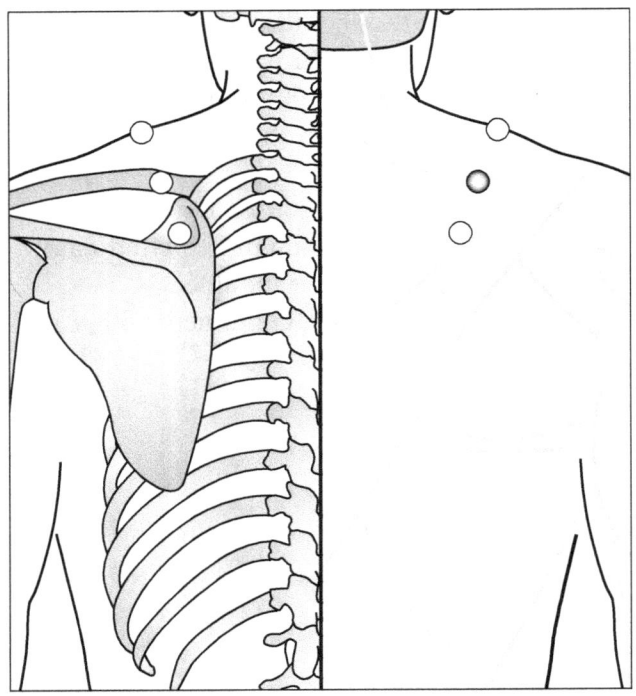

Location: On the back, at the midpoint on the line connecting GB-21 Gyeonjeong and SI-13 Quyuan on the superior angle of the scapula.

Functions: Activates the channel, relieves pain in the shoulder and neck, extinguishes wind-damp.

Indications: Pain in the shoulder and neck, stiffness of the neck.

Notes

_____

_____

_____

_____

_____

_____

_____

_____

Point Combinations

_____

_____

_____

_____

_____

_____

_____

SJ 16
TIANYOU

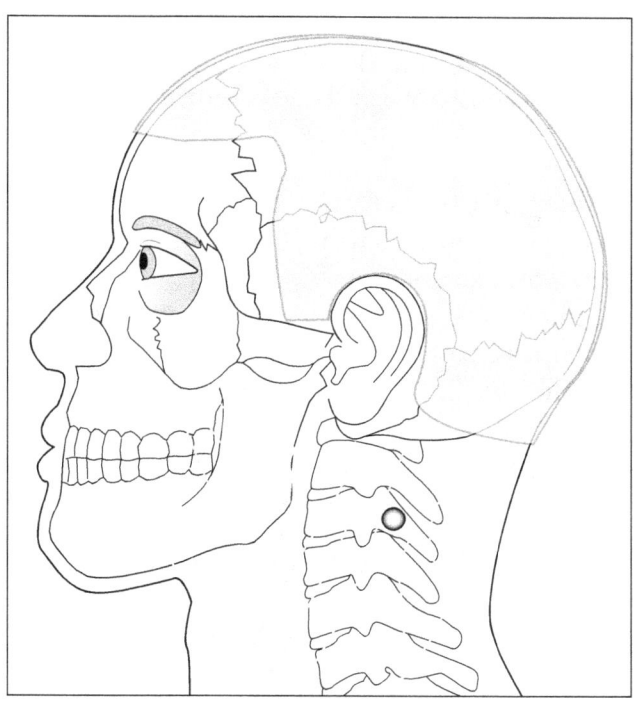

Location: On the lateral side of the neck, level with the angle of the mandible, on the posterior border of the sternocleidomastoid muscle.

Functions: Clears heat, benefits the head and sensory organs, relieves pain.

Indications: Deafness, loss of vision, headache, dizziness, stiffness of the neck, swelling of the face.

Notes

_____
_____
_____
_____
_____
_____
_____
_____
_____

Point Combinations

_____
_____
_____
_____
_____
_____
_____

SJ 17
YIFENG

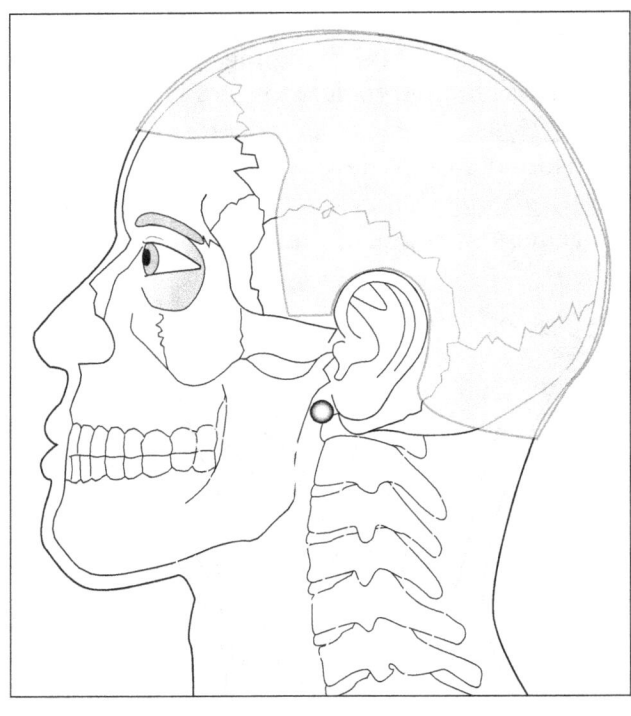

Location: On the lateral side of the neck, posterior to the lobule of the ear, in the depression between the angle of the mandible and the mastoid process.

Functions: Activates the channel, relieves pain, extinguishes wind, benefits the ears, head and face, clears heat.

Indications: Disorders of the ear (tinnitus, deafness, pain, itching and swelling), swelling of the cheek, Bell's palsy, toothache, lock jaw, scrofula.

Attributes: Meeting point of the San Jiao and Gall Bladder channels.

Notes

Point Combinations

SJ 18
QIMAI

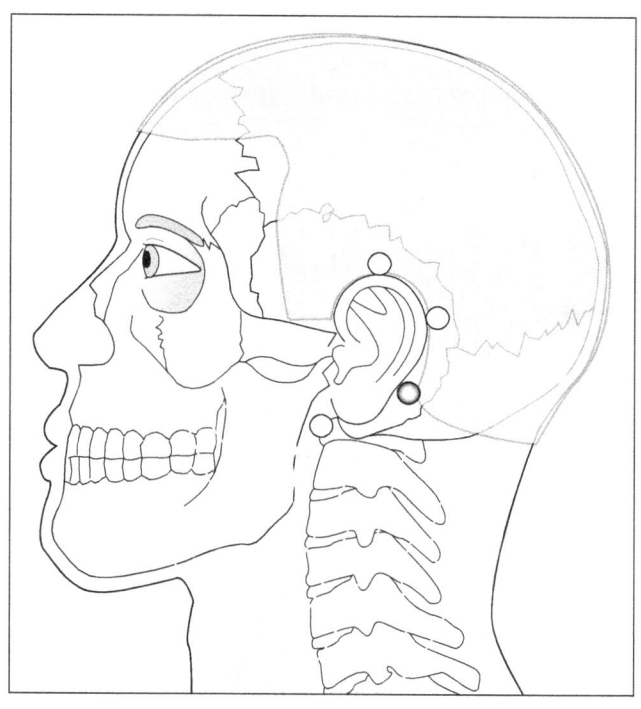

Location: On the head, posterior to the ear in the center of the mastoid process, at the junction of the middle and lower 3rd of the curve on the line connecting SJ-20 Jiaosun and SJ-17 Yifeng.

Functions: Benefits the ears, extinguishes wind, relieves pain.

Indications: Disorders of the ear (tinnitus, deafness, pain behind the ear), headache, infantile convulsions.

Notes

_____
_____
_____
_____
_____
_____
_____
_____
_____

Point Combinations

_____
_____
_____
_____
_____
_____
_____

SJ 19
LUXI

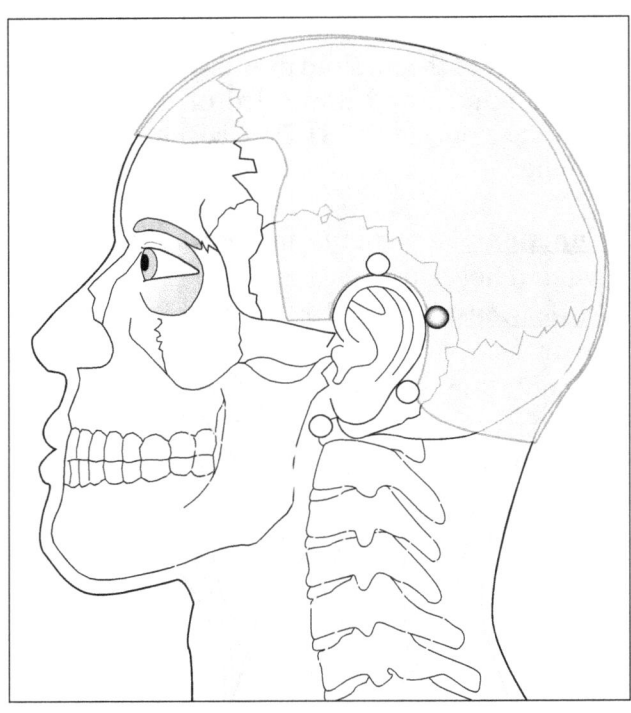

Location: On the head, posterior to the ear in the center of the mastoid process, at the junction of the upper and middle 3rd of the curve on the line connecting SJ-20 Jiaosun and SJ-17 Yifeng.

Functions: Benefits the ears and head, extinguishes wind, relieves pain.

Indications: Disorders of the ear (tinnitus, deafness, pain behind the ear), headache, infantile convulsions.

Notes

Point Combinations

SJ 20
JIAOSUN

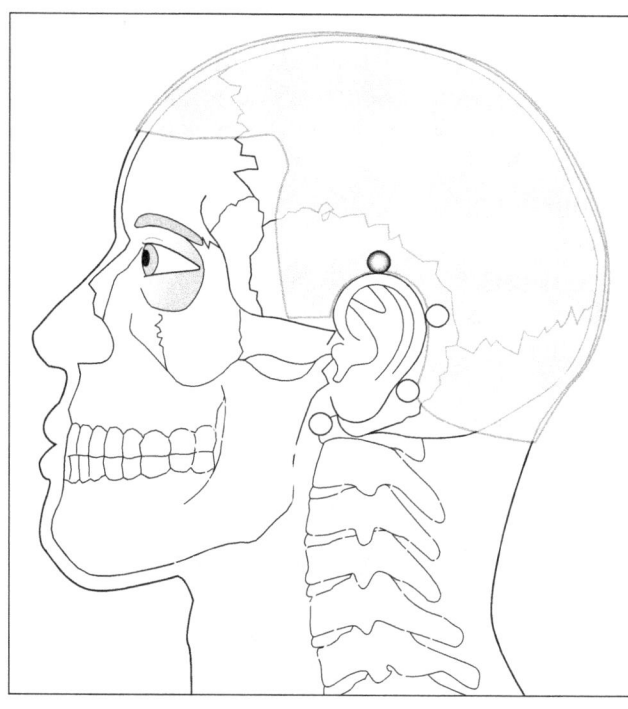

Location: On the head, directly above the apex of the ear within the hairline.

Functions: Benefits the ears, teeth and gums, clears heat, relieves pain.

Indications: Disorders of the ear (tinnitus, deafness, ear pain, swelling), toothache, swelling and pain of the gums.

Attributes: Meeting point of the San Jiao, Gall Bladder and Small Intestine channels.

Notes

Point Combinations

SJ 21
ERMEN

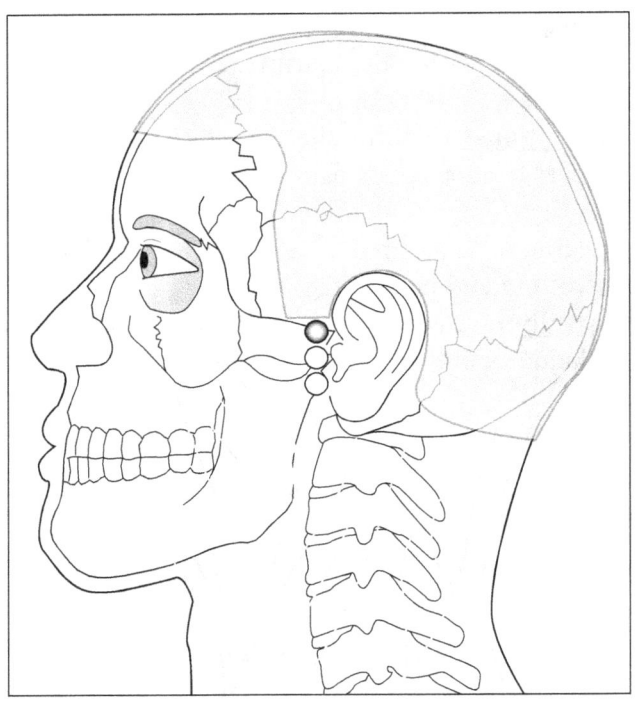

Location: On the face, anterior to the supratragus notch and on the posterior border of the condyloid process of the mandible, in the depression formed when the mouth is opened.

Functions: Benefits the ears, clears heat, relieves pain.

Indications: Disorders of the ear (tinnitus, deafness, ear pain, swelling, itching of the ear), toothache.

Notes

Point Combinations

SJ 22
ERHELIAO

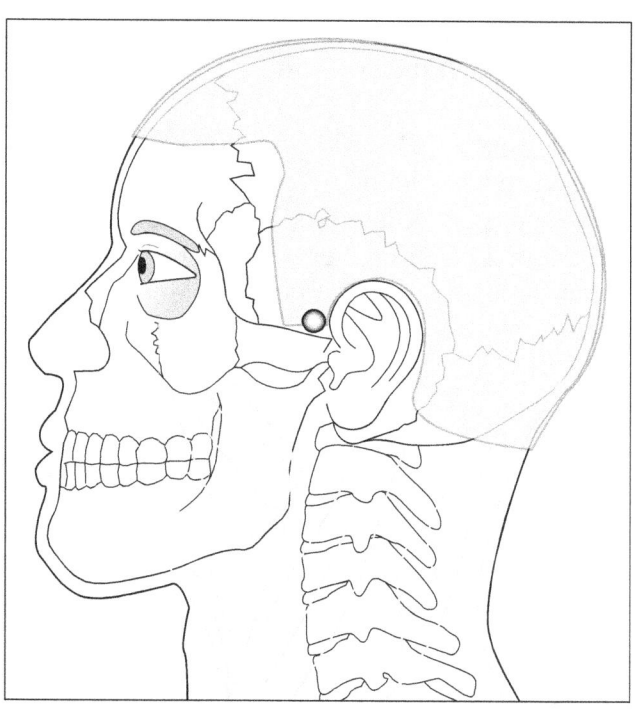

Location: On the face, anterior and superior to SJ-21 Ermen, level with the root of the auricle on the posterior border of hairline of the temple where superficial temporal artery passes.

Functions: Benefits the ears, extinguishes wind, relieves pain.

Indications: Disorders of the ear (tinnitus, deafness, ear pain), headache.

Attributes: Meeting point of the San Jiao, Gall Bladder and Small Intestine channels.

Notes

Point Combinations

SJ 23
SIZHUKONG

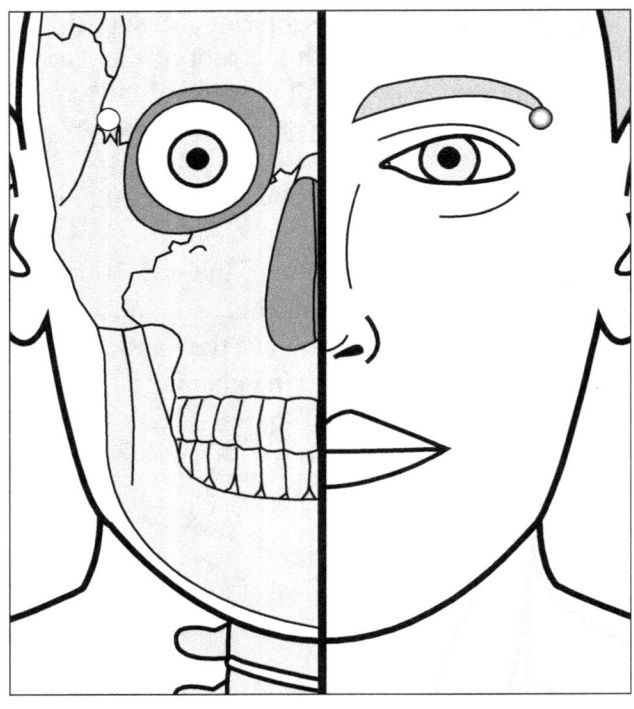

Location: On the face, in the depression at the lateral end of the eyebrow.

Functions: Benefits the eyes, extinguishes wind, relieves pain.

Indications: Disorders of the eye (eye pain, redness, swelling, twitching of the eye), headache, dizziness, epilepsy, mania.

Notes

_____
_____
_____
_____
_____
_____
_____
_____

Point Combinations

_____
_____
_____
_____
_____
_____
_____
_____

GB 1
TONGZILIAO

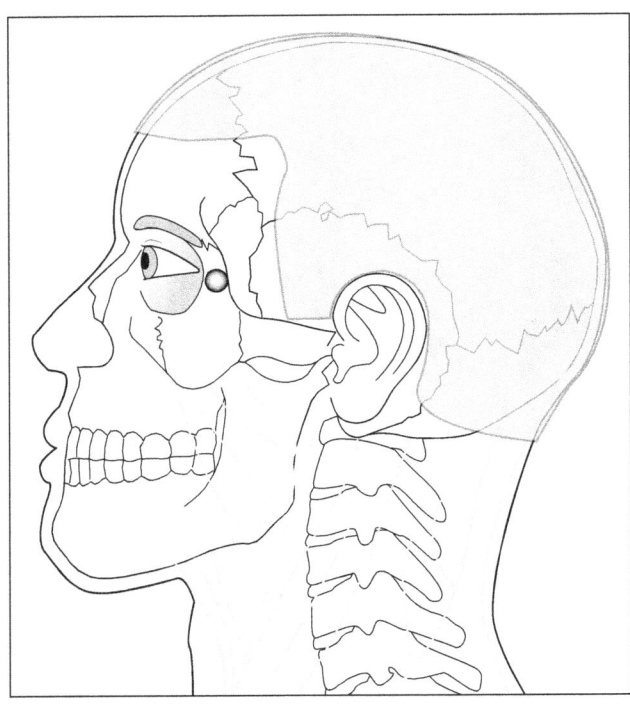

Location: On the face, 0.5 cun lateral to the outer canthus, on the lateral border of the orbit.

Functions: Benefits the eyes, extinguishes wind, clears heat.

Indications: Disorders of the eye (eye pain, redness, swelling, loss of vision), headache.

Attributes: Meeting point of the San Jiao, Gall Bladder and Small Intestine channels.

Notes

Point Combinations

GB 2
TINGHUI

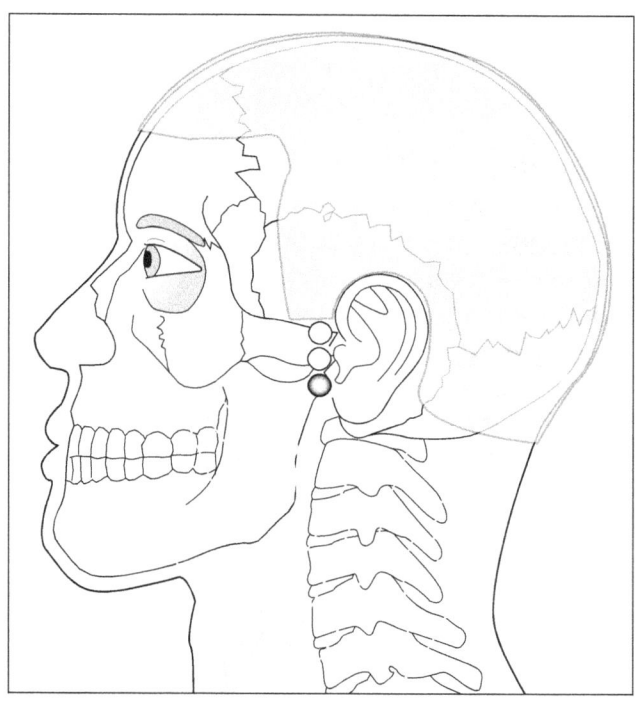

Location: On the face, anterior to the intertragic notch, in the depression posterior to the condyloid process of the mandible when the mouth is open.

Functions: Benefits the eyes, extinguishes wind, clears heat, relieves pain.

Indications: Disorders of the ear (tinnitus, deafness, ear pain), toothache, deviation of the mouth and eye, Bell's palsy.

Notes

Point Combinations

GB 3
SHANGGUAN

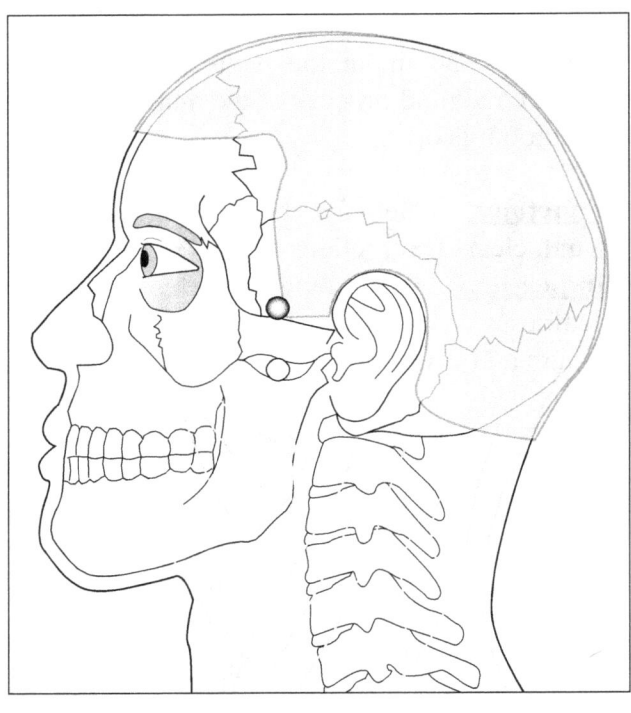

Location: On the face, on the upper border of the zygomatic arch, directly above ST-7 Xiaguan.

Functions: Benefits the ears, extinguishes wind, relieves pain.

Indications: Disorders of the ear (tinnitus, deafness, ear pain), toothache, headache, deviation of the mouth and eye, Bell's palsy.

Attributes: Meeting point of the San Jiao, Gall Bladder and Stomach channels.

Notes
_____
_____
_____
_____
_____
_____
_____
_____
_____

Point Combinations
_____
_____
_____
_____
_____
_____
_____
_____

GB 4
HANYAN

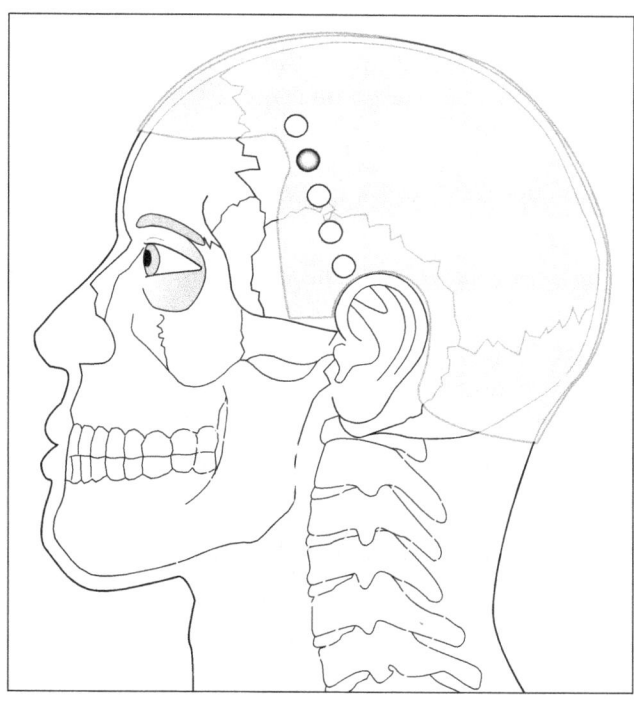

Location: On the head, within the hairline of the temporal region, at the junction of the upper 1/4th and lower 3/4th of the curve on the line connecting ST-8 Touwei and GB-7 Qubin.

Functions: Extinguishes wind, relieves pain, clears heat.

Indications: Headache, tinnitus, toothache, deviation of the mouth and eye, Bell's palsy, lockjaw, dizziness, epilepsy.

Attributes: Meeting point of the San Jiao, Gall Bladder and Stomach channels.

Notes

_____
_____
_____
_____
_____
_____
_____
_____

Point Combinations

_____
_____
_____
_____
_____
_____
_____

GB 5
XUANLU

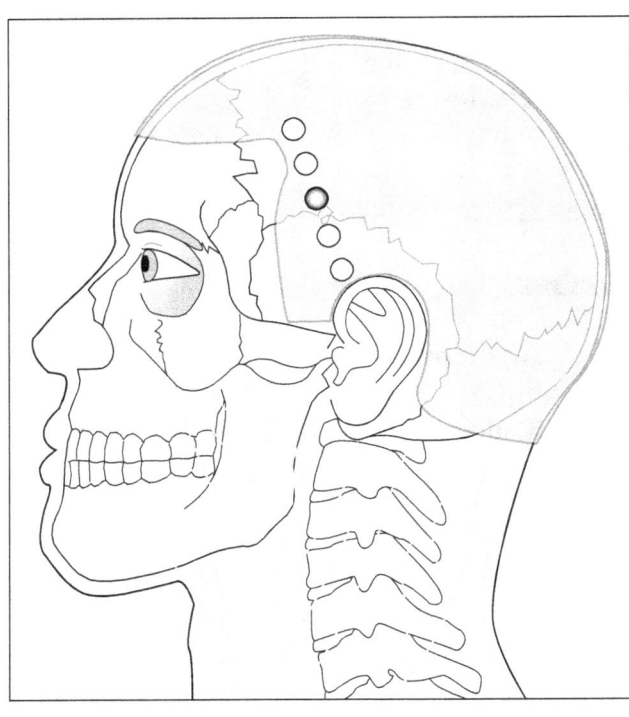

Location: On the head, within the hairline of the temporal region, at the midpoint along the curve on the line connecting ST-8 Touwei and GB-7 Qubin.

Functions: Extinguishes wind, relieves pain, clears heat.

Indications: Headache, toothache, pain in the eye, redness and swelling of the eye.

Attributes: Meeting point of the San Jiao, Gall Bladder, Stomach and Large Intestine channels.

Notes

_____
_____
_____
_____
_____
_____
_____
_____

Point Combinations

_____
_____
_____
_____
_____
_____

GB 6
XUANLI

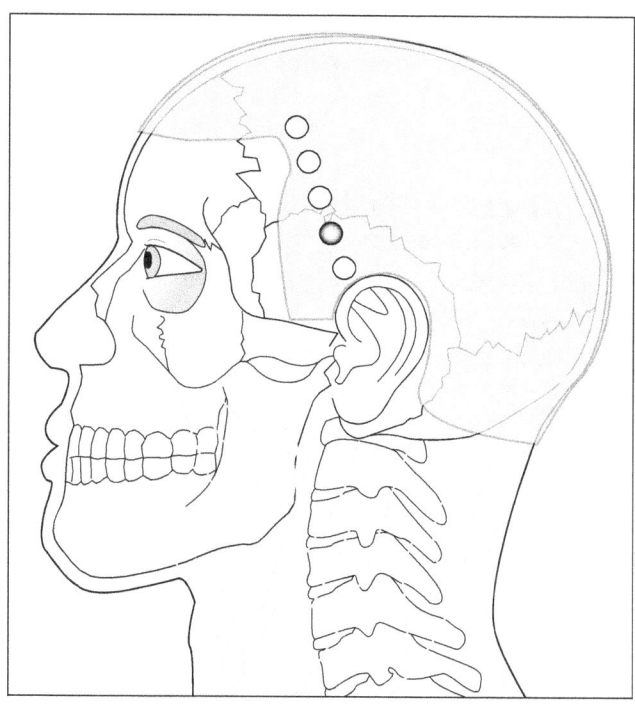

Location: On the head, within the hairline of the temporal region, at the junction of the lower 1/4th and upper 3/4th of the curve on the line connecting ST-8 Touwei and GB-7 Qubin.

Functions: Extinguishes wind, relieves pain, clears heat.

Indications: Headache, tinnitus, pain in the eye, redness and swelling of the eye.

Attributes: Meeting point of the San Jiao, Gall Bladder, Stomach and Large Intestine channels.

Notes

Point Combinations

GB 7
QUBIN

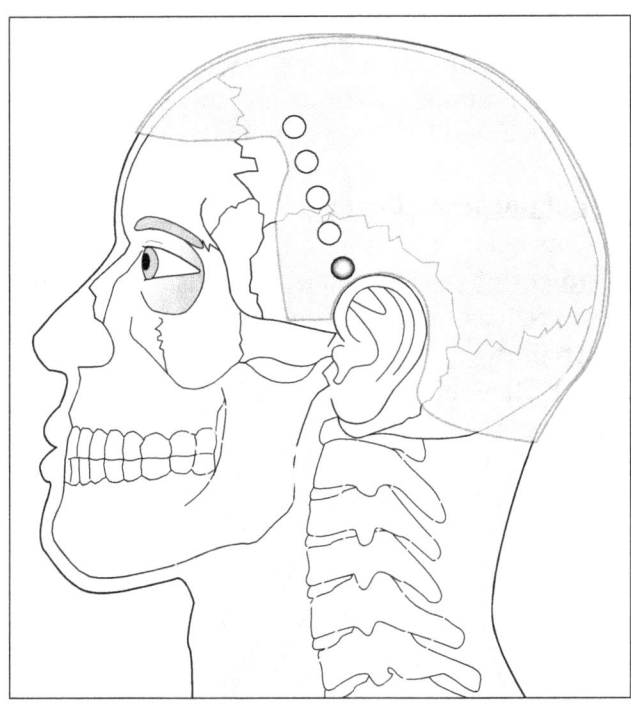

Location: On the head, within the hairline of the temporal region, at the junction of the upper 3/4th and lower 3/4th of the curve on the line connecting ST-8 Touwei and GB-7 Qubin.

Functions: Extinguishes wind, relieves pain, clears heat, benefits the mouth and jaw.

Indications: Headache, toothache, loss of voice, swelling of the cheek.

Attributes: Meeting point of the Gall Bladder and Urinary Bladder channels.

Notes

Point Combinations

GB 8
SHUAIGU

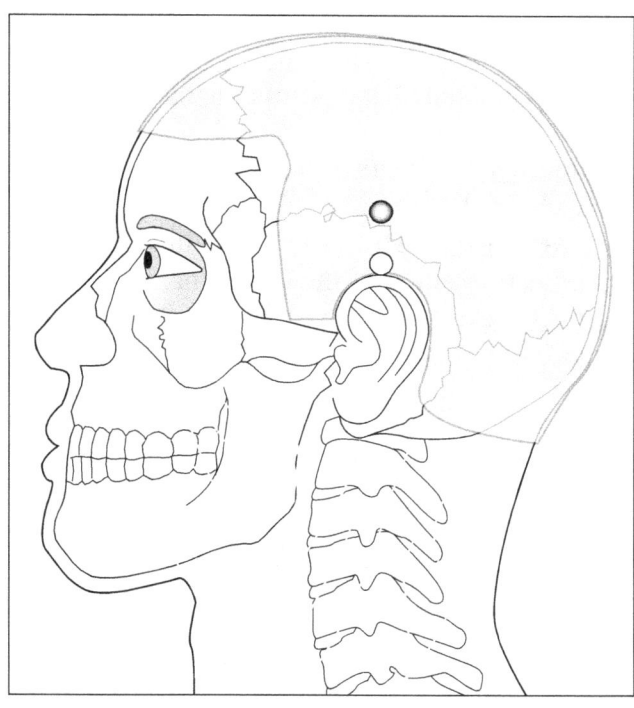

Location: On the head, directly above the apex of the ear (SJ-20 Jiaosun), 1.5 cun within the hairline.

Functions: Extinguishes wind, relieves pain, benefits the head, relieves vomitting.

Indications: Headache, vomiting, childhood convulsions.

Attributes: Meeting point of the Gall Bladder and Urinary Bladder channels.

Notes

_____
_____
_____
_____
_____
_____
_____
_____

Point Combinations

_____
_____
_____
_____
_____
_____
_____

GB 9
TIANCHONG

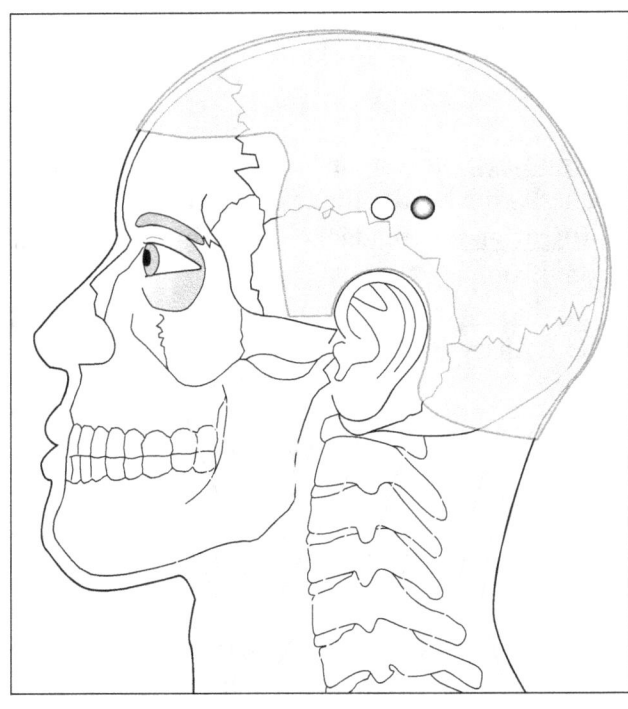

Location: On the head, directly above the posterior border of the ear, 0.5 cun posterior to GB-8 Shuaigu, 2 cun within the hairline.

Functions: Clears heat, calms shen, activates the channel.

Indications: Headache, tinnitus, deafness, pain and swelling of the gums, mania.

Attributes: Meeting point of the Gall Bladder and Urinary Bladder channels.

Notes

Point Combinations

GB 10
FUBAI

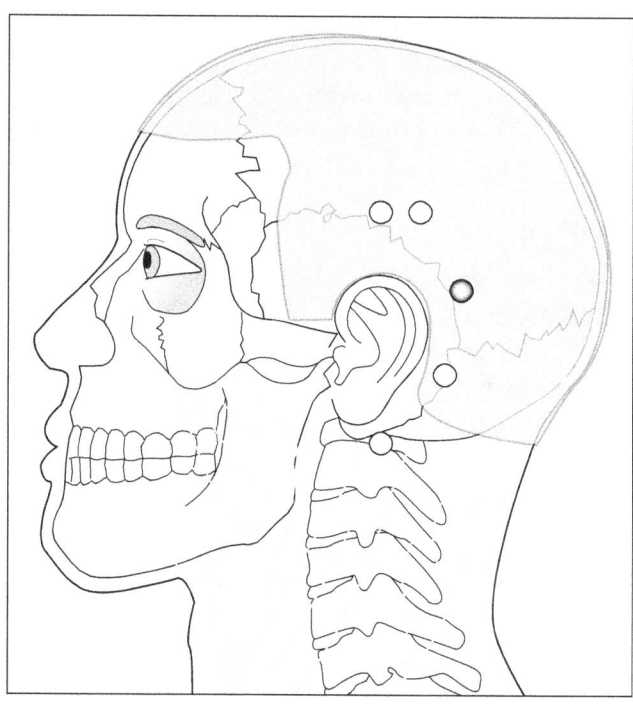

Location: On the head, directly above the posterior border of the ear, at the midpoint along the curve on the line connecting GB-9 Tianchong and GB-11 TouQiaoyin, at the junction of the middle 1/3rd and upper 1/3rd on the curve on the line connecting GB-9 Tianchong and GB-12 Wangu.

Functions: Clears heat, activates the channel, relieves pain, benefits the neck.

Indications: Headache, tinnitus, deafness, pain and swelling of the neck, goiter.

Attributes: Meeting point of the Gall Bladder and Urinary Bladder channels.

Notes

_____

_____

_____

_____

_____

_____

_____

_____

_____

Point Combinations

_____

_____

_____

_____

_____

_____

_____

GB 11
TouQiaoyin

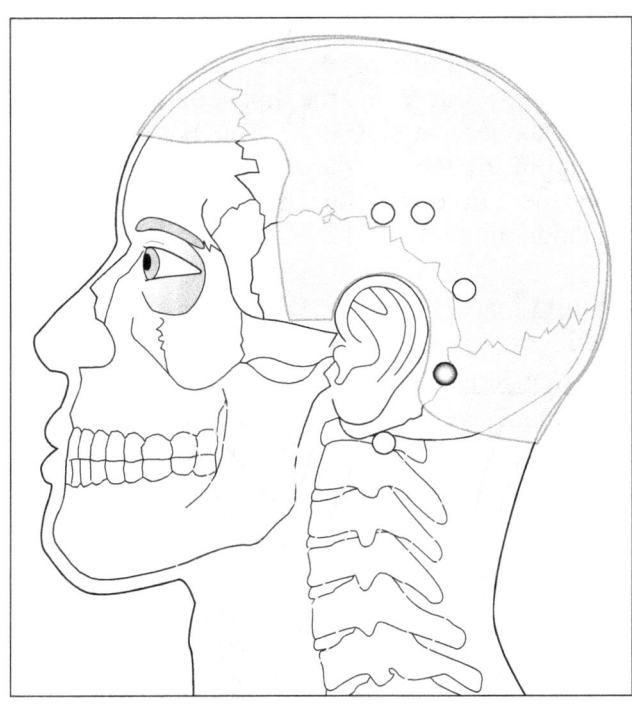

Location: On the head, directly above the posterior border of the ear, at the junction of the middle 1/3rd and lower 1/3rd on the curve on the line connecting GB-9 Tianchong and GB-12 Wangu.

Functions: Clears heat, activates the channel, relieves pain, benefits the neck.

Indications: Headache, tinnitus, deafness, pain and swelling of the neck, goiter.

Attributes: Meeting point of the Gall Bladder, Urinary Bladder, San Jiao and Small Intestine channels.

Notes

_____

_____

_____

_____

_____

_____

_____

_____

Point Combinations

_____

_____

_____

_____

_____

_____

GB 12
WANGU

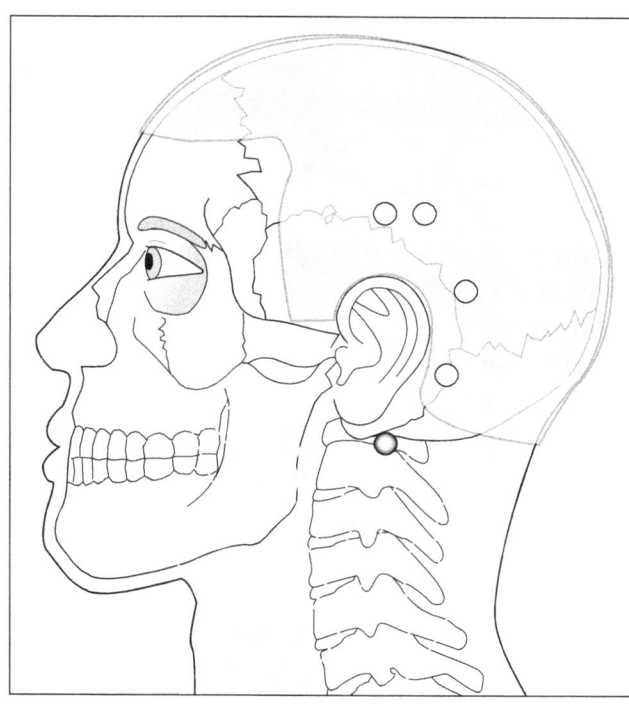

Location: On the head, directly above the posterior border of the ear, in the depression posterior and inferior to the mastoid process.

Functions: Extinguishes wind, activates the channel, relieves pain, benefits the head, calms shen.

Indications: Headache, toothache, swelling of the cheek, pain and stiffness of the neck, mania.

Attributes: Meeting point of the Gall Bladder and Urinary Bladder channels.

Notes
_____
_____
_____
_____
_____
_____
_____
_____

Point Combinations
_____
_____
_____
_____
_____
_____

GB 13
BENSHEN

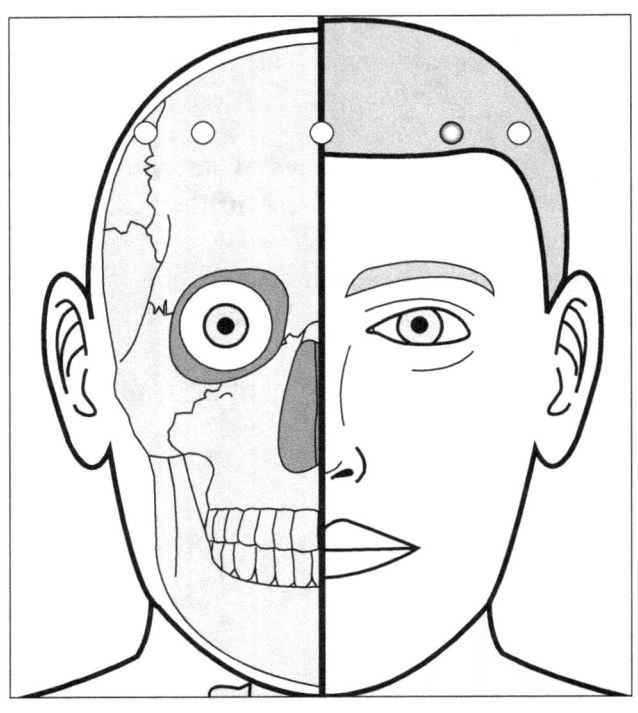

Location: On the head, 0.5 cun above the anterior hairline, 3 cun lateral to DU-24 Shenting, at the junction of the medial two thirds and lateral third of the line connecting DU-24 Shenting and ST-8 Touwei.

Functions: Extinguishes wind, transforms phlegm, calms shen.

Indications: Headache, dizziness, pain and stiffness of the neck, mania, childhood convulsions.

Attributes: Meeting point of the Gall Bladder channel and Yang Wei Vessel.

Notes

Point Combinations

GB 14
YANGBAI

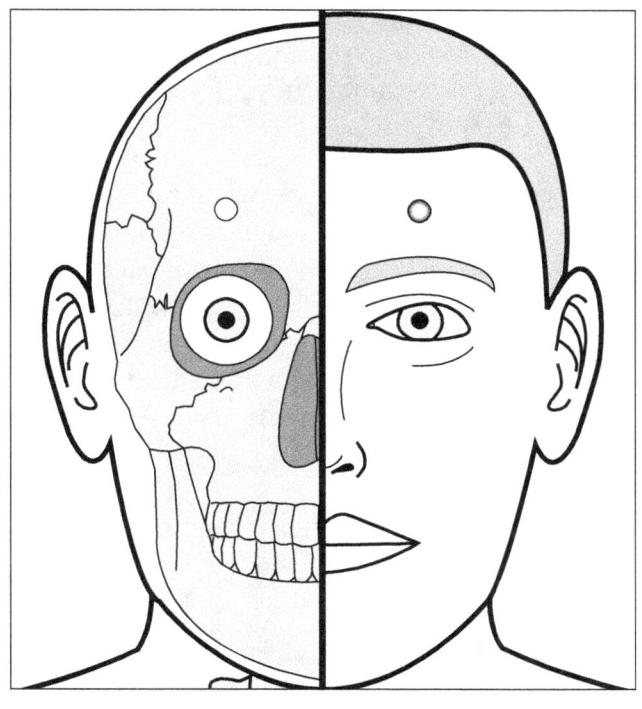

Location: On the forehead, directly above the pupil, 1 cun above the midpoint of the eyebrow.

Functions: Extinguishes wind, relieves pain, benefits the eyes and head.

Indications: Headache, dizziness, pain and stiffness of the face, Bell's palsy, eye pain, difficulty closing the eyes, forehead pain.

Attributes: Meeting point of the Gall Bladder channel and Yang Wei Vessel.

Notes

Point Combinations

GB 15
TOULINQI

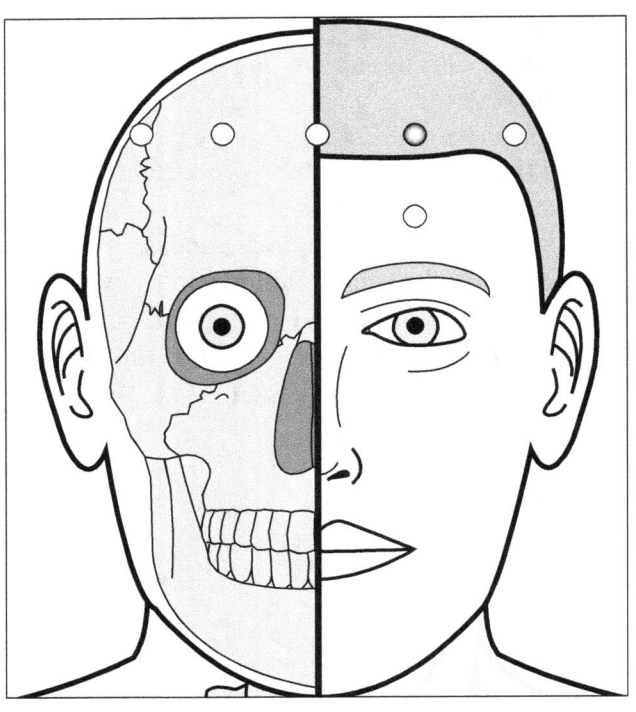

Location: On the head, directly above the pupil, 0.5 cun posterior to the anterior hairline, at the midpoint on the line joining DU-24 Shenting and ST-8 Touwei.

Functions: Extinguishes wind, relieves pain, benefits the eyes, nose and head, calms shen.

Indications: Headache, dizziness, occiput and forehead pain, nasal congestion, redness and pain of the eyes, Bell's palsy.

Attributes: Meeting point of the Gall Bladder, Urinary Bladder channels and Yang Wei Vessel.

Notes

Point Combinations

GB 16
MUCHUANG

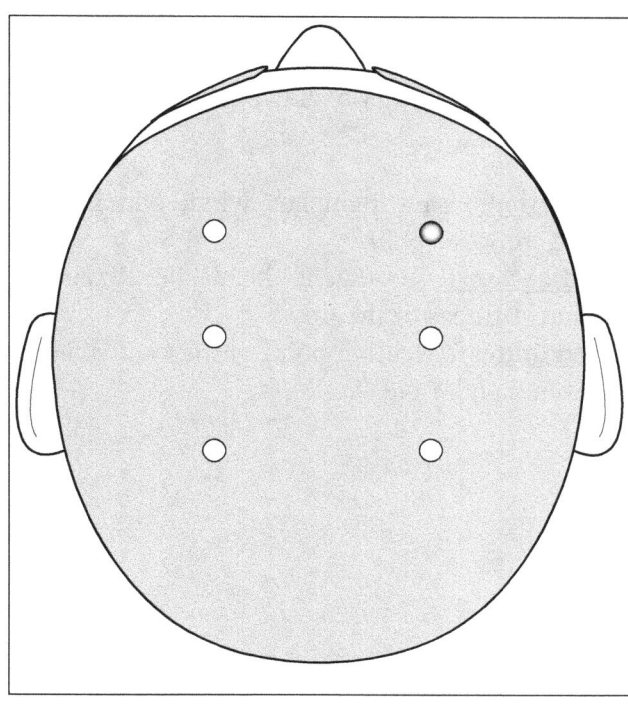

Location: On the head, 2 cun posterior to the anterior hairline, 2.25 cun lateral to the anterior midline (1.5 cun posterior to GB-15 Toulingi).

Functions: Extinguishes wind, benefits the eyes and head, relieves pain.

Indications: Headache, nasal congestion, swelling of the facial region, epilepsy, blurred vision, glaucoma, redness, swelling and pain of the eye.

Attributes: Meeting point of the Gall Bladder channel and the Yang Wei Vessel.

Notes

_____
_____
_____
_____
_____
_____
_____
_____
_____

Point Combinations

_____
_____
_____
_____
_____
_____
_____

GB 17
ZHENGYING

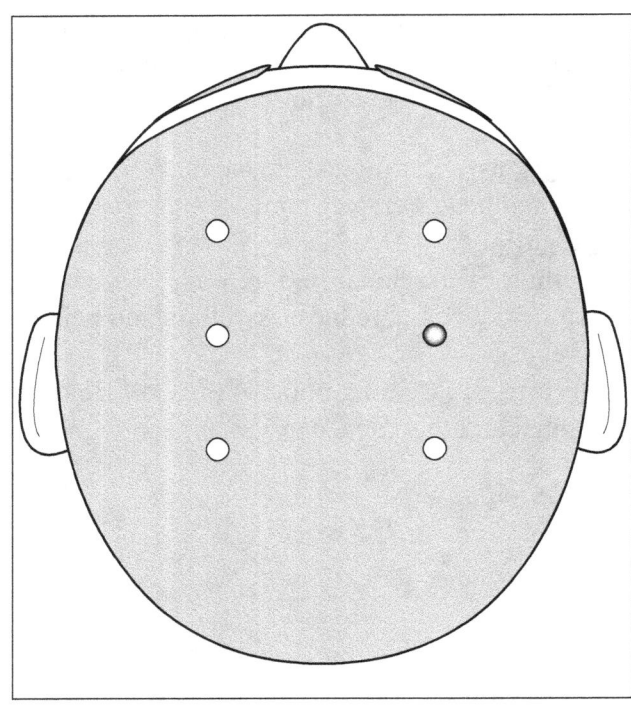

Location: On the head, 3.5 cun posterior to the anterior hairline, 2.25 cun lateral to the anterior midline (1.5 cun posterior to GB-16 Muchuang).

Functions: Extinguishes wind, benefits the head, relieves pain.

Indications: Toothache, headache, dizziness, acute stiffness of the lips.

Attributes: Meeting point of the Gall Bladder channel and Yang Wei Vessel.

Notes

_____

_____

_____

_____

_____

_____

_____

_____

Point Combinations

_____

_____

_____

_____

_____

_____

GB 18
CHENGLING

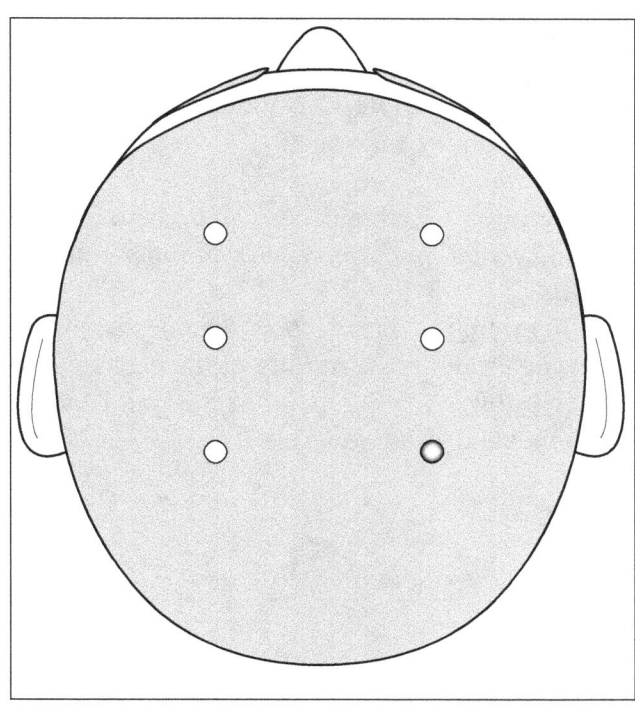

Location: On the head, 5 cun posterior to the anterior hairline, 2.25 cun lateral to the anterior midline (1.5 cun posterior to GB-17 Zhengying).

Functions: Extinguishes wind, benefits the head, clears heat, relieves pain.

Indications: Nasal congestion, headaches, dizziness, epistaxis, eye pain

Attributes: Meeting point of the Gall Bladder channel and the Yang Wei Vessel.

Notes
_____
_____
_____
_____
_____
_____
_____
_____
_____

Point Combinations
_____
_____
_____
_____
_____
_____

GB 19
NAOKONG

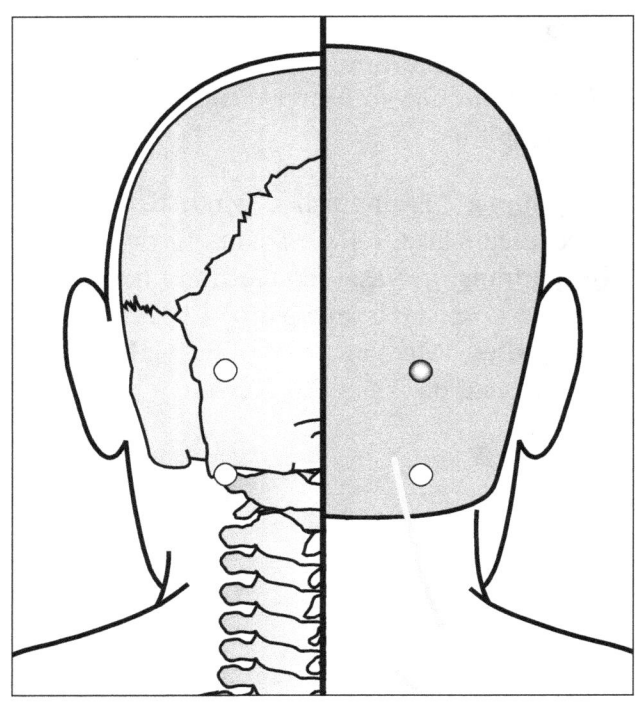

Location: On the head and on the level of the upper border of the external occipital protuberance or DU-17 Naohu, 2.25 cun lateral to the midline of the head.

Functions: Extinguishes wind, benefits the head, clears fire, opens the portals, relieves pain.

Indications: Headache, dizziness, manic psychosis, epilepsy, rigidity of the neck.

Attributes: Meeting point of the Gall Bladder channel and Yang Wei Vessel.

Notes _____

_____

_____

_____

_____

_____

_____

_____

Point Combinations _____

_____

_____

_____

_____

_____

_____

GB 20
FENGCHI

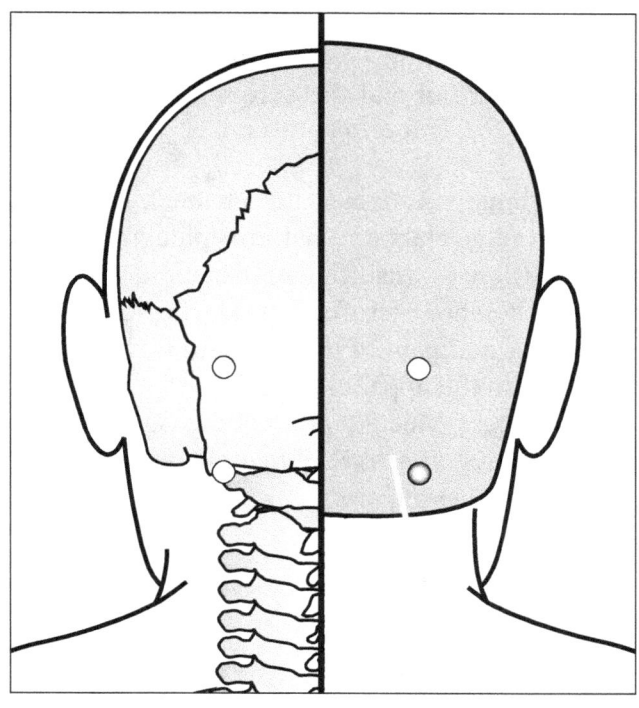

Location: On the nape, below the occipital bone, on the level of DU-16 Fengfu, in the depression between the upper ends of the sternocleidomastoid and trapezius muscles.

Functions: Extinguishes interior and exterior wind, clears the head, benefits the eyes, subdues Liver yang, activates the channel, relieves pain.

Indications: Common cold, nasal congestion, headaches, pain, redness and swelling of the eye, rhinorrhea, epistaxis, rigidity and pain of the neck, limited range of motion of the shoulder, dizziness, vertigo, hemiplegia, epilepsy.

Attributes: Meeting point of the Gall Bladder channel and the Yang Wei Vessel.

Notes
_____
_____
_____
_____
_____
_____
_____
_____

Point Combinations
_____
_____
_____
_____
_____
_____

GB 21
JIANJING

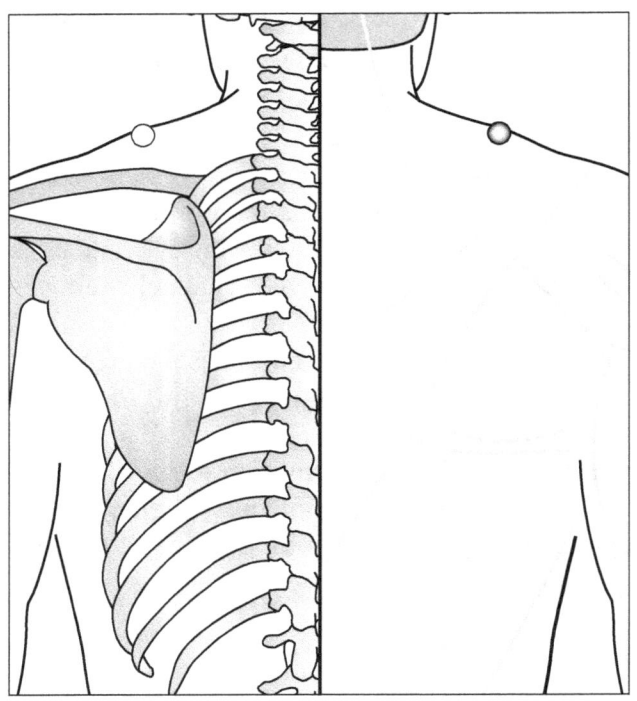

Location: On the shoulder, directly above the nipple, at the midpoint on the line connecting DU-14 Dazhui and the acromion (at the high point of the Trapezius muscle).

Functions: Activates the channel, descends Qi, promotes labor, transforms phlegm.

Indications: Insufficient lactation, mastitis, difficult labor, scrofula, headache, dizziness, stiffness and pain of the neck, limited range of motion in the upper extremities.

Attributes: Meeting point of the Gall Bladder, San Jiao, Stomach, San Jiao channels and the Yang Wei Vessel.

Notes

_____
_____
_____
_____
_____
_____
_____
_____

Point Combinations

_____
_____
_____
_____
_____
_____
_____

GB 22
YUANYE

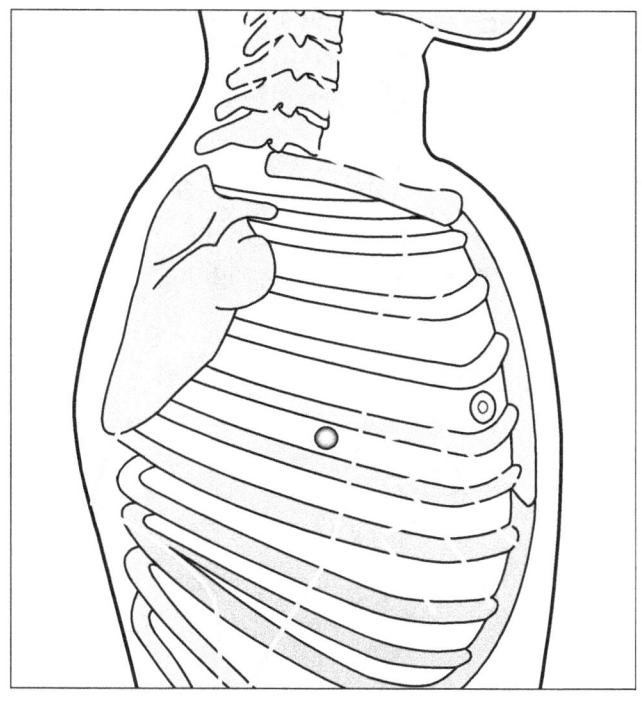

Location: On the lateral side of the chest and on the middle axillary line, in the 5th intercostal space, 3 cun below the axilla.

Functions: Relaxes the sinews, opens the chest.

Indications: Spasm and pain in the upper extremities, chest congestion, pain in the hypochondrium.

Notes

_____
_____
_____
_____
_____
_____
_____
_____
_____

Point Combinations

_____
_____
_____
_____
_____
_____
_____
_____

GB 23
ZHEJIN

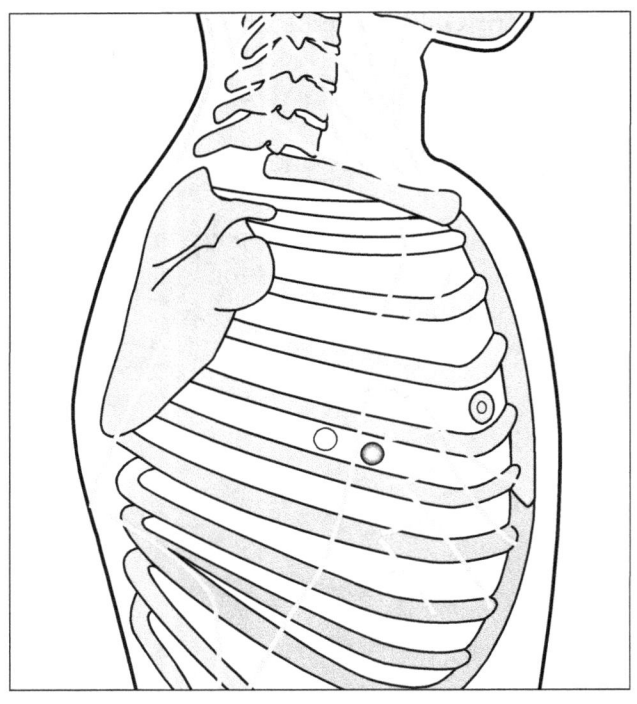

Location: On the lateral side of the chest at the level of the nipple in the 5th intercostal space, 1 cun anterior to GB-22 Yuanye.

Functions: Subdues rebellious Qi, opens the chest.

Indications: Asthma, pain in the hypochondrium, chest congestion.

Notes

_____

_____

_____

_____

_____

_____

_____

_____

Point Combinations

_____

_____

_____

_____

_____

_____

_____

GB 24
ZHEJIN

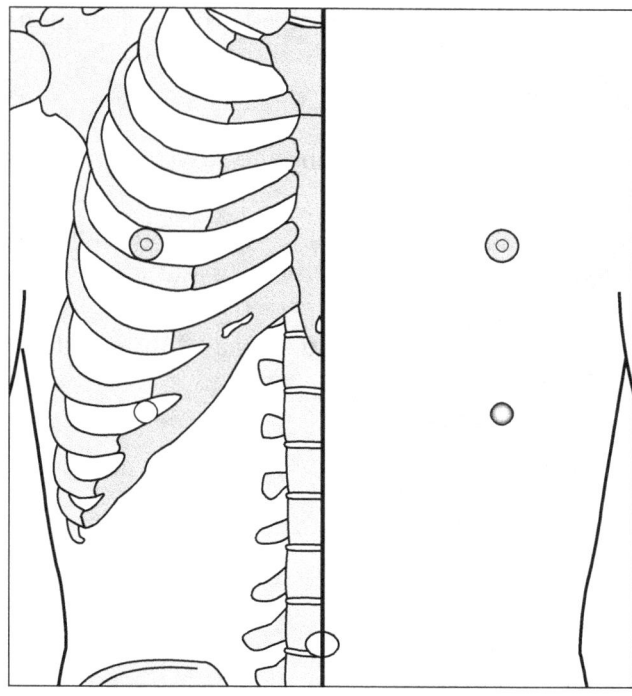

Location: On the upper abdomen, directly below the nipple, in the 7th intercostal space, 4 cun lateral to the anterior midline.

Functions: Resolves damp-heat, regulates the Gall Bladder and Liver Qi, subdues rebellious Qi, regulates the middle jiao.

Indications: Vomiting, hiccups, acid reflux, jaundice, swelling and pain in the hypochondrium.

Attributes: Front-Mu point of the Gall Bladder, meeting point of the Gall Bladder and Urinary Bladder channel.

Notes

Point Combinations

GB 25
JINGMEN

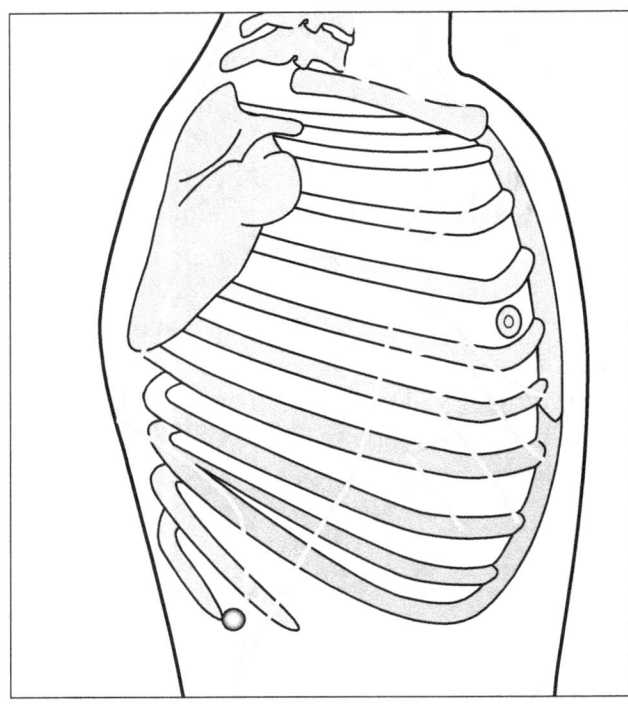

Location: On the lateral side of the abdomen, on the lower border of the free end of the 12th floating rib.

Functions: Strengthens the low back, opens the water passages.

Indications: Pain in the hypochondrium, abdominal pain, diarrhea, dysuria, edema, lumbar pain.

Attributes: Front-Mu point of the Kidney channel.

Notes
_____
_____
_____
_____
_____
_____
_____
_____
_____

Point Combinations
_____
_____
_____
_____
_____
_____
_____
_____

GB 26
DAIMAI

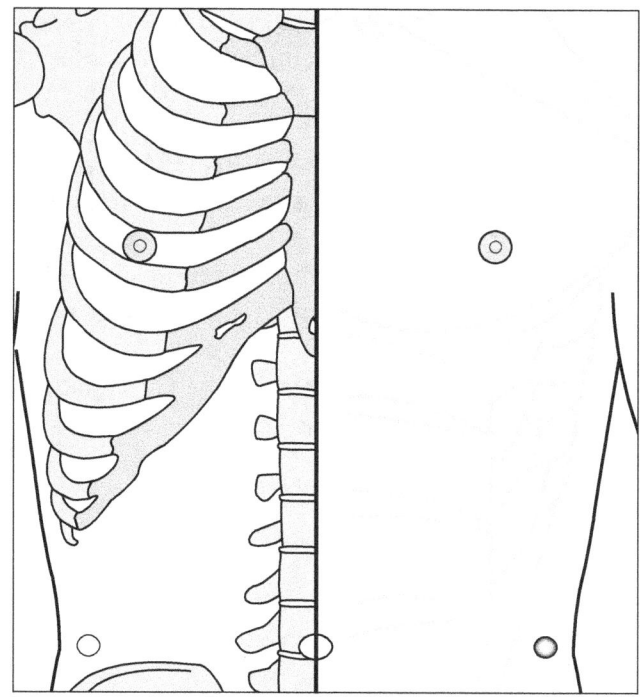

Location: On the lateral side of the abdomen, 1.8 cun below LR-13 Zhangmen, at the meeting point of a vertical line through free end of the 11th rib and a horizontal line through umbilicus.

Functions: Regulates the Dai Mai Vessel, regulates menstruation, relieves pain, activates the channel, resolves damp.

Indications: Irregular menstruation, amenorrhea, morbid leukorrhea, abdominal pain, hernia, pain in the lumbar and hypochondrium.

Attributes: Meeting point of the Gall Bladder channel and the Dai Mai Vessel.

Notes

Point Combinations

GB 27
WUSHU

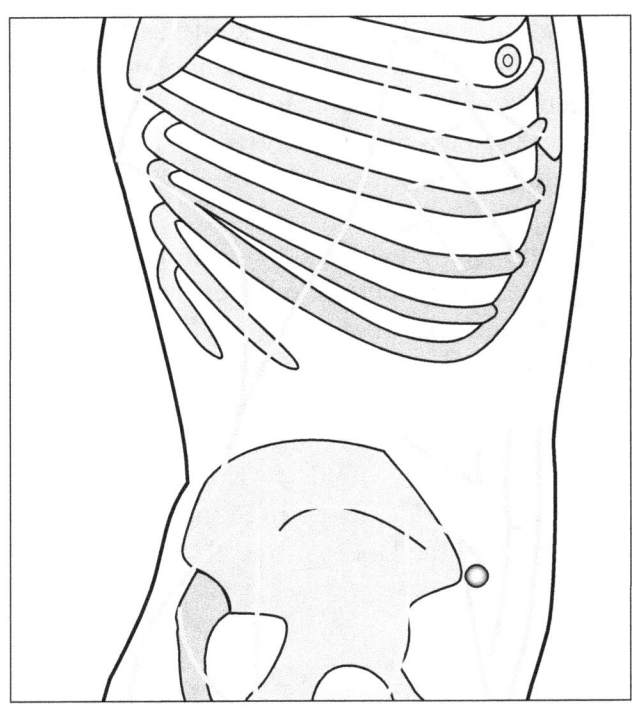

Location: On the lateral side of the abdomen, anterior to the ASIS, 3 cun below the center of the umbilicus.

Functions: Regulates the Dai Mai Vessel, resolves damp, moves stagnant Qi, regulates the lower jiao.

Indications: Constipation, prolapse of the Uterus, morbid leukorrhea, abdominal pain, hernia.

Attributes: Meeting point of the Gall Bladder channel and the Dai Mai Vessel.

Notes

_____
_____
_____
_____
_____
_____
_____
_____
_____

Point Combinations

_____
_____
_____
_____
_____
_____

GB 28
WEIDAO

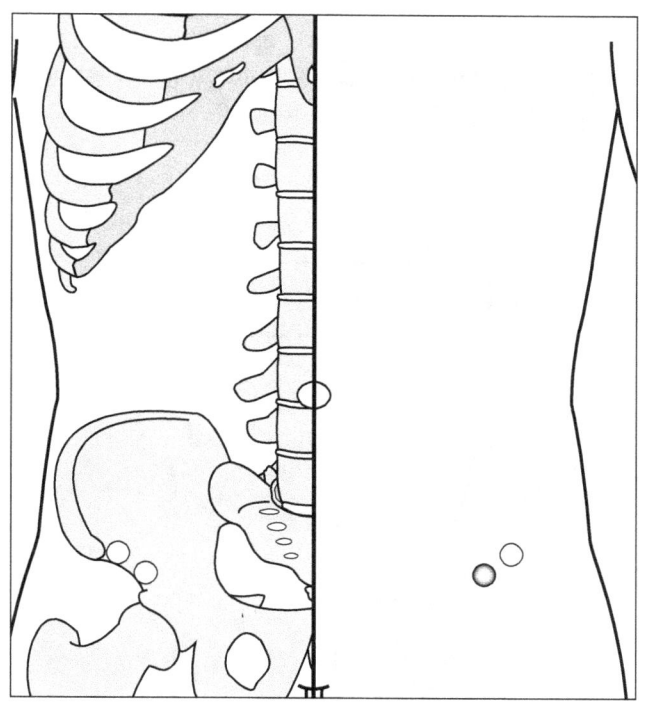

Location: On the lateral side of the abdomen, anterior and inferior to the ASIS, 0.5 cun anterior and inferior to GB-27 Wushu.

Functions: Regulates the Dai Mai Vessel, regulates the lower jiao.

Indications: Morbid leukorrhea, prolapse of the Uterus, abdominal pain, hernia.

Attributes: Meeting point of the Gall Bladder channel and the Dai Mai Vessel.

Notes

_____
_____
_____
_____
_____
_____
_____
_____
_____

Point Combinations

_____
_____
_____
_____
_____
_____
_____

GB 29
JULIAO

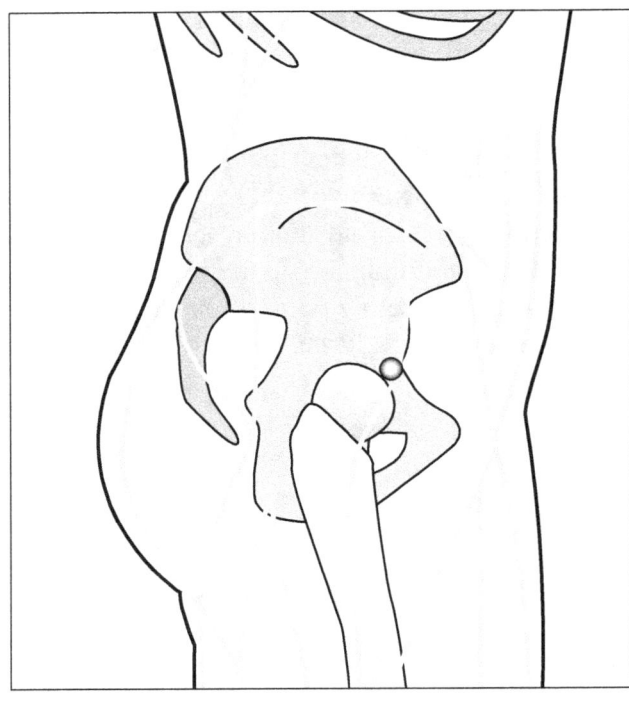

Location: On the lateral aspect of the hip, at the midpoint on the line connecting the greater trochanter of the femur and the ASIS.

Functions: Removes obstructions in the channel, activates the channel, benefits the lower extremities and hips, relieves pain.
Indications: Weakness, numbness and pain of the lower extremities, lumbar pain, difficulty in rotating the body.
Attributes: Meeting point of the Gall Bladder channel and the Yang Qiao Vessel.

Notes

Point Combinations

GB 30
HUANTIAO

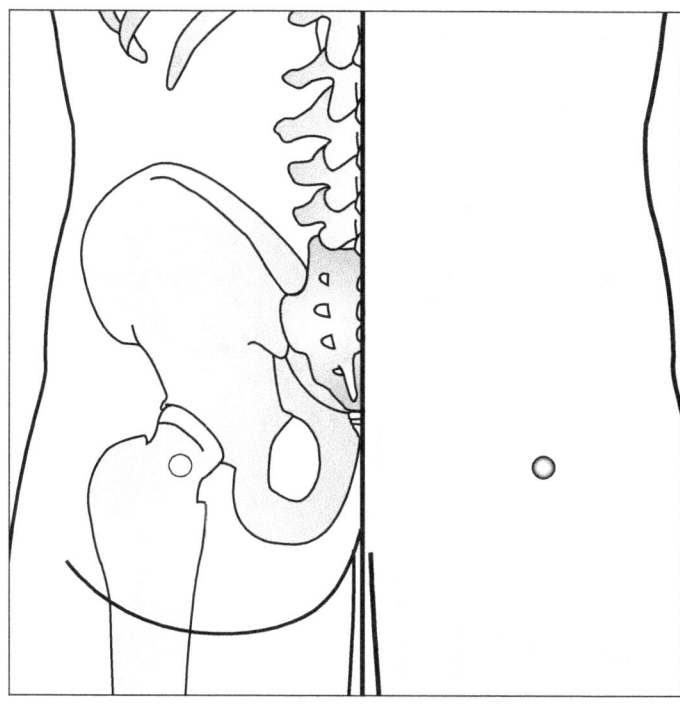

Location: On the lateral side of the buttocks, at the junction of the middle 1/3rd and lateral 1/3rd of the line connecting the prominence of the great trochanter and the sacral hiatus when the patient is in a lateral recumbent position with the thigh flexed.

Functions: Removes obstructions, activates the channel, benefits the lower extremities and hips, resolves wind-damp, relieves pain,
Indications: Pain of the lumbar and leg, sciatica, hemiplegia, weakness and pain of the lower extremities.
Attributes: Meeting point of the Gall Bladder and Urinary Bladder channel.

Notes
_____
_____
_____
_____
_____
_____
_____
_____

Point Combinations
_____
_____
_____
_____
_____
_____

GB 31
FENGSHI

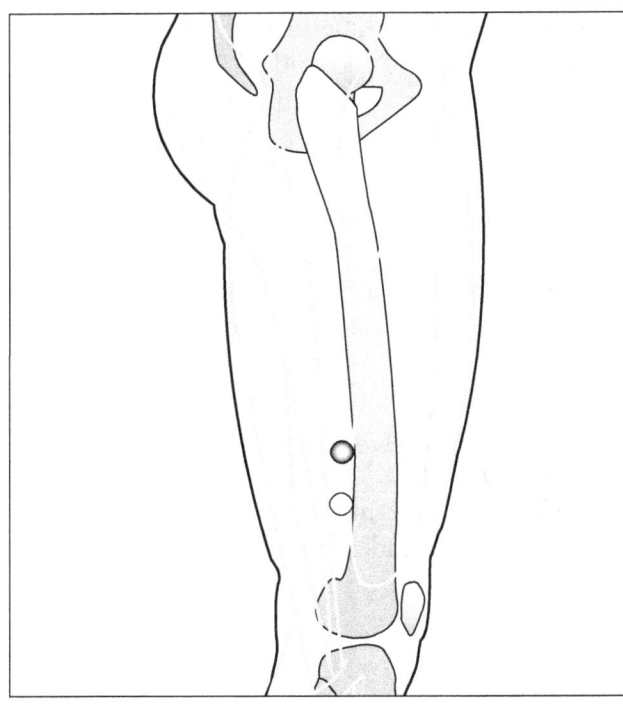

Location: On the lateral side of the thigh, directly below the greater trochanter, 7 cun above the transverse popliteal crease.

Functions: Extinguishes wind, relieves itching, relieves pain, activates the channel.

Indications: Weakness, beriberi, sudden deafness, general pruritis, numbness and pain of the lower extremities.

Attributes: Empirical point to treat itching.

Notes

Point Combinations

GB 32
ZHONGDU

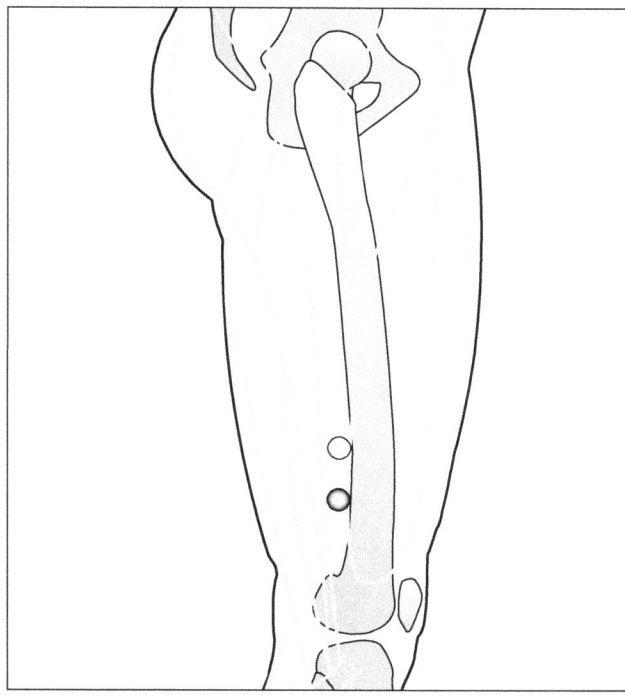

Location: On the lateral side of the thigh, directly below the greater trochanter, 5 cun above the transverse popliteal crease (2 cun below GB-31 Fengshi).

Functions: Activates the channel, relieves pain, resolves wind-damp and expels cold.
Indications: Pain, numbness and weakness of the lower extremities, hemiplegia.

Notes

Point Combinations

GB 33
XIYANGGUAN

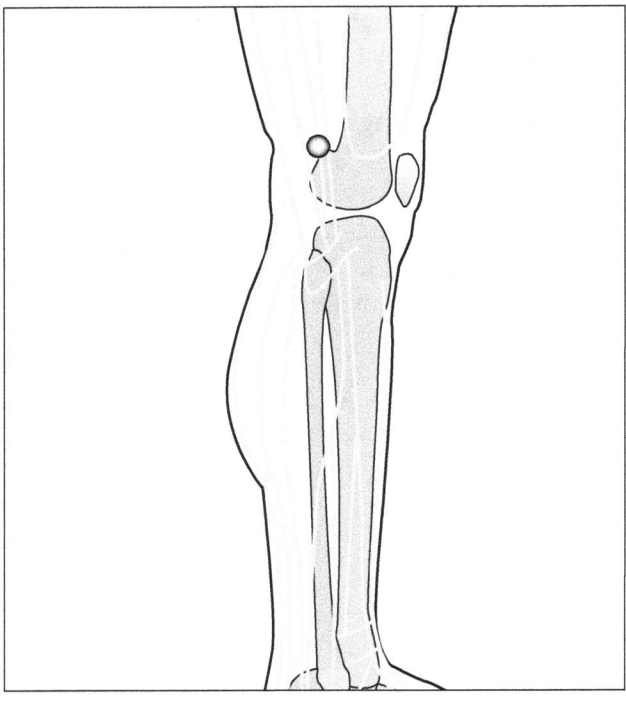

Location: On the lateral side of the knee, 3 cun above GB-34 Yanglingquan in the depression above the lateral epicondyle of the femur.

Functions: Activates the channel, relieves pain, resolves wind-damp.

Indications: Pain, numbness and swelling of the knees.

Notes
_____
_____
_____
_____
_____
_____
_____
_____

Point Combinations
_____
_____
_____
_____
_____
_____

GB 34
YANGLINGQUAN

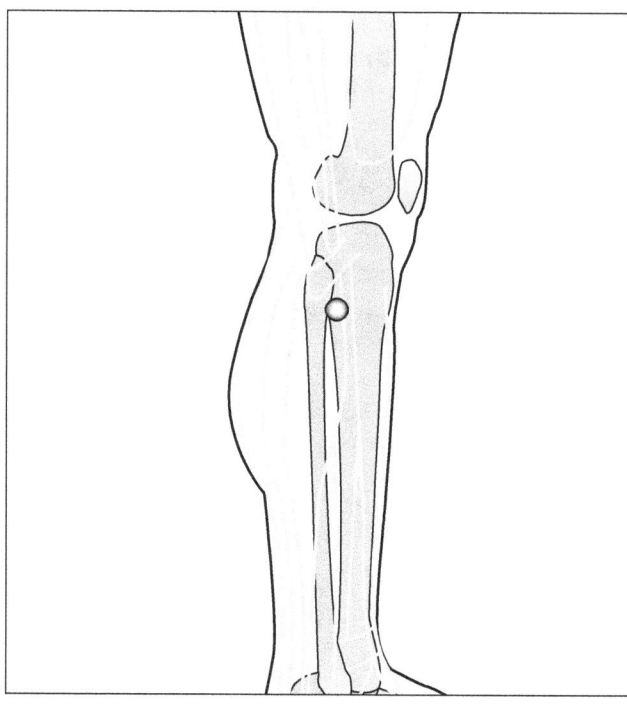

Location: On the lateral side of the leg, in the depression anterior and inferior to the head of the fibula.

Functions: Activates the channel, relieves pain, moves Liver Qi, harmonizes Shaoyang, benefits the joints and sinews.

Indications: Pain, weakness and numbness in the lower extremities, pain and distention of the hypochondrium, mania, pain and swelling of the knees, hemiplegia, disorders of the sinews (stiffness, contraction, tightness), bitter taste in the mouth, jaundice, malaria, chills and fever.

Attributes: Earth point, He-Sea point, Converging point of the Sinews.

Notes

Point Combinations

GB 35
YANGJIAO

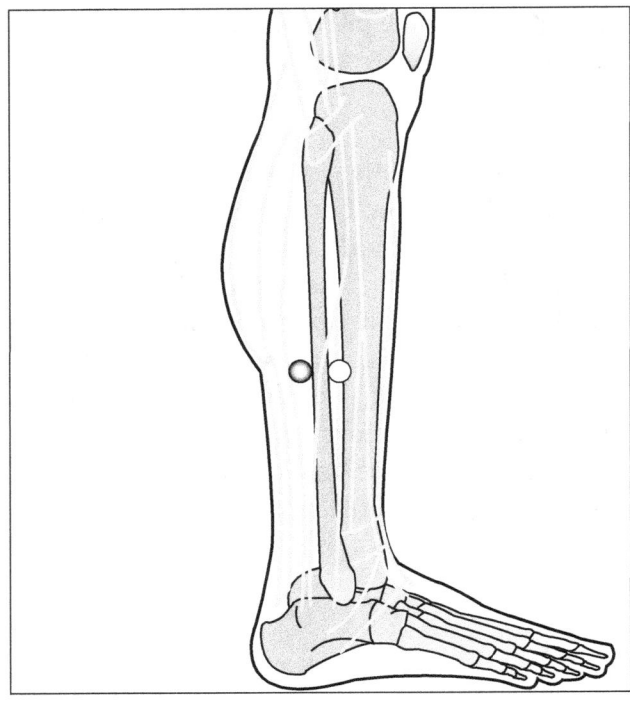

Location: On the lateral side of the leg, 7 cun above the tip of the external malleolus, on the posterior border of the fibula.

Functions: Activates the channel, relieves pain, relaxes sinews, calms shen.
Indications: Pain, weakness and numbness in the lower extremities, pain and distention of the hypochondrium, mania.
Attributes: Xi-Cleft point of the Yang Wei Vessel.

Notes

Point Combinations

GB 36
WaiQiu

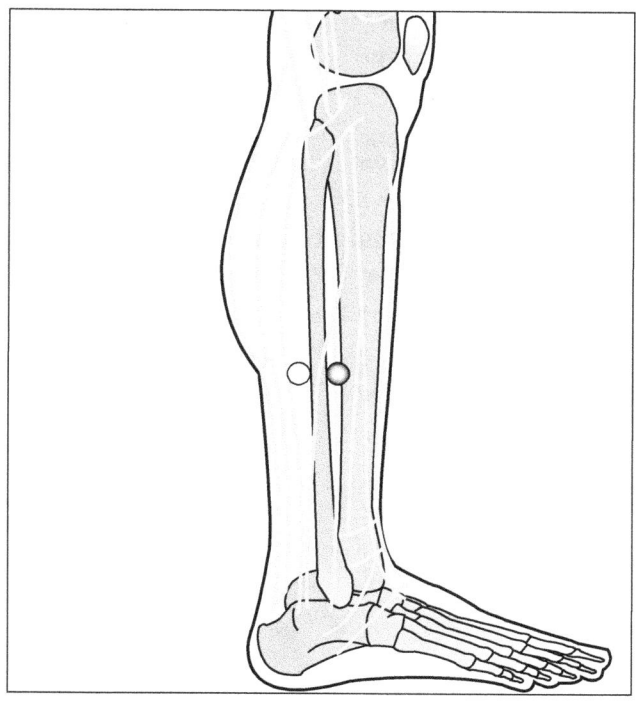

Location: On the lateral side of the leg, 7 cun above the tip of the external malleolus, on the anterior border of the fibula.

Functions: Activates the channel, relieves pain, clears heat, relaxes sinews.

Indications: Pain, weakness and numbness in the lower extremities, neck pain, pain and distention of the hypochondrium.

Attributes: Xi-Cleft point.

Notes

Point Combinations

GB 37
GUANGMING

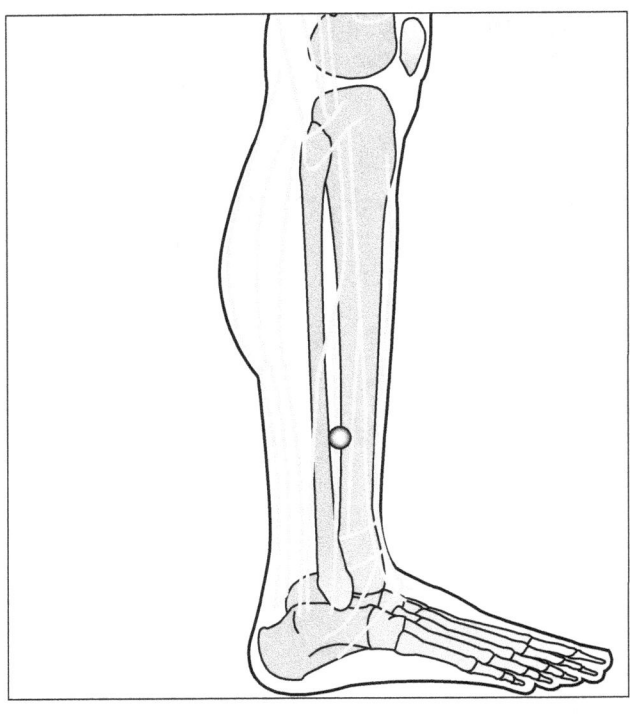

Location: On the lateral side of the leg, 5 cun above the tip of the external malleolus, on the posterior border of the fibula.

Functions: Activates the channel, benefits the eyes, extinguishes wind.

Indications: Pain, weakness and numbness in the lower extremities, knee pain, eye pain, night blindness, headache, pain and distention of the breast.

Attributes: Luo-Connecting point.

Notes

Point Combinations

GB 38
YANGFU

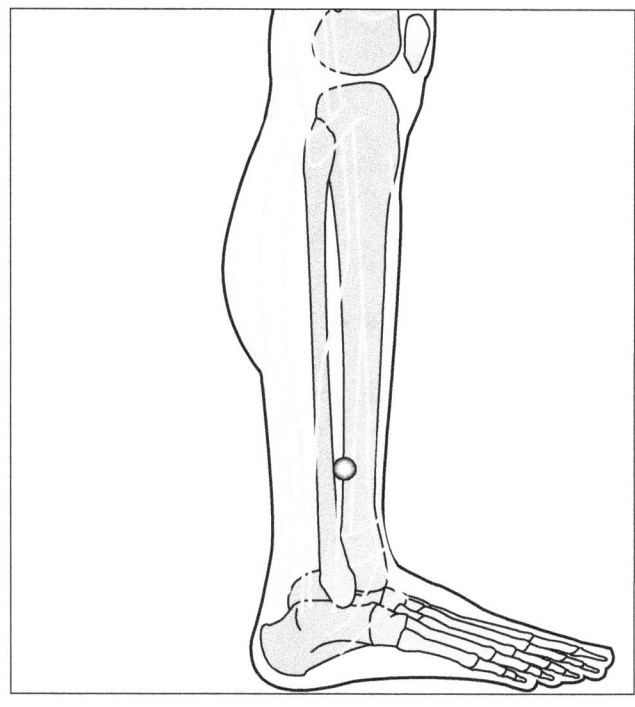

Location: On the lateral side of the leg, 4 cun above the tip of the external malleolus, slightly anterior to the anterior border of the fibula.

Functions: Activates the channel, relieves pain, clears heat, benefits the sinews and bones, harmonizes Shaoyang.

Indications: Headache, pain in the outer canthus, pain and swelling in the hypochondrium and axillary region, pain, weakness and numbness in the lower extremities, scrofula, malaria, hemiplegia,

Attributes: Fire point, Jing River point.

Notes

Point Combinations

GB 39
XUANZHONG

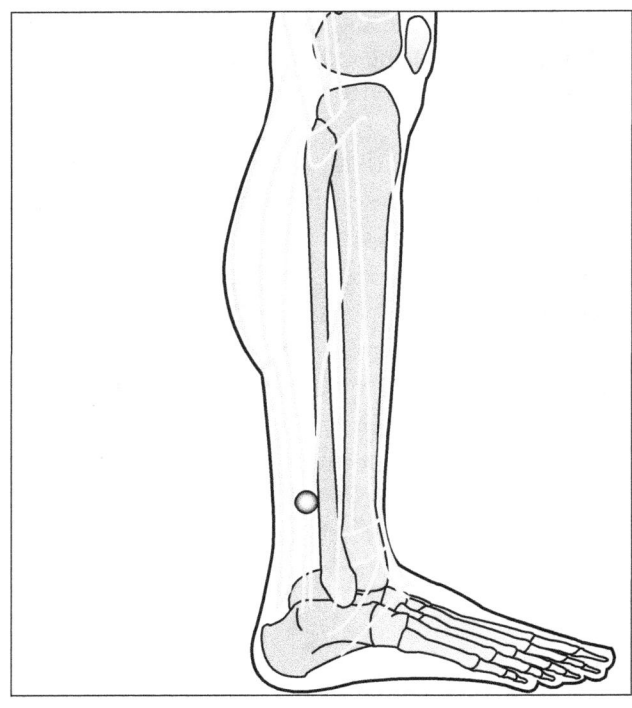

Location: On the lateral side of the leg, 3 cun above the tip of the external malleolus, on the anterior border of the fibula.

Functions: Activates the channel, relieves pain, benefits the sinews, bones and neck, nourishes marrow, resolves wind-damp, clears fire in the channel.

Indications: Pain and stiffness in the neck, pain in the hypchondrium, pain and numbness in the lower extremities, hemiplegia.

Attributes: Converging point of Marrow.

Notes

Point Combinations

GB 40
QIUXU

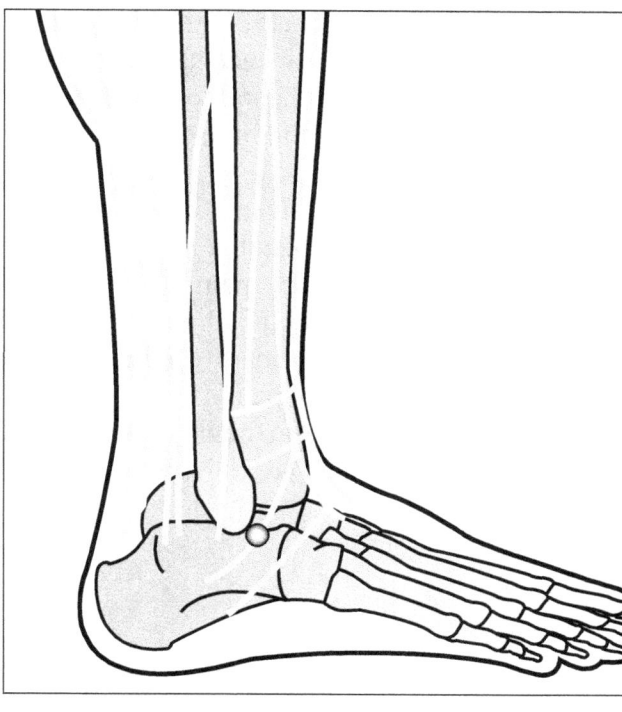

Location: On the lateral side of the leg, anterior and inferior to the external malleolus, in the depression lateral to the tendon of the long extensor muscle of the toes.

Functions: Moves Liver Qi, benefits the hypochondrium and eyes, regulates the Dai Mai Vessel.

Indications: Headache, pain and swelling of the eye, pain in the hypchondrium, breast distention, scrofula, pain in the hip and lower leg, pain and swelling of the feet and toes, irregular menstruation.

Attributes: Yuan-Source point.

Notes

_____
_____
_____
_____
_____
_____
_____
_____
_____

Point Combinations

_____
_____
_____
_____
_____
_____
_____

GB 41
ZULINQI

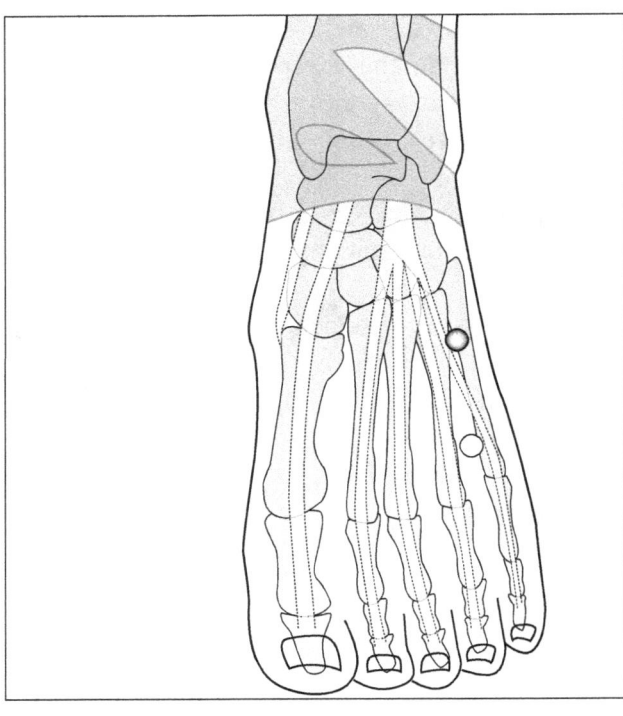

Location: On the lateral side of the instep of the foot, posterior to the 4th metatarsophalangeal joint, in the depression lateral to the tendon of the extensor muscle of the little toe.

Functions: Moves Liver Qi, activates the channel, relieves pain, benefits joints.

Indications: Headache, pain and swelling of the eye, pain in the hypochondrium, pain, swelling and numbness of the external malleolus, malaria, neck pain.

Attributes: Shu Stream point, Wood point, Confluent point of the Dai Mai Vessel.

Notes

_____
_____
_____
_____
_____
_____
_____
_____

Point Combinations

_____
_____
_____
_____
_____
_____

GB 42
DIWUHUI

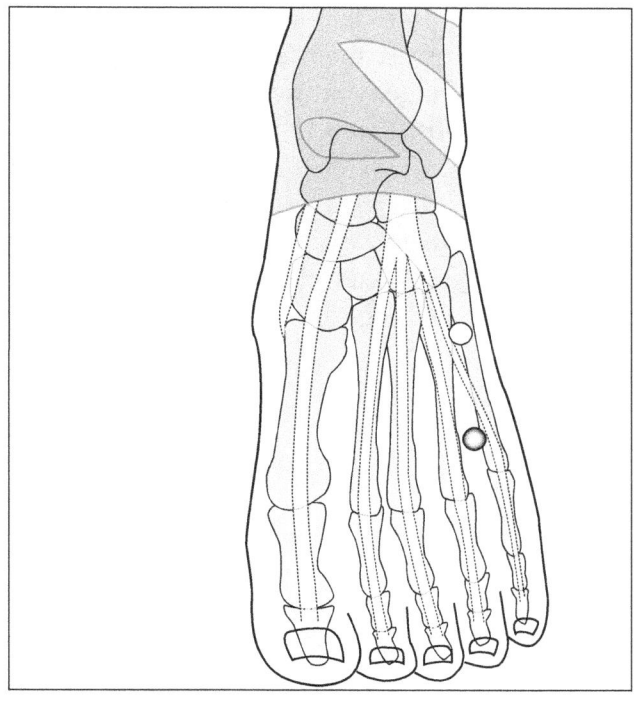

Location: On the lateral side of the instep of the foot, posterior to the 4th metatarsophalangeal joint, between the 4th and 5th toes, on the medial side of the tendon of the extensor digiti minimi muscle.

Functions: Clears heat in the channel, moves Liver Qi.

Indications: Headache, tinnitus, deafness, pain and swelling of the eye, pain in the hypochondrium, pain and swelling of the dorsum of the foot.

Notes

Point Combinations

GB 43
XIAXI

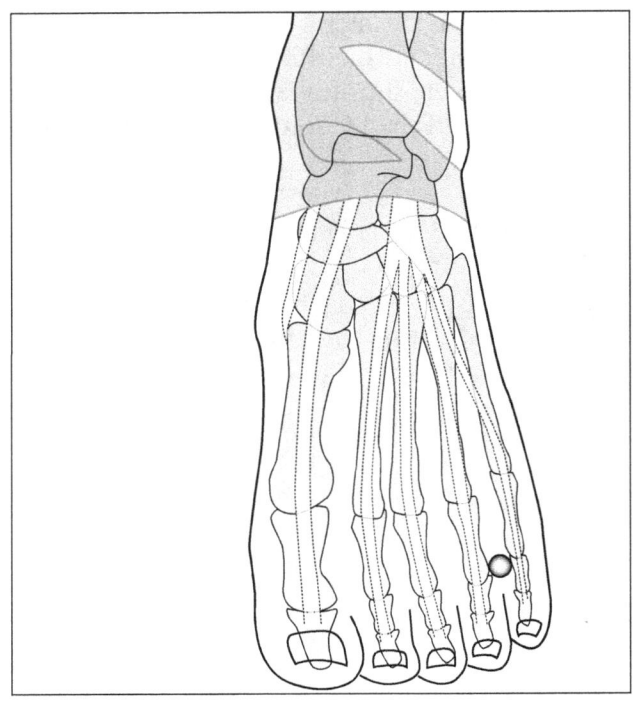

Location: On the lateral side of the instep of the foot, between the 4th and 5th toes, at the junction of the red and white skin, proximal to the margin of the web.

Functions: Clears heat, calms shen, benefits the eyes and head,

Indications: Headache, tinnitus, deafness, pain and swelling of the eye, pain in the hypochondrium.

Attributes: Water point, Ying Spring point.

Notes

_____

_____

_____

_____

_____

_____

_____

_____

Point Combinations

_____

_____

_____

_____

_____

_____

GB 44
ZuQIAOYIN

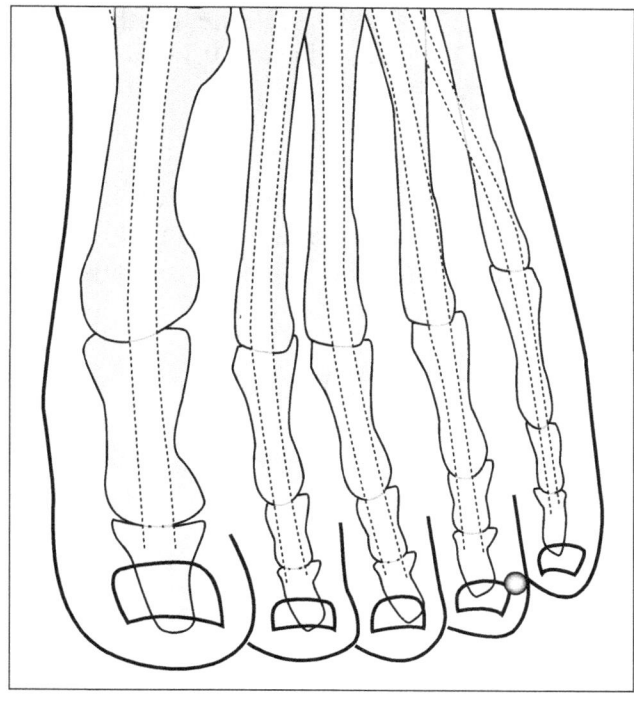

Location: On the lateral side of the distal segment of the 4th toe, 0.1 cun from the corner of the nail.

Functions: Clears heat, benefits the eyes, ears and head, resolves damp-heat in the channel

Indications: Headache, tinnitus, deafness, pain and swelling of the eye, pain in the hypochondrium, nightmares and insomnia.

Attributes: Metal point, Jing Well point.

Notes

_____

_____

_____

_____

_____

_____

_____

_____

Point Combinations

_____

_____

_____

_____

_____

_____

LV 1
DADUN

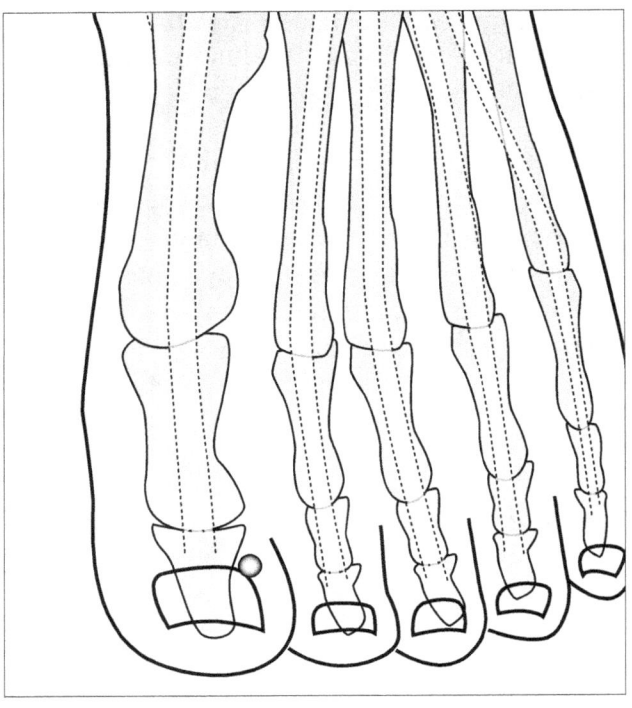

Location: On the lateral side of the distal segment of the great (big) toe, 0.1 cun from the corner of the nail.

Functions: Manages Qi in lower jiao, relieves pain, moves Liver Qi, stops menstrual bleeding (with moxa), nourishes menstrual blood, assists the Kidneys, Spleen, genitals and regulates urination, calms shen and revives consciousness.

Indications: Irregular menstruation, abnormal uterine bleeding, urinary incontinence, hematuria, pain from hernia, swelling or retraction of the genitals, uterine prolapse, loss of consciousness, epilepsy.

Attributes: Wood point, Jing Well point.

Notes

_____
_____
_____
_____
_____
_____
_____
_____

Point Combinations

_____
_____
_____
_____
_____
_____
_____

LV 2
XINGJIAN

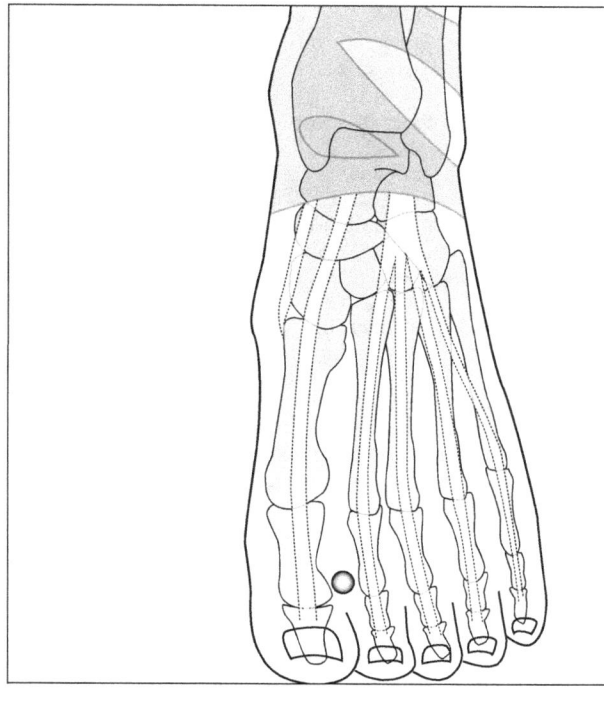

Location: On the instep of the foot, between the 1st and 2nd toes, at the junction of the red and white skin proximal to the margin of the web.

Functions: Courses Qi and blood, drains Liver fire, cools blood, clears heat, extinguishes wind, and stops bleeding, assists lower jiao.

Indications: Headache, dizziness, vertigo, seizures, diseases and symptoms of the eye, nosebleeds, dry or sore throat, hemoptysis, chest distention, lumbar pain, colic, infantile convulsions, night sweats, insomnia, anger, sadness, shingles, intercostal neuralgia, lower abdominal distention, hernia, genital pain, abnormal uterine bleeding, cloudy urine.

Attributes: Fire point, Ying Spring point.
*Good point for muscle cramps and spasms.
**Main point for hypertensive headache (or headache from Liver fire, stagnant menstrual blood.
***Caution during pregnancy.

Notes
_____
_____
_____
_____
_____
_____
_____
_____
_____

Point Combinations
_____
_____
_____
_____
_____
_____
_____

LV 3
TAICHONG

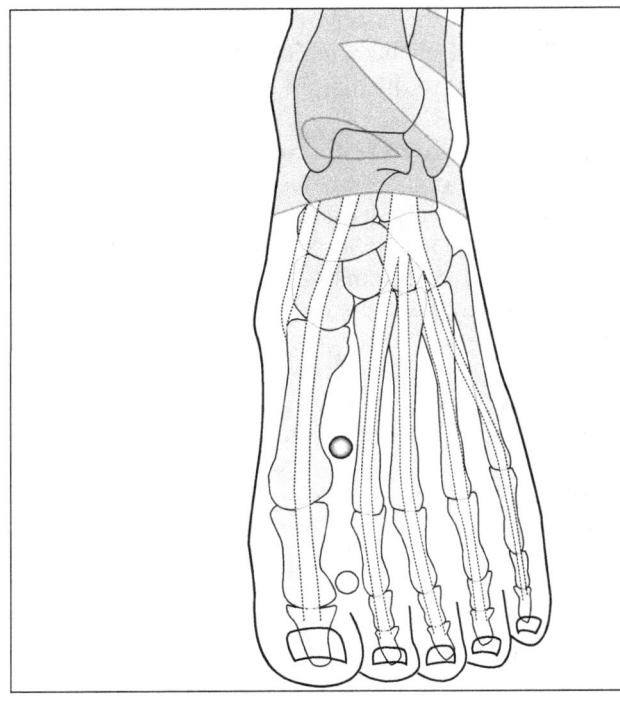

Location: On the instep of the foot, in between the 1st and 2nd toes, in the depression on the posterior end of the 1st interosseous metatarsal space.

Functions: Removes blockages from the channel, opens the head and eyes, sedates the Liver, supports Liver yin and blood, nourishes Qi, blood, yin and courses Liver Qi, anchors Liver yang, clears Liver heat, blood heat and extinguishes wind, resolves damp-heat in Liver and Gall Bladder, promotes lactation, supports vision, manages Qi, menstruation and the lower jiao, relieves pain, calms the fetus.

Indications: Headache, dizziness, vertigo, eye pain, blurred vision, cracked or swollen lips, sore throat, deviation of the mouth, swelling of the axillary area, swelling, pain or abscess of the breast, distention or pain in the chest, lateral costal region or abdomen, low back pain, cold sensations in the lower extremities, jaundice, hepatitis, nausea, vomiting of blood, constipation, dysentery, diarrhea with undigested food or blood, urinary retention, seminal emission, low sperm count, menstrual irregularities, uterine prolapse, Insomnia, seizures, epilepsy, sighing.

Attributes: Earth point, Shu Stream point, Yuan-Source point, Heavenly Star point.

* Good point for cirrhosis, muscle cramps and visual disturbances.

**Main point for headache, vertigo and detoxification.

***Caution during pregnancy.

Notes

_____

_____

_____

_____

_____

_____

_____

_____

Point Combinations

_____

_____

_____

_____

_____

_____

LV 4
ZHONGFENG

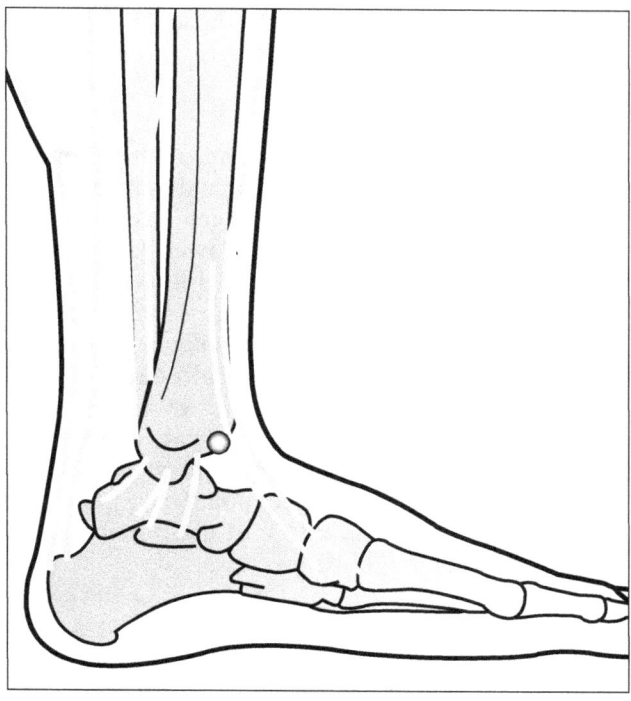

Location: On the medial side of the foot, at the midpoint along the line connecting SP-5 ShangQiu and ST-41 Jiexi in the depression on the medial side of the tendon of the tibialis anterior muscle.

Functions: Removes blockages from the channel, resolves damp-heat in the Liver and Gall Bladder, disperses Liver Qi, clears heat clears fire, resolves damp.

Indications: Colic, goiter, malaria, pain, swelling or issues of the ankle, foot, and local areas including the knees, urinary difficulty or retention, genital pain or retraction, seminal or nocturnal emission, low back pain, hepatitis, jaundice, hernia, lower abdominal pain, nocturnal emissions.

Attributes: Metal point, Jing River point.
*Good point for hepatitis.
**Main point for urinary retention.

Notes

Point Combinations

LV 5
LIGOU

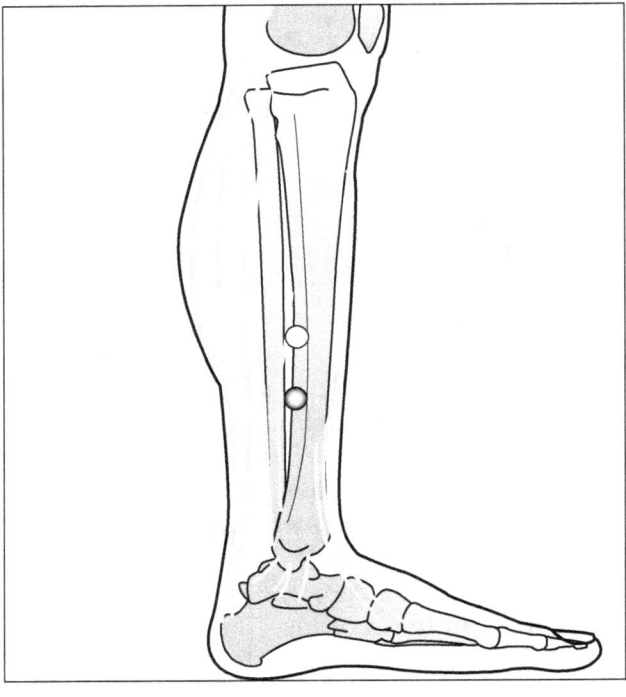

Location: On the medial side of the leg, 5 cun above the tip of the medial malleolus, on the midline of the medial surface of the tibia.

Functions: Removes blockages from the channel, disperses Liver Qi, manages and supports Qi, Liver yin, Liver blood, and genitals, manages menstruation, resolves damp in lower jiao.

Indications: Low back pain and difficulty turning, hernia, urinary retention or difficulty, swelling, pain, and itchiness of the genitals, impotence and sexual dysfunction, abnormal uterine bleeding, vaginal discharge, menstrual irregularities or pain, uterine prolapse, pain and coldness of the lower extremities, fear, fright, palpitations, worry, depression.

Attributes: Luo-Connecting point.

*Good point for plum pit Qi of the throat, genital herpes and itching of the genitals.

Notes
_____
_____
_____
_____
_____
_____
_____
_____

Point Combinations
_____
_____
_____
_____
_____
_____
_____

LV 6
ZHONGDU

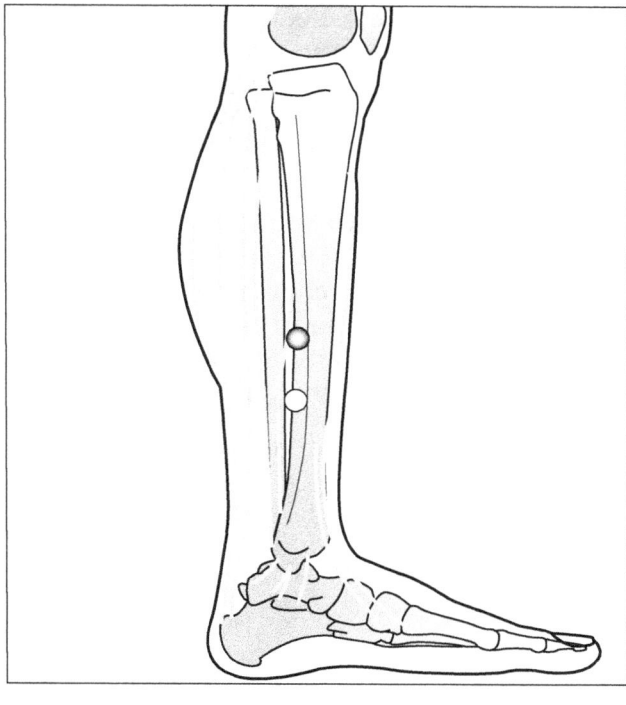

Location: On the medial side of the leg, 7 cun above the tip of the medial malleolus, on the midline of the medial surface of the tibia.

Functions: Removes blockages from the channel, courses Liver Qi, stimulates the connecting vessel, tendons and ligaments, calms muscles and tendons, manages Qi and blood, the manages the lower jiao, Qi and blood, resolves damp, extinguishes wind-cold, resolves damp-heat, relieves pain.

Indications: Acute hepatitis, numbness of the hands, pain of the lower abdomen, diarrhea, abnormal uterine bleeding, damp Bi syndrome, cold sensations, numbness, or muscular atrophy of lower extremities, weakness of the legs, hot sensation of the feet.

Attributes: Xi-Cleft point.

* Upon palpation, this point will be tender on patients with hepatitis.

Notes

_____
_____
_____
_____
_____
_____
_____
_____

Point Combinations

_____
_____
_____
_____
_____
_____

LV 7
XIGUAN

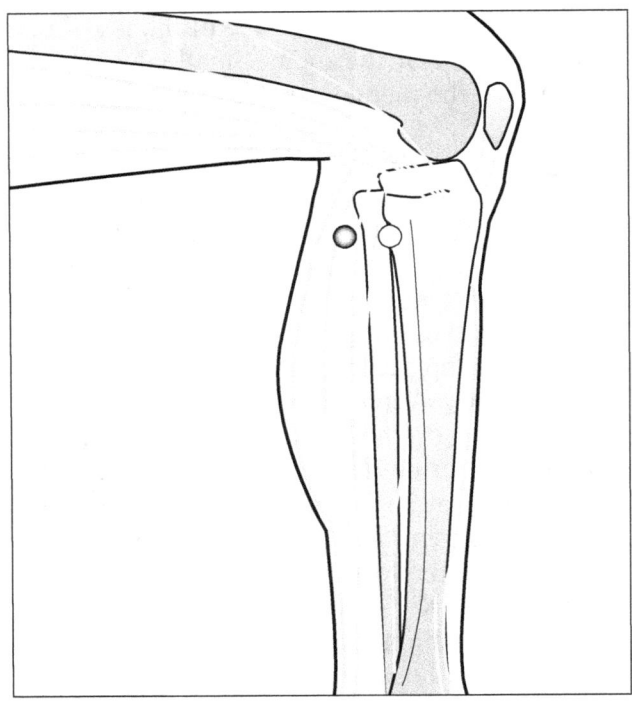

Location: On the medial side of the leg, posterior and inferior to the medial condyle of the tibia, in the upper portion of the medial head of the gastrocnemius muscle, 1 cun posterior to SP-9 Yinlingquan.

Functions: Removes blockages from the channel, calms muscles and tendons, assists the knees and joints, relieves pain, extinguishes wind and resolves damp.

Indications: Headache, throat and abdominal pain, welling, pain, and arthritis of the knee.

Notes
_____
_____
_____
_____
_____
_____
_____
_____

Point Combinations
_____
_____
_____
_____
_____
_____

LV 8
QUQUAN

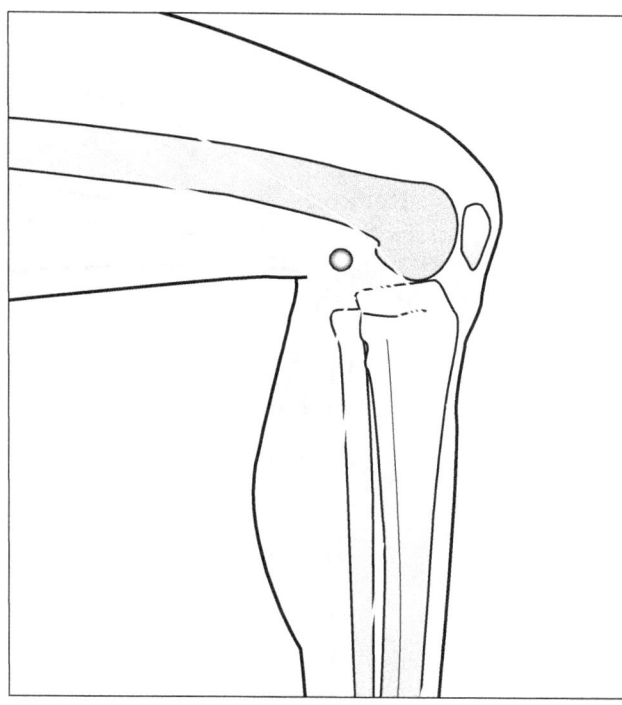

Location: On the medial end of the transverse popliteal crease, posterior to the medial epicondyle of the tibia, in a depression on the anterior border of the insertions of the tendons of the semimembranosus muscle and semitendinosus muscle, with the knee flexed.

Functions: Supports the bladder, cools and resolves damp-heat in lower jiao and Liver fire, supports the genitals and the uterus, manages and supports Yin, Liver Qi and blood, manages menses and courses blood, supports the knees, relieves pain in the Liver channel channel, calms muscles and tendons.

Indications: Headache, dizziness, pain and swelling of the eyes, nosebleed, lateral costal and abdominal pain and swelling, abdominal masses, diarrhea containing blood, puss or undigested food, nephritis, hernia, swelling, itching and pain of the genitals, urinary difficulty or retention, impotence, infertility, amenorrhea, uterine prolapse, pain and coldness of the knee and lower leg.

Attributes: Water point, He-Sea point.

*Good point for genital herpes and vaginitis.

**Main point for prostatitis or blood in the stools.

Notes

_____
_____
_____
_____
_____
_____
_____
_____

Point Combinations

_____
_____
_____
_____
_____
_____
_____

LV 9
YINBAO

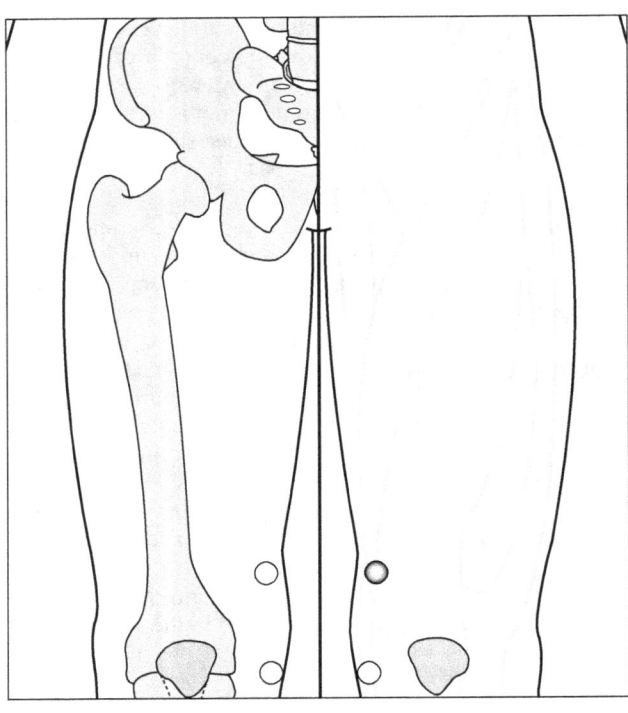

Location: On the medial side of the thigh, 4 cun above the medial epicondyle of the femur, between the vastus medialis muscle and sartorius muscle.

Functions: Removes blockages from the channel, courses Liver Qi, supports the Liver and Kidneys, cools and resolves damp-heat in the lower jiao, regulates menses, promotes interaction with Penetrating and Ren channels.

Indications: Lower back and abdominal pain, enuresis, retention of urine, irregular menstruation.

Notes

Point Combinations

LV 10
ZUWULI

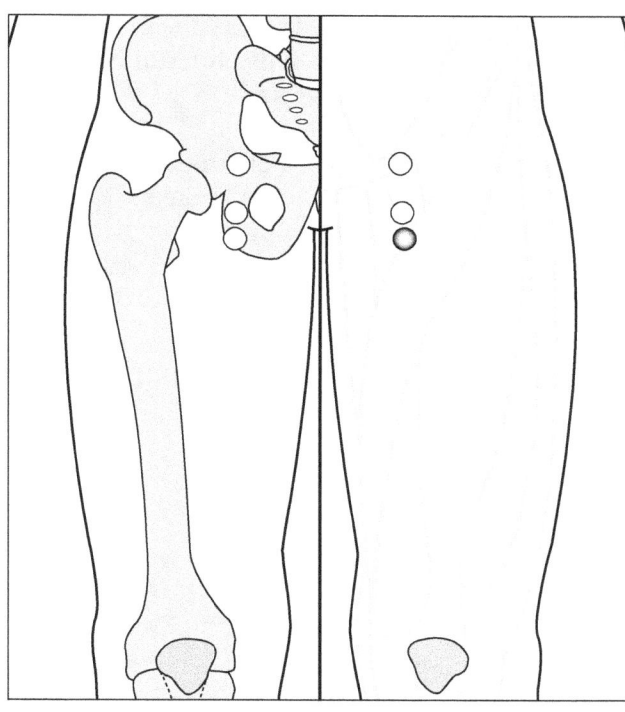

Location: On the medial side of the thigh, 3 cun below ST-30 Qichong, on the anterior border of the adductor longus muscle.

Functions: Removes blockages from the channel, relaxes muscles and tendons, resolves damp-heat and supports the Kidneys and lower jiao.

Indications: Lassitude, labored breathing, cough, abdominal distention and fullness, swelling, pain, and itchiness of the genitals, incontinence, enuresis, urinary difficulty and retention, local pain.

Notes

Point Combinations

LV 11
YINLIAN

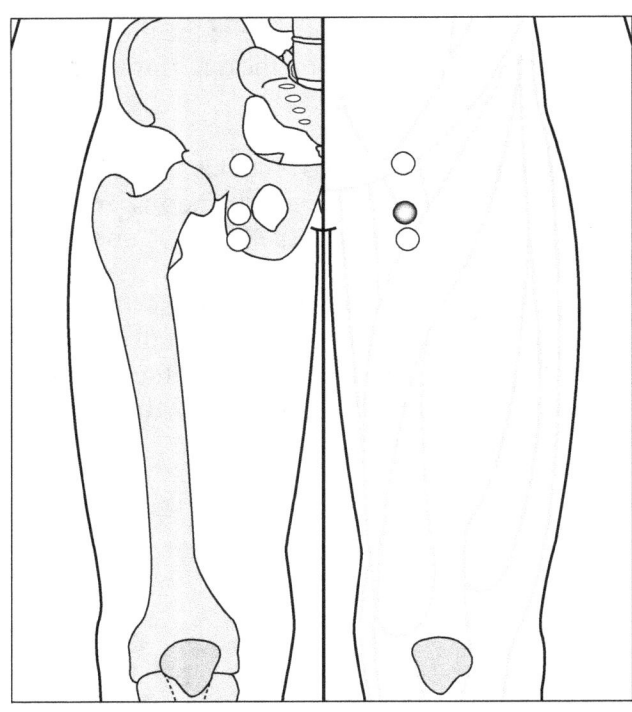

Location: On the medial side of the thigh, 2 cun below ST-30 Qichong, on the anterior border of the adductor longus muscle.

Functions: Manages Penetrating and Ren channels, assists the uterus, relaxes muscles and tendons, stimulates blood circulation.
Indications: Hernia, pain of knee and thigh, infertility, irregular menstruation.
*Good point for sterility.

Notes _____

_____

_____

_____

_____

_____

_____

_____

_____

Point Combinations _____

_____

_____

_____

_____

_____

_____

LV 12
JIMAI

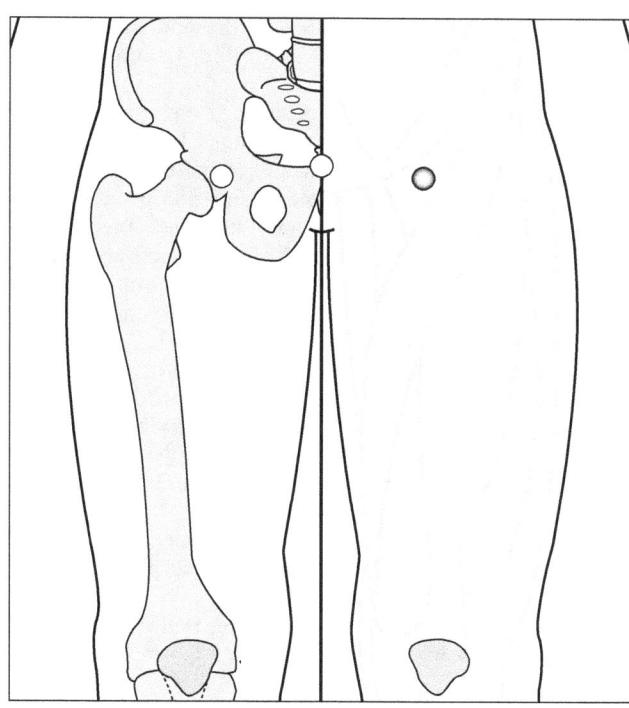

Location: On the lateral side of the pubic tubercle, lateral and inferior to ST 30 Qichong in the inguinal groove where the femoral artery is palpable, 2.5 cun lateral to the anterior midline.

Functions: Removes blockages from the channel, manages Qi, supports the lower jiao, expels cold from Liver channel.

Indications: Hypogastric pain, hernia, inner thigh pain, uterine prolapse, pain or swelling of the penis or testicles.

Notes
_____
_____
_____
_____
_____
_____
_____
_____
_____

Point Combinations
_____
_____
_____
_____
_____
_____
_____

LV 13
ZHANGMEN

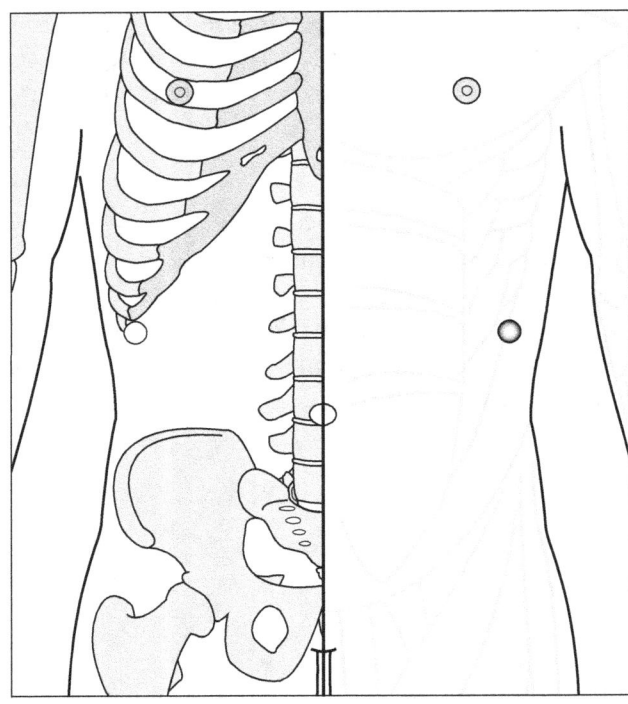

Location: On the lateral side of the abdomen, on the lower border of the free end of the 11th floating rib.

Functions: Removes blockages from the channel, courses Liver Qi and blood, manages Liver Qi, blood, and yin, resolves damp-heat and transforms phlegm in the Liver, Gall Bladder, Spleen and Stomach, reduces hard masses, manages organs, manages the middle and lower jiao, stimulates Spleen, Stomach and blood, supports Spleen in transformation and transportation functions, expels cold in the yin organs, balances Liver and Spleen interactions.

Indications: Epilepsy, labored breathing or shortness of breath, cough, fullness of the chest, chest distention or presence of lumps in the chest, chest or rib pain, weak or cold extremities, enlarged Liver or Spleen, vomiting, running piglet syndrome, enteritis, jaundice, hepatitis, lower back pain, diarrhea, cloudy urine.

Attributes: Front Mu point of the Spleen, Influential point for all Zang (Yin) Organs, meeting point of Liver and Gall Bladder channels.

*Good point for exhaustion, fatigue, malabsorption, or diseases of the yin organs.

Notes _____

_____

_____

_____

_____

_____

_____

_____

Point Combinations _____

_____

_____

_____

_____

_____

_____

LV 14
QIMEN

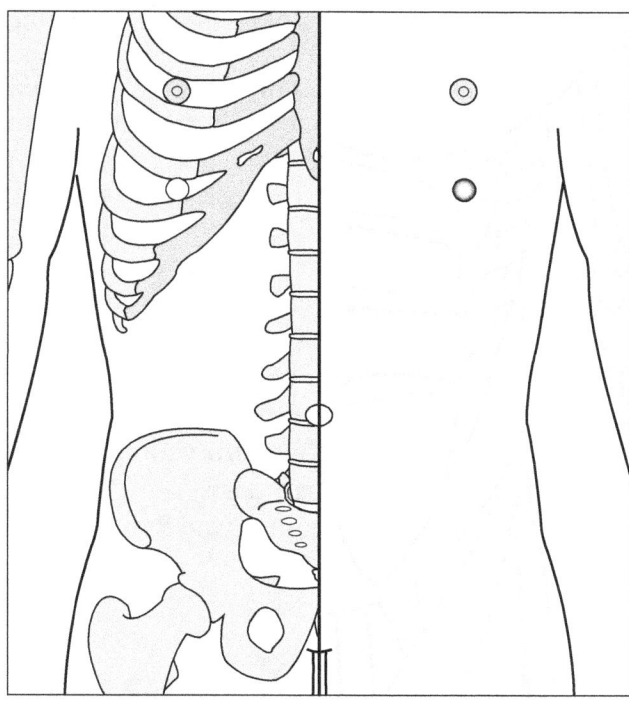

Location: On the chest, directly below the nipple, in the 6th intercostal space, 4 cun lateral to the anterior midline.

Functions: Removes blockages from the channel, courses Liver Qi, supports Spleen and Stomach, manages Gall Bladder Qi and resolves Liver, Gall Bladder damp-heat, balances Liver and Stomach, courses blood, softens masses, opens the chest and promotes lactation.

Indications: Head and neck pain and stiffness, dizziness, pain, distention, and fullness of the chest and abdomen, pleurisy, cough, dyspnea, vomiting and hiccup, sharp pain of the Heart, intercostal neuralgia, acid regurgitation, watery diarrhea, alternating chills and fever, tidal fever, red face, hepatitis, malaria, jaundice, gallstones, "running piglet Qi", enlarged Liver of Spleen or Gall Bladder, abnormal uterine bleeding, failure to discharge the placenta and post-partum disorders, sighing.

Attributes: Front Mu point of the Liver, meeting point of Liver, Spleen and Yin Wei (linking) channels.

*Main point for shingles and intercostal neuralgia.

Notes

Point Combinations

CV 1
HUIYIN

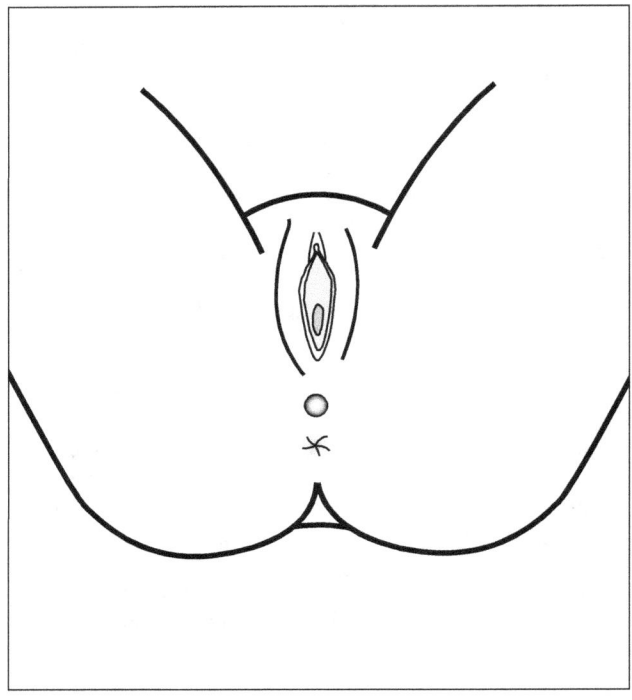

Location: On the center of the perineum, at the midpoint between the root of the scrotum and the anus in males, and at the midpoint between the posterior labial commissure and the anus in females.

Functions: Nourishes Kidney yin, resuscitates, treats prolapse, resolves damp-heat.

Indications: Constipation and dysuria, or incontinence of feces and urine, amenorrhea, irregular menstruation, hemorrhoids, prolapse of rectum, spermatorrhea, impotence, pruritus vulva, asphyxiation from drowning, loss of consciousness, manic psychosis.

Attributes: Meeting point of the Ren, DU and Penetrating channels.

Notes

Point Combinations

CV 2
QUGU

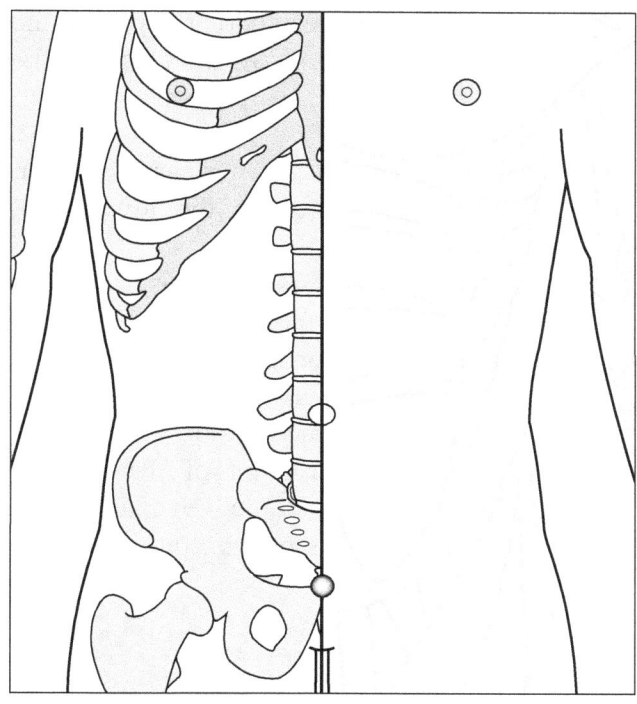

Location: On the lower abdomen and on the anterior midline, 5 cun below the umbilicus, at the midpoint of the upper boarder of the pubic symphysis.

Functions: Regulates the lower jiao, clears heat, resolves damp, tonifies the Kidneys, regulates menstruation.

Indications: Dysuria, enuresis, frequent urination, genital pain (itching, redness, dampness, pain) spermatorrhea, impotence, irregular menstruation, leukorrhea.

Attributes: Meeting point of the Ren and Liver channels.

Notes

_____
_____
_____
_____
_____
_____
_____
_____
_____

Point Combinations

_____
_____
_____
_____
_____
_____
_____

CV 3
ZHONGJI

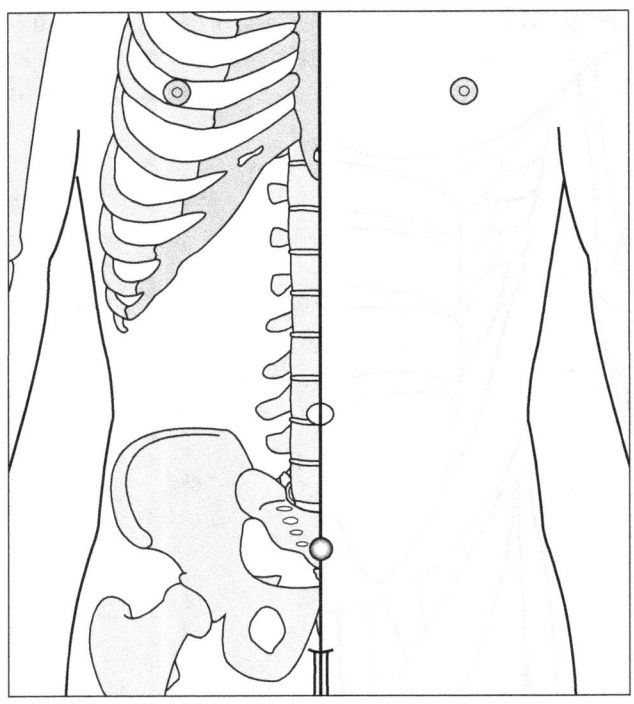

Location: On the lower abdomen and on the anterior midline, 4 cun below the center of the umbilicus.

Functions: Benefits the Urinary Bladder, benefits urination, regulates the lower jiao, resolves damp-heat.

Indications: Enuresis, dysuria, cystitis, spermatorrhea, impotence, irregular menstruation, metrorrhagia, leukorrhea, prolapse of the uterus, infertility, hernia, fibroids, running piglet syndrome.

Attribues: Front-Mu point of the Urinary Bladder, Meeting point of the Ren channel and the Three Yin channels of the Foot - (Spleen, Liver and Kidney).

Notes

Point Combinations

CV 4
GUANYUAN

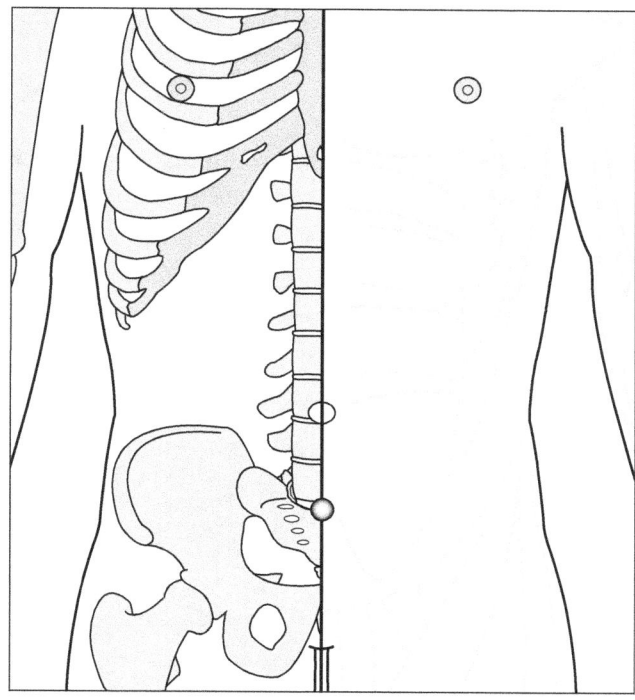

Location: On the lower abdomen and on the anterior midline, 3 cun below the center of the umbilicus.

Functions: Strengthens, nourishes the Kidneys (Qi, yin and yang), nourishes essence, benefits original Qi, calms shen, benefits menstruation and the uterus.

Indications: Impotence, spermatorrhea, enuresis, frequent micturition, retention of urine, irregular menstruation, metrorrhagia, morbid leukorrhea, dysmenorrhea, prolapse of the uterus, infertility, postpartum hemorrhage, flaccidity of apoplexy, emaciation due to consumptive disease, chronic fatigue, diarrhea, prolapse of rectum, dyspepsia, low back pain, shortness of breath.

Attributes: Front-Mu point of the Small Intestine, Meeting point of the Ren channel and the Three Yin channels of the Foot - (Spleen, Liver and Kidney).

Notes

Point Combinations

CV 5
SHIMEN

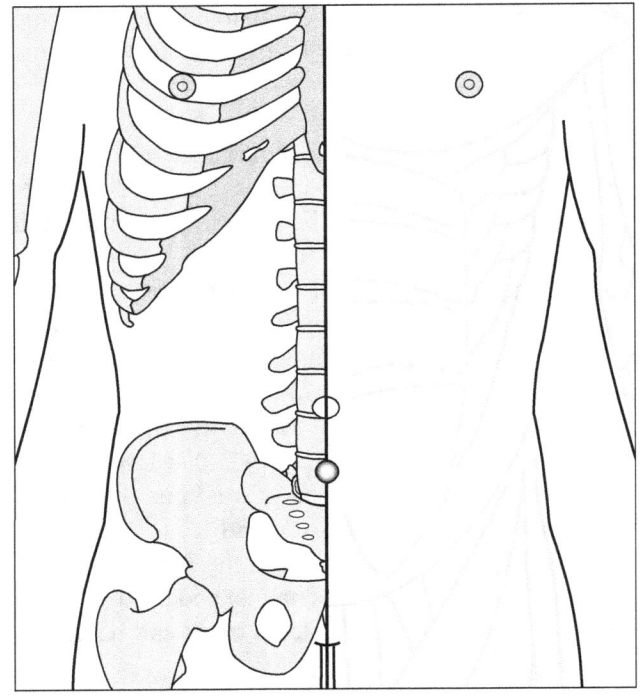

Location: On the lower abdomen and on the anterior midline, 2 cun below the center of the umbilicus.

Functions: Opens and regulates the water passages, promotes the function of the San Jiao, regulates Qi.

Indications: Dysuria, edema, hernia, abdominal pain, diarrhea, amenorrhea, morbid leukorrhea, metrorrhagia, undigested food in the stool, poor appetite, urinary tract disorder.

Attributes: Front-Mu point of the San Jiao.

Notes _____

_____

_____

_____

_____

_____

_____

_____

Point Combinations _____

_____

_____

_____

_____

_____

CV 6
QIHAI

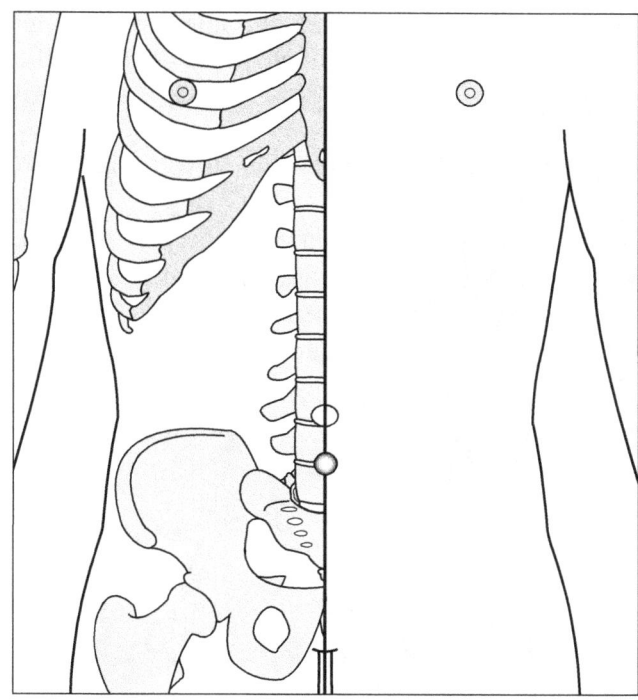

Location: On the lower abdomen and on the anterior midline, 1.5 cun below the center of the umbilicus.

Functions: Strengthens Kidney Qi and yang, regulates Qi, benefits original Qi, treats prolapse.

Indications: Abdominal pain, diarrhea, constipation, enuresis, hernia, spermatorrhea, impotence, irregular menstruation, uterine bleeding, leukorrhea, amenorrhea, emaciation due to consumptive disease, prolapse of any type, genital swelling, stroke, loss of consciousness, weakness of the muscles, asthma, shortness of breath, general fatigue.

Notes

_____

_____

_____

_____

_____

_____

_____

_____

Point Combinations

_____

_____

_____

_____

_____

_____

CV 7
YINJIAO

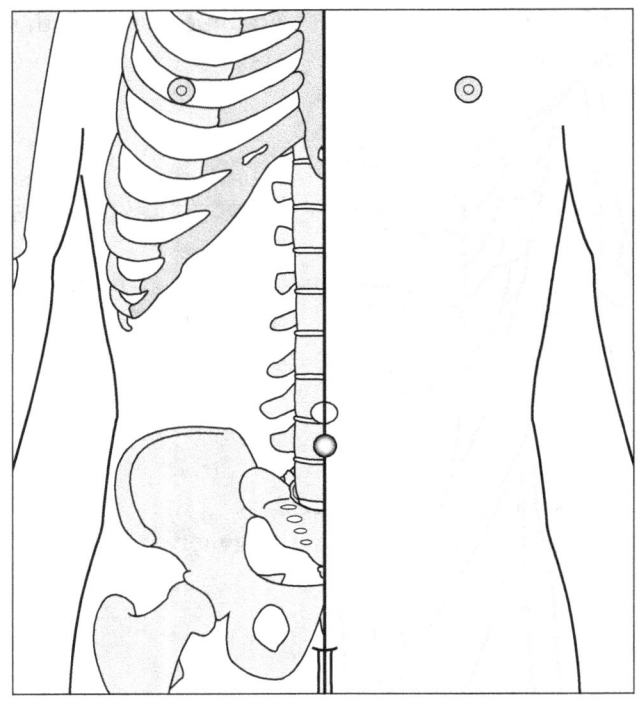

Location: On the lower abdomen and on the anterior midline, 1 cun below the center of the umbilicus.

Functions: Regulates the lower jiao and menstruation.

Indications: Dysuria, edema, hernia, abdominal pain, irregular menstruation, morbid leukorrhea, metrorrhagia, pruritus vulva, postpartum hemorrhage, genital pain, running piglet syndrome.

Attributes: Meeting point of the Ren and Penetrating channels.

Notes

_____

_____

_____

_____

_____

_____

_____

Point Combinations

_____

_____

_____

_____

_____

_____

CV 8
SHENQUE

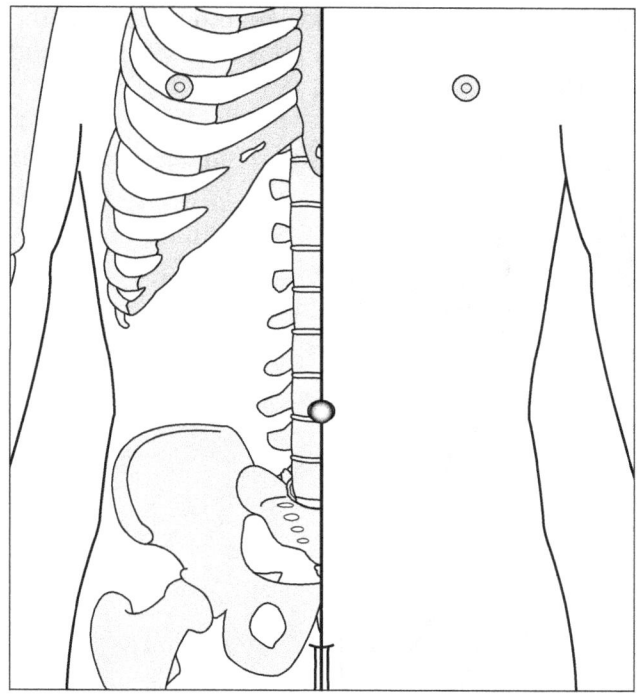

Location: On the lower abdomen and on the anterior midline, in the center of the umbilicus.

Functions: Rescues yang collapse, resuscitates, warms yang, regulates the intestines.

Indications: Flaccidity of apoplexy, coldness of the four extremities, chronic diarrhea, hemihidrosis (sweating on only one side of the body), edema, chronic illness, exhaustion, stroke, epilepsy, digestive disorders.

Notes

Point Combinations

CV 9
SHUIFEN

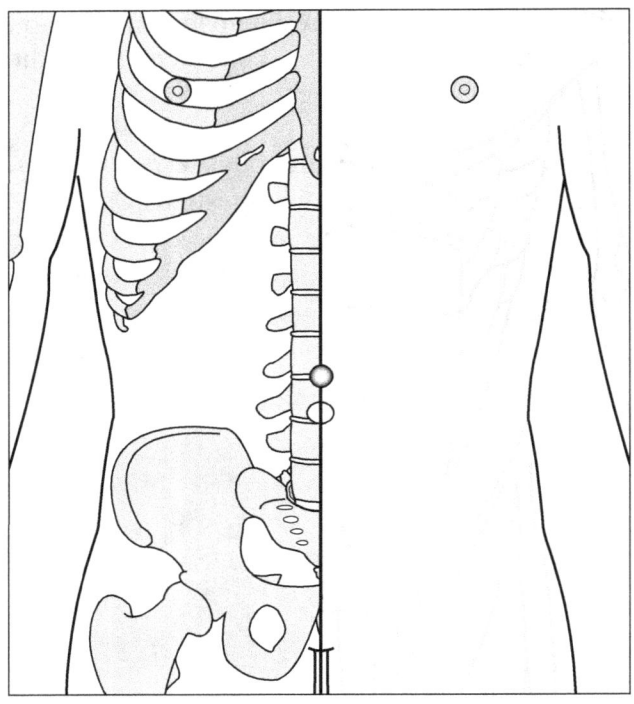

Location: On the upper abdomen and on the anterior midline, 1 cun above the center of the umbilicus.

Functions: Opens and regulates the water passages, treats edema.

Indications: Edema, retention of urine, abdominal pain, diarrhea, regurgitation of food from Stomach, weight loss, borborygmus, GERD.

Notes

Point Combinations

CV 10
XIAWAN

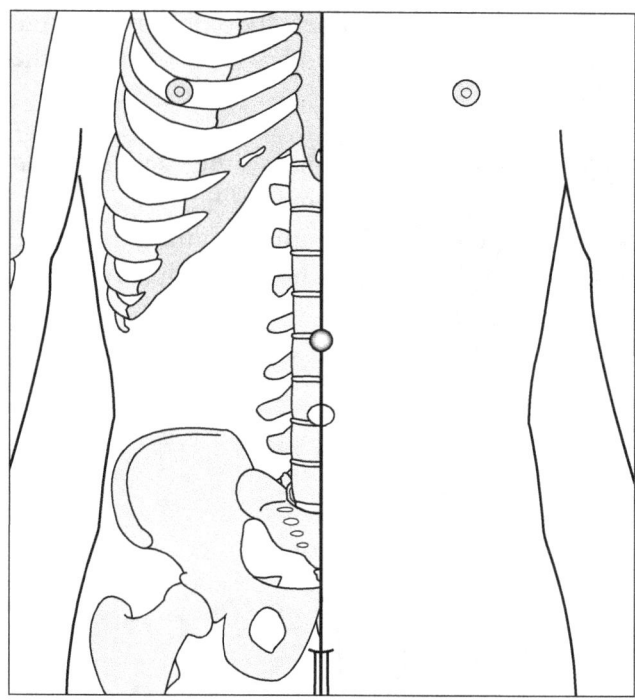

Location: On the upper abdomen and on the anterior midline, 2 cun above the center of the umbilicus.

Functions: Descends Stomach Qi, relieves food stagnation, harmonizes the middle jiao.

Indications: Epigastric pain, abdominal distention, bloating, diarrhea, hiccup, undigested food in the stool, vomiting, borborygmus.

Attributes: Meeting point of the Ren and the Urinary Bladder channels.

Notes

_____

_____

_____

_____

_____

_____

_____

_____

Point Combinations

_____

_____

_____

_____

_____

_____

CV 11
JIANLI

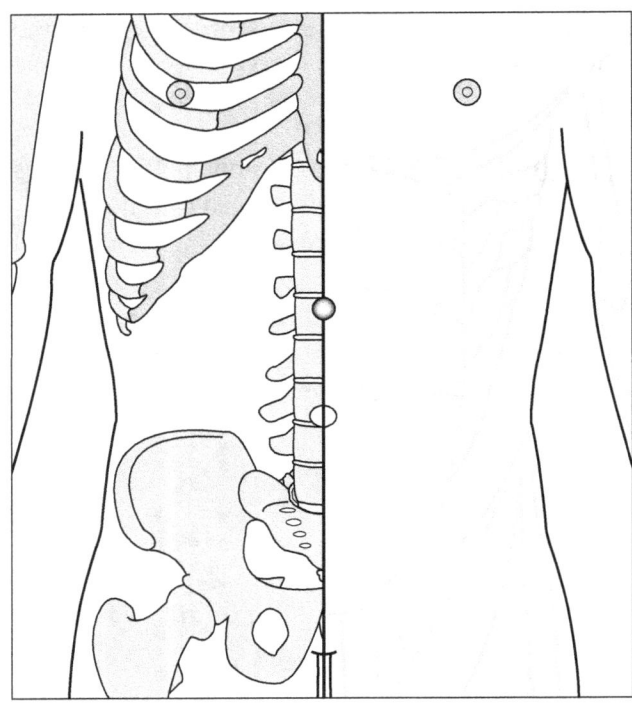

Location: On the upper abdomen and on the anterior midline, 3 cun above the center of the umbilicus.

Functions: Harmonizes the Spleen and Stomach, descends Stomach Qi.

Indications: Gastric pain, vomiting, anorexia, abdominal distention, borborygmus bloating, poor appetite.

Notes

_____
_____
_____
_____
_____
_____
_____
_____

Point Combinations

_____
_____
_____
_____
_____
_____

CV 12
ZHONGWAN

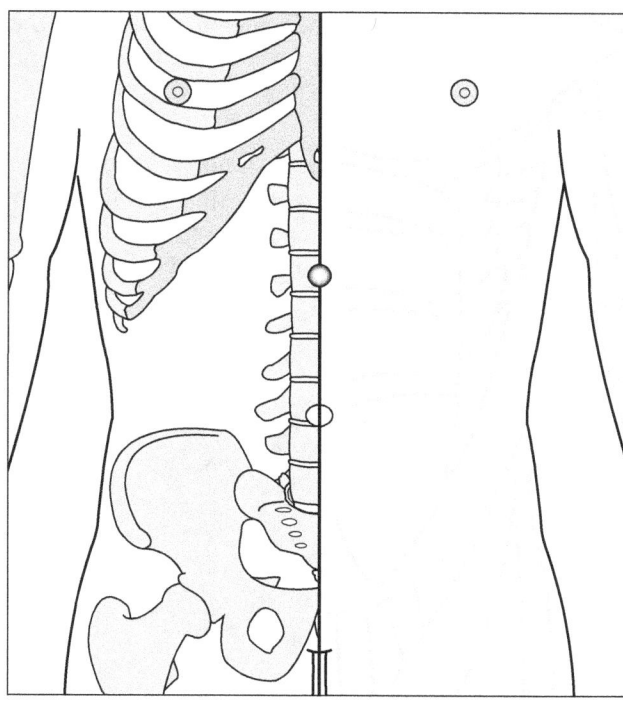

Location: On the upper abdomen and on the anterior midline, 4 cun above the center of the umbilicus.

Functions: Strengthens and harmonizes the Spleen and Stomach, resolves damp, relieves pain.

Indications: Epigastric pain, vomiting, hiccup, acid regurgitation, abdominal distention, diarrhea, dyspepsia, cough, copious phlegm, jaundice, insomnia, nervous Stomach, over thinking, insomnia, anxiety, weight loss, esophagus issues.

Attributes: Front-Mu point of the Stomach, Converging point of the Fu-Organs, Meeting point of the Ren, Small Intestine, San Jiao and Stomach channels.

Notes

Point Combinations

CV 13
SHANGWAN

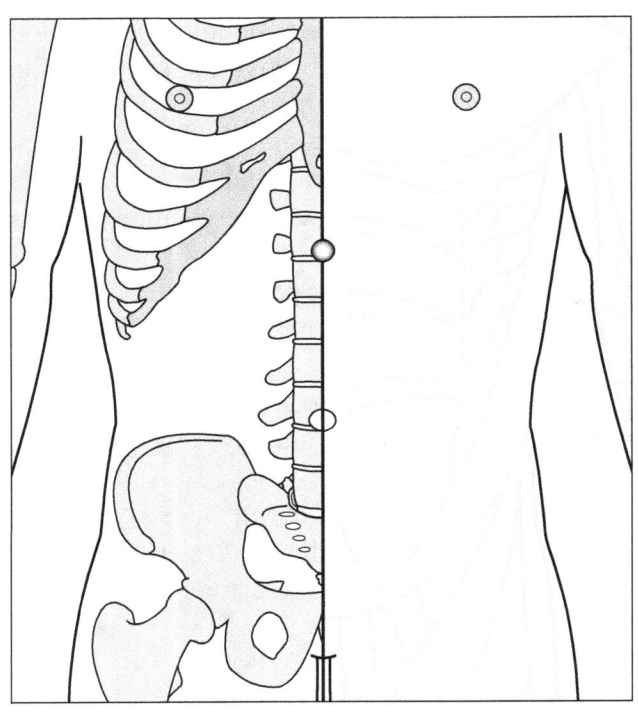

Location: On the upper abdomen and on the anterior midline, 5 cun above the center of the umbilicus.

Functions: Harmonizes and regulates the middle jiao, descends rebellious Qi, stops vomiting.

Indications: Gastric pain, vomiting, abdominal distention, epilepsy, hiatal hernia, hiccups, running piglet syndrome, palpitations, insomnia, anxiety.

Attributes: Meeting point of the Ren, Small Intestine and Stomach channels.

Notes

_____
_____
_____
_____
_____
_____
_____
_____

Point Combinations

_____
_____
_____
_____
_____
_____
_____

CV 14
JUQUE

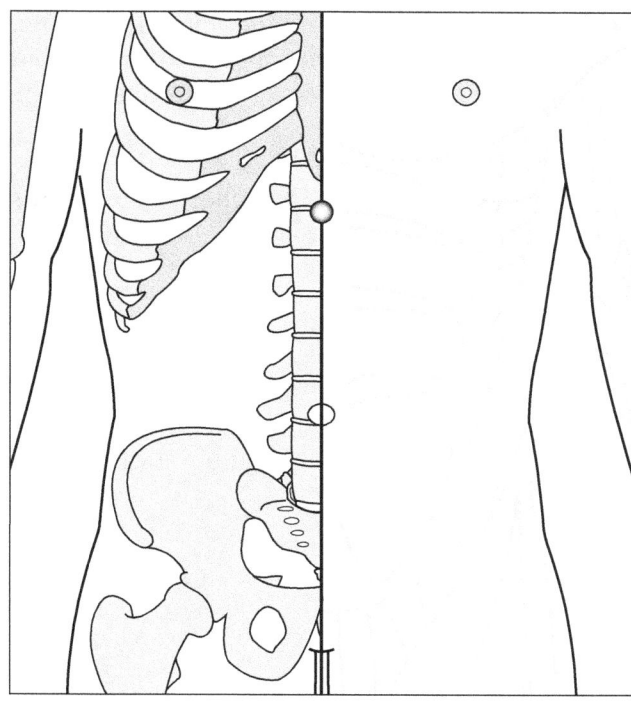

Location: On the upper abdomen and on the anterior midline, 6 cun above the center of the umbilicus.

Functions: Opens the chest, transforms phlegm, regulates the Heart, calms shen, subdues rebellious Qi.

Indications: Pain in the cardiac region and chest, palpitations, manic psychosis, epilepsy, gastric pain, vomiting, nausea, acid regurgitation, shen disturbances from phlegm, anxiety, palpitations, panic attacks, epilepsy.

Attributes: Front-Mu point of the Heart.

Notes
_____
_____
_____
_____
_____
_____
_____
_____
_____

Point Combinations
_____
_____
_____
_____
_____
_____

CV 15
JIUWEI

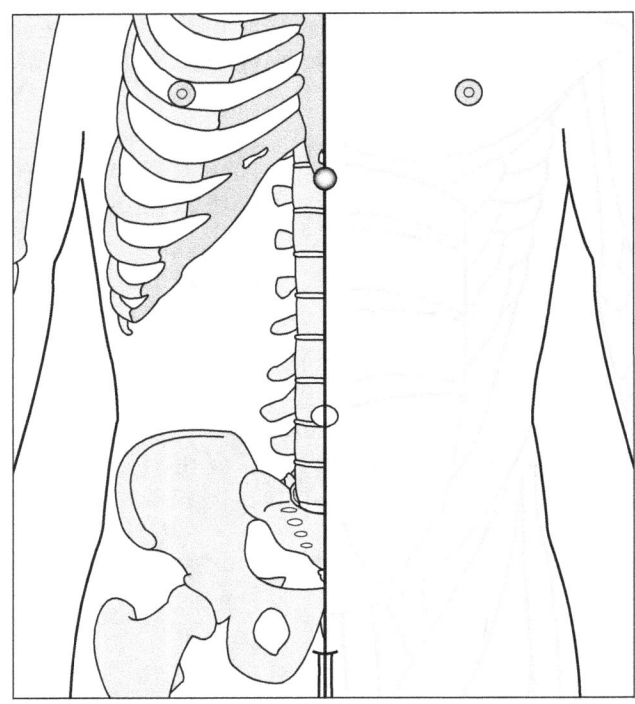

Location: On the upper abdomen and on the anterior midline, 1 cun below the xiphoid process or 7 cun above the center of the umbilicus.

Functions: Opens the chest, transforms phlegm, regulates the Heart, calms shen, subdues rebellious Qi.

Indications: Manic depression, epilepsy, chest pain, palpitations, abdominal distention, digestive issues, nausea, reflux, sore throat, wheezing.

Attributes: Luo-Connecting point of the Ren channel.

Notes

Point Combinations

CV 16
ZHONGTING

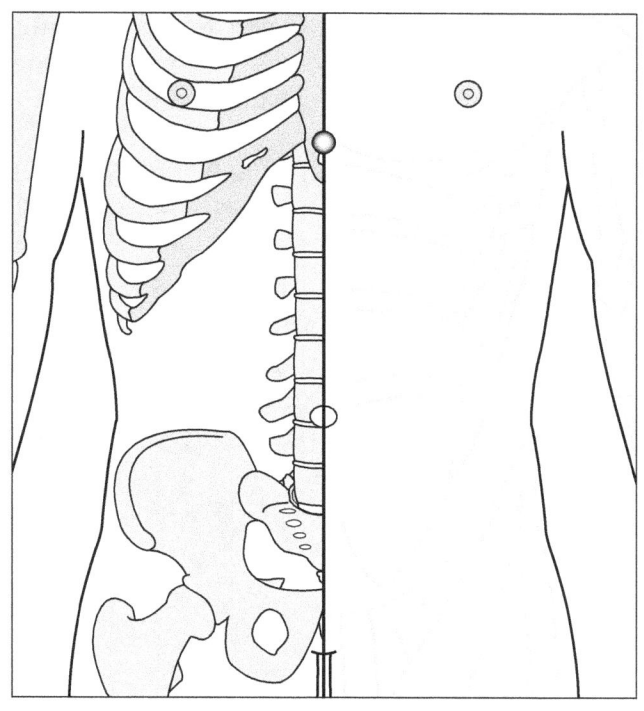

Location: On the chest and on the anterior midline at the 5th intercostal space.

Functions: Opens the chest, subdues rebellious Qi, regulates the middle jiao.

Indications: Distention and fullness in the chest and costal region, cardiac pain, vomiting, infantile milk regurgitation.

Notes
_____
_____
_____
_____
_____
_____
_____
_____
_____

Point Combinations
_____
_____
_____
_____
_____
_____
_____

CV 17
SHANZHONG

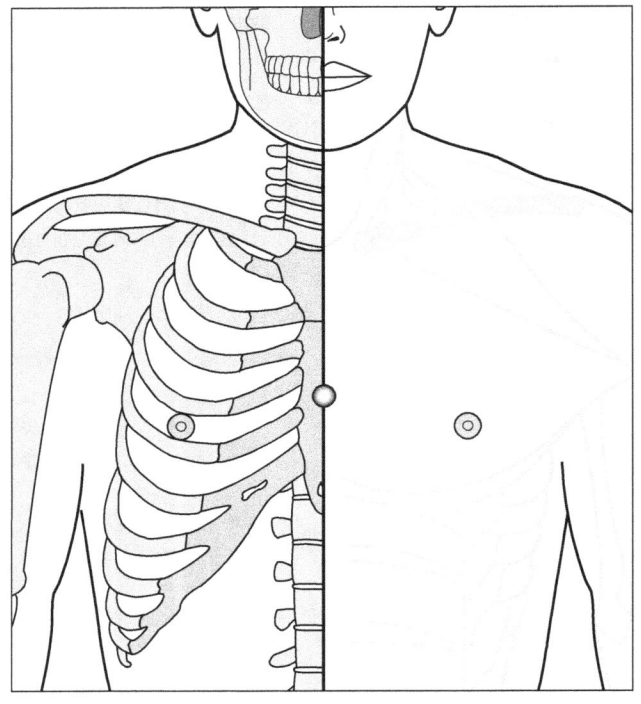

Location: On the chest and on the anterior midline at the 4th intercostal space, at the midpoint of the line connecting both nipples.

Functions: Opens the chest, tonifies and regulates Lung Qi, subdues rebellious Lung Qi, benefits the breasts.

Indications: Asthma, pain and oppression of the chest, cardiac pain, palpitations, insufficient lactation, hiccup, dysphagia, chronic lung issues, cough, mastitis, difficulty swallowing.

Attributes: Front-Mu point of the Pericardium, Converging point of Qi.

Notes
_____
_____
_____
_____
_____
_____
_____
_____

Point Combinations
_____
_____
_____
_____
_____
_____

CV 18
YUTANG

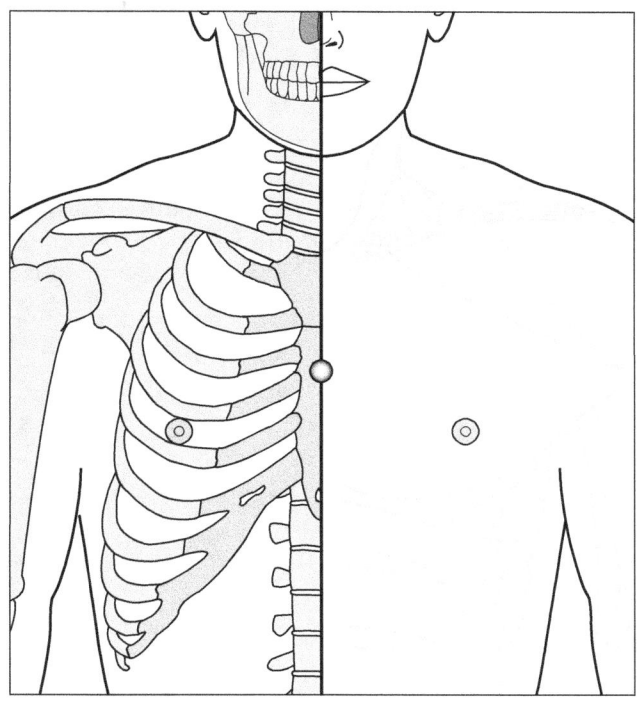

Location: On the chest and on the anterior midline at the 3rd intercostal space.

Functions: Opens the chest, regulates and subdues rebellious Lung Qi, stops cough.

Indications: Cough, asthma, chest pain, pain of the breast, sore throat.

Notes

Point Combinations

CV 19
ZIGONG

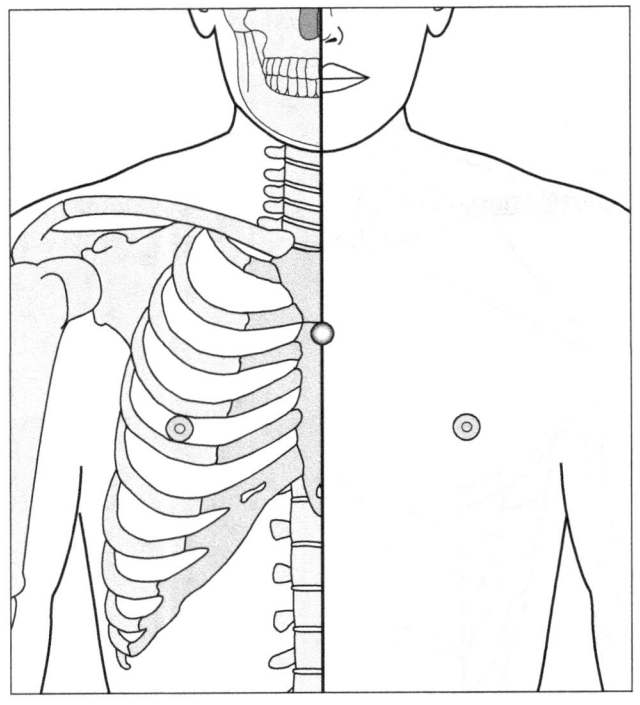

Location: On the chest and on the anterior midline at the 2nd intercostal space.

Functions: Opens the chest, regulates and subdues rebellious Lung Qi, stops cough.

Indications: Cough, chest pain, asthma, vomiting, difficulty ingesting.

Notes

Point Combinations

CV 20
HUAGAI

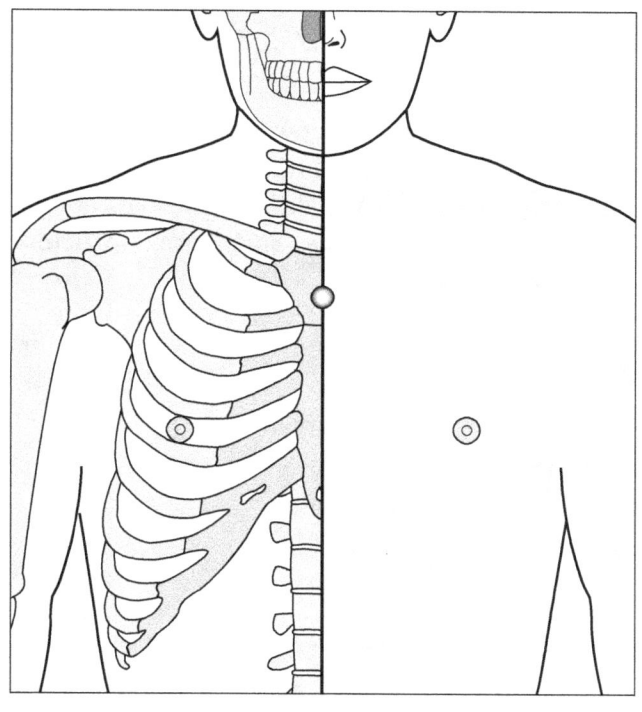

Location: On the chest and on the anterior midline at the 1st intercostal space.

Functions: Opens the chest, regulates and subdues rebellious Lung Qi, stops cough.

Indications: Cough, distention and pain in the chest and hypochondrium, asthma, wheezing, difficulty ingesting.

Notes

_____
_____
_____
_____
_____
_____
_____
_____
_____

Point Combinations

_____
_____
_____
_____
_____
_____
_____

CV 21
ZUANJI

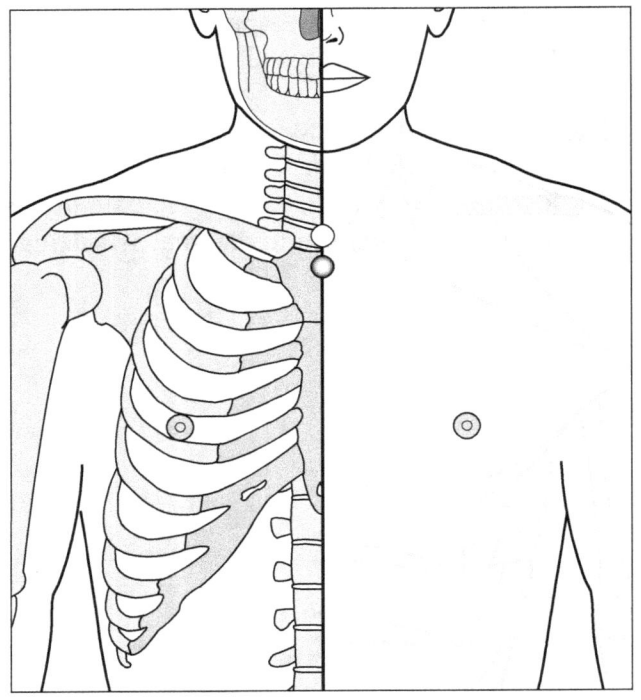

Location: On the neck and on the anterior midline, 1 cun below CV-22 Tiantu.

Functions: Opens the chest, subdues rebellious Lung Qi, benefits the throat.

Indications: Chest pain, sore throat, cough, asthma, wheezing, food stagnation, difficulty ingesting.

Notes _____

_____

_____

_____

_____

_____

_____

_____

Point Combinations _____

_____

_____

_____

_____

_____

CV 22
TIANTU

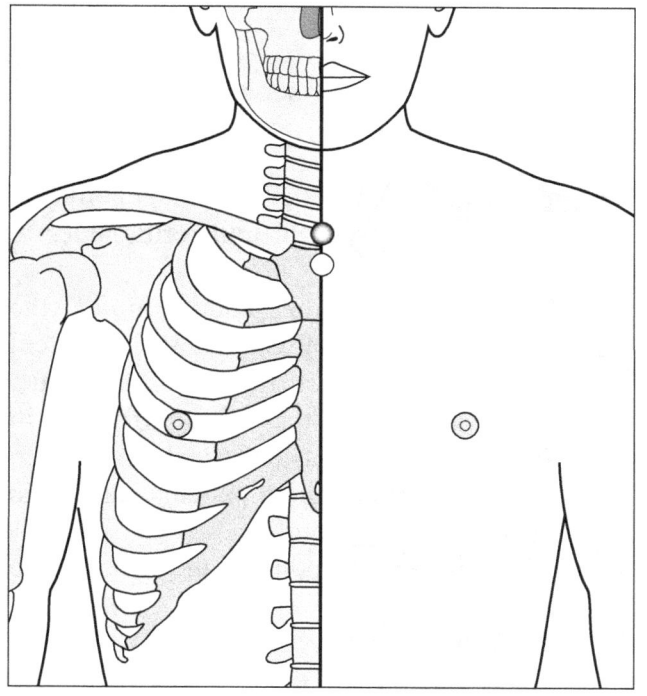

Location: On the neck and on the anterior midline, 0.5 cun superior to the suprasternal notch, at the center of the suprasternal fossa.

Functions: Subdues rebellious Lung Qi, benefits the throat, transforms phlegm, stops cough.

Indications: Sore throat, swallowing issues, sudden hoarseness of the voice, vocal cord disorders, goiter, cough, asthma, chest pain, plum pit sensation.

Attributes: Window of the Sky point.

Notes

Point Combinations

CV 23
LIANQUAN

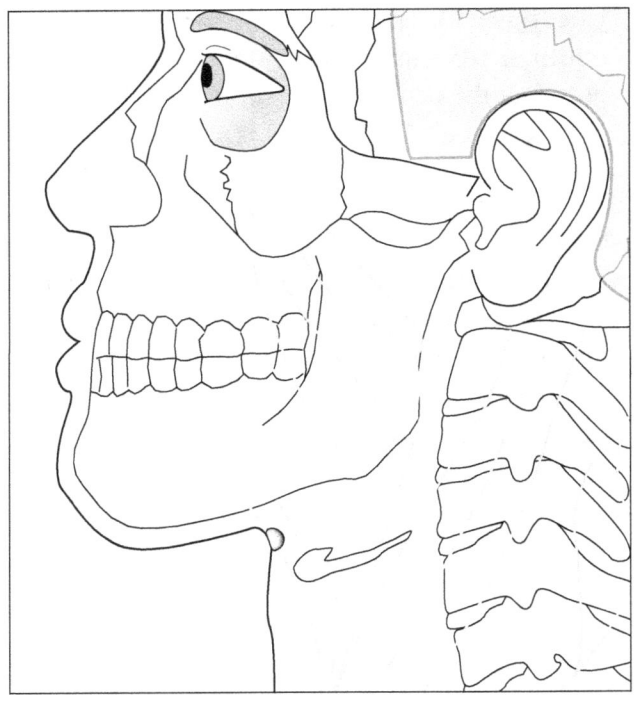

Location: On the neck and on the anterior midline, above the throat prominence, in the depression above the upper border of the hyoid bone.

Functions: Subdues rebellious Qi, benefits the tongue throat and speech, transforms phlegm, stops cough.

Indications: Swelling and pain of the subglossal region, salivation with flaccid tongue, aphasia with stiffness of the tongue, sudden hoarseness of the voice, difficulty in swallowing, main point for speech and mouth disorders, used with stroke patients, excessive drooling and/or dry mouth.

Attributes: Meeting point of the Ren and the Yin Wei channels.

Notes

Point Combinations

CV 24
CHENGJIANG

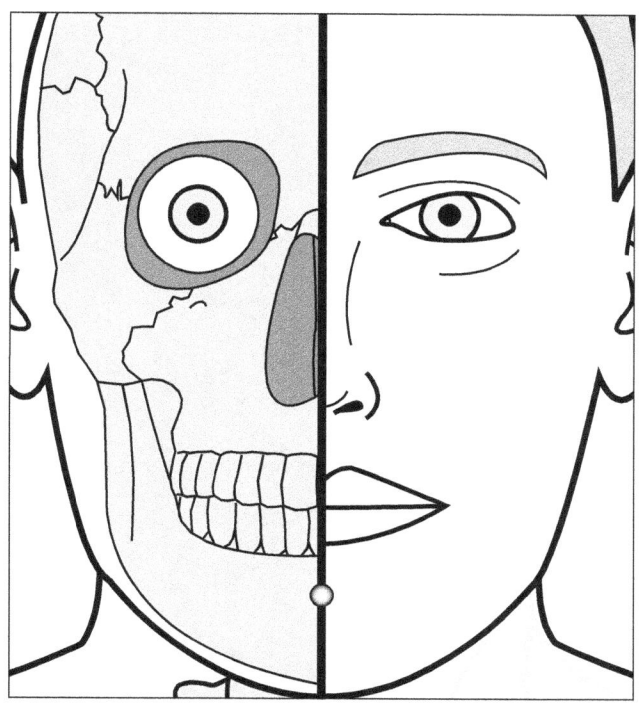

Location: On the face, in the depression at the midpoint of the mentolabial sucus.

Functions: Extinguishes Wind.

Indications: Facial pain/paralysis, Bell's palsy, swelling and pain of the gums, pain in the teeth, salivation, epilepsy, enuresis, dry mouth/wasting thirst disorders.

Attributes: Meeting point of the Ren and the Stomach channels.

Notes

Point Combinations

DU 1
CHANGQIANG

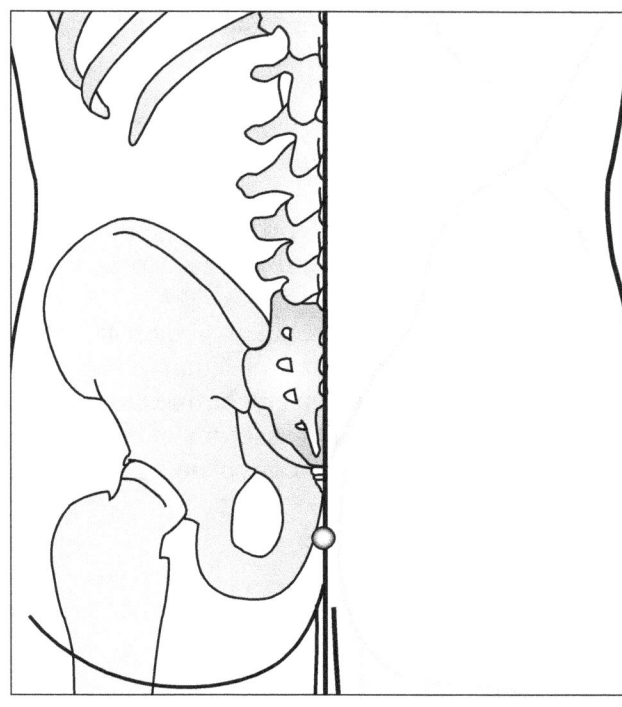

Location: Below the tip of the coccyx, at the midpoint of the line connecting the tip of the occcyx and anus.

Functions: Manages DU and Ren channels, courses Qi, harmonizes the intestines, yin, and yang, resolves damp-heat, clears blood-heat, calms shen, stimulates the channel and relieves pain, swelling and spasm, supports the lower back, stops diarrhea.

Indications: Impotence, low sperm count, eczema of the scrotum, cloudy or turbid urine, constipation, diarrhea, rectal bleeding, hemorrhoids, prolapsed anus, pain of the coccyx, low back pain, infantile convulsions, induce labor, eyes fixed upward, mania, psychosis.

Attributes: Intersecting point of Ren, DU, Liver, Gall Bladder and Kidney channels.
Luo-Connecting point of DU channel.
* Main point for hemorrhoids.
**Good point for stiffness of the spine.

Notes
_____
_____
_____
_____
_____
_____
_____
_____
_____

Point Combinations
_____
_____
_____
_____
_____
_____
_____
_____

DU 2
YAOSHO

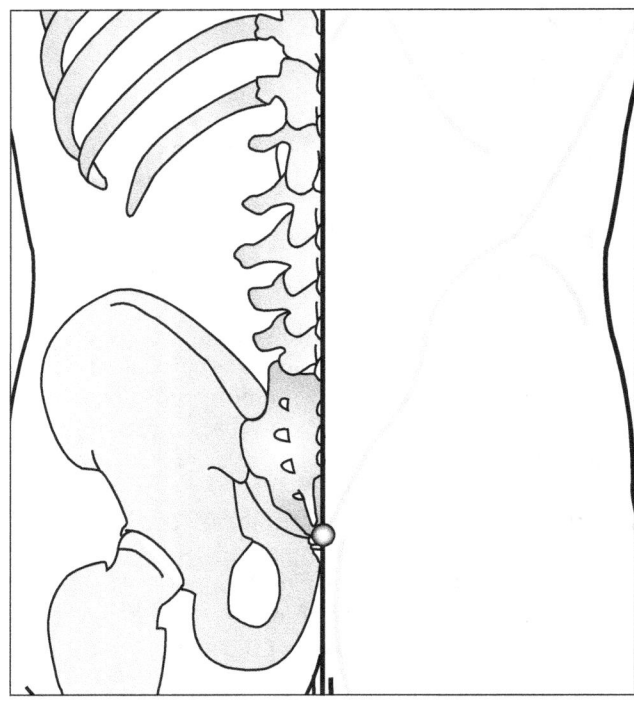

Location: On the sacrum and on the posterior midline, in the sacral hiatus.

Functions: Extinguishes internal wind and wind-damp, removes blockages in the channel and stimulates the connecting vessel, nourishes Kidney and warms the lower jiao, calms shen, supports lower back and knees, stops spasm and convulsions.

Indications: Irregular menstruation, leukorrhea, paralysis or muscular atrophy of the lower limbs, enuresis, incontinence (related to paraplegia), pain of the sacrum and low back, hemorrhoids, spasms, convulsions, seizures, epilepsy.

Notes

Point Combinations

DU 3
YAOYANGGUAN

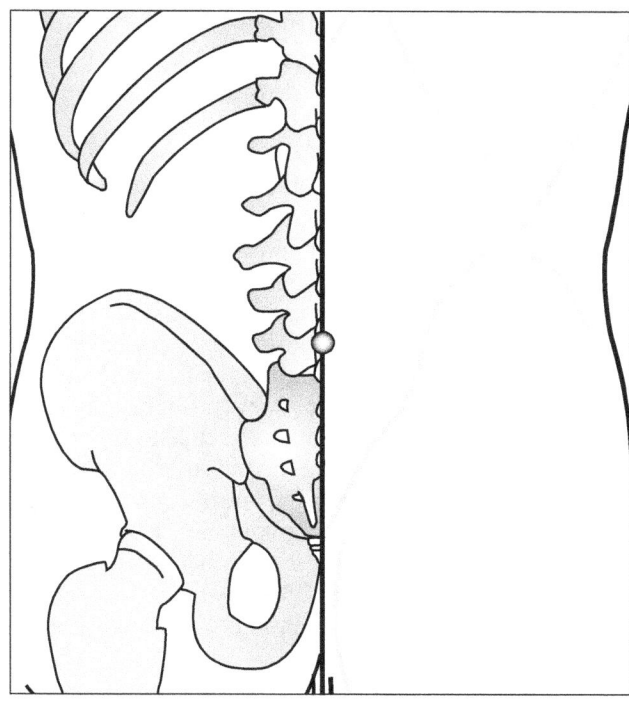

Location: On the low back and on the posterior midline, in the depression below the spinous process of the 4th lumbar vertebra.

Functions: Manages and grasps Kidney Qi, manages Penetrating, Ren and the lower jiao resolves damp-cold, strengthens lower back and legs, warms blood, yang, essence and semen.

Indications: Scrofula, vomiting, diarrhea, chronic enteritis, lower abdominal distention, lower back pain, irregular menstruation, leukorrhea, spermatorrhea, impotence, seminal emission, knee pain or stiffness, numbness or paralysis of the lower limbs.

Attributes: *Main point for premature ejaculation, low back pain, knee pain.

Notes
_____
_____
_____
_____
_____
_____
_____
_____
_____

Point Combinations
_____
_____
_____
_____
_____
_____
_____

DU 4
MINGMEN

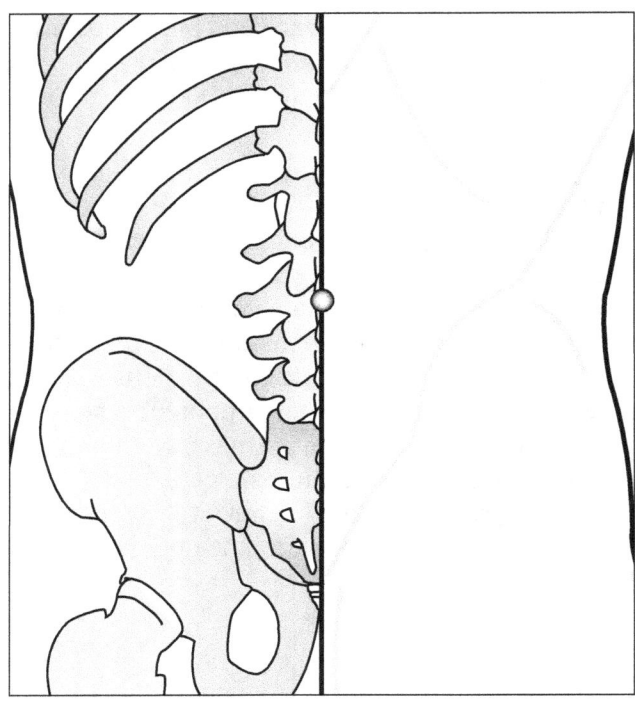

Location: On the low back and on the posterior midline, in the depression below the spinous process of the 2nd lumbar vertebra.

Functions: Manages the DU channel, supports Yuan Qi, Jing, yang and Kidneys, removes blockages from the channel and stimulates the connecting vessels, nourishes lumbar spine, manages the water pathways, resolves damp-heat, calms the fetus.

Indications: Dizziness, tinnitus, headache, asthma, peritonitis, nephritis, abdominal and low back pain, intestinal colic, low back sprain or limited range of motion of lower back, tidal fever, nephritis, spinal myelitis, sciatica, daybreak diarrhea, endometriosis, irregular menstruation, leukorrhea, uterine bleeding, spermatorrhea, impotence, hemorrhoids, prolapsed anus, enuresis, infantile convulsions or paralysis.

Attributes: *Good point for low back pain, lumbar issues, and to build fire of vitality.

**Main point for issues relating to sexual organs or desire and vitality.

Notes

_____

_____

_____

_____

_____

_____

_____

_____

Point Combinations

_____

_____

_____

_____

_____

_____

_____

DU 5
XUANSHU

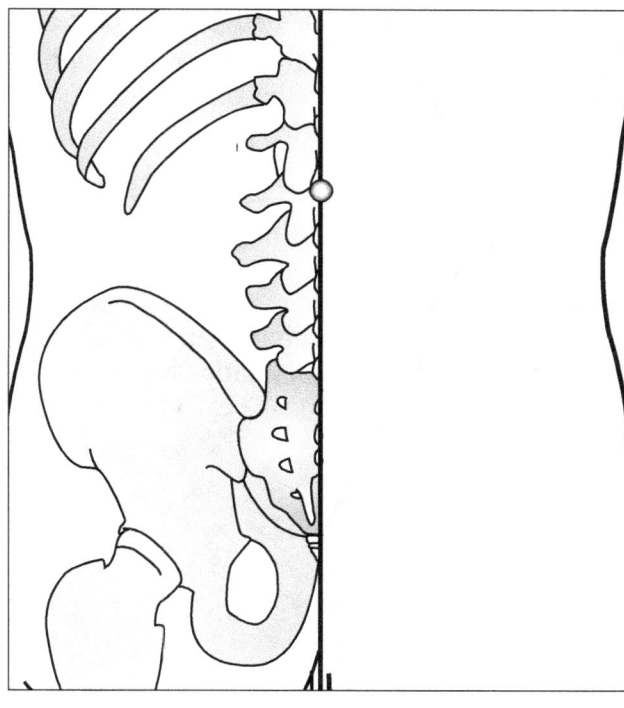

Location: On the low back and on the posterior midline, in the depression below the spinous process of the 1st lumbar vertebra.

Functions: Nourishes the Spleen and Stomach, manages and builds Spleen Qi and yang, encourage Yuan Qi, supports lumbar spine, knees and lower jiao.

Indications: Limited range of motion, stiffness and pain of the lumbar spine, running piglet Qi, indigestion, dysentery, diarrhea, abdominal pain, prolapse of the anus, retraction of the testicles.

Notes

Point Combinations

DU 6
JIZHONG

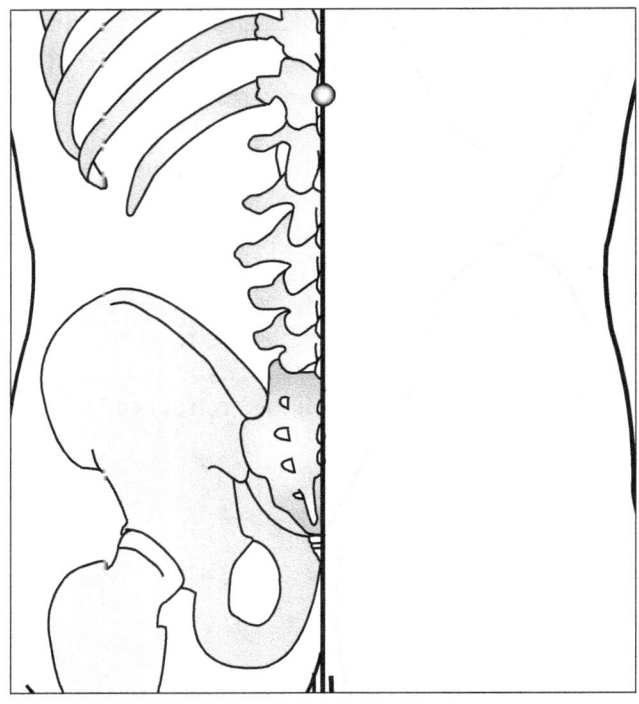

Location: On the back and on the posterior midline, in the depression below the spinous process of the 11th thoracic vertebra.

Functions: Nourishes the Spleen, Stomach, Kidneys, Liver, lower jiao and lumbar spine, encourage Jing Qi, resolves damp, retract prolapse.

Indications: Jaundice, hepatitis, loss of appetite, intestinal bleeding, diarrhea, stiffness and pain of the lumbar spine, hemorrhoids, rectal prolapse, paralysis or lower limbs, seizures, epilepsy.

Notes

Point Combinations

DU 7
ZHONGSHU

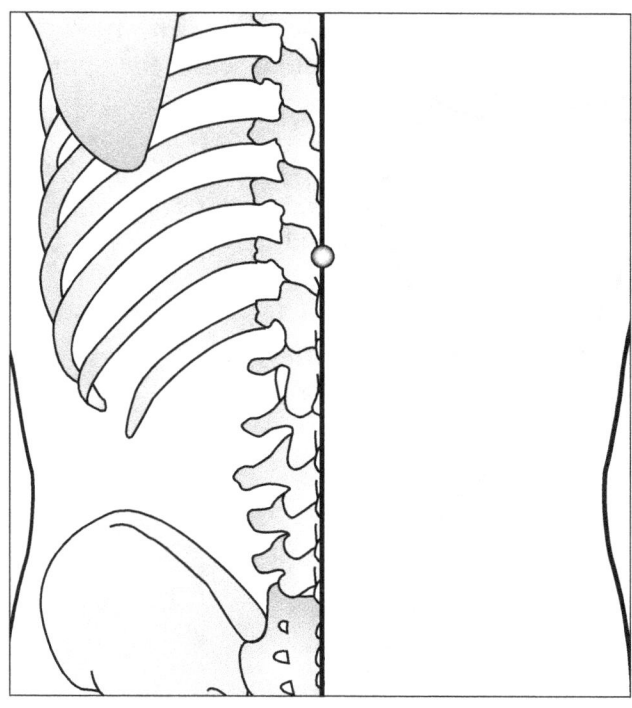

Location: On the back and on the posterior midline, in the depression below the spinous process of the 10th thoracic vertebra.

Functions: Nourishes the Stomach, Liver, Gall Bladder, lumbar spine and middle jiao, manages Spleen, Stomach, and Stomach Qi, supports Kidney, relieves pain.

Indications: Stomach ache, abdominal fullness, loss of appetite, low back pain and stiffness, cholecystitis, decline in vision.

Notes

_____
_____
_____
_____
_____
_____
_____
_____

Point Combinations

_____
_____
_____
_____
_____
_____

DU 8
JINSUO

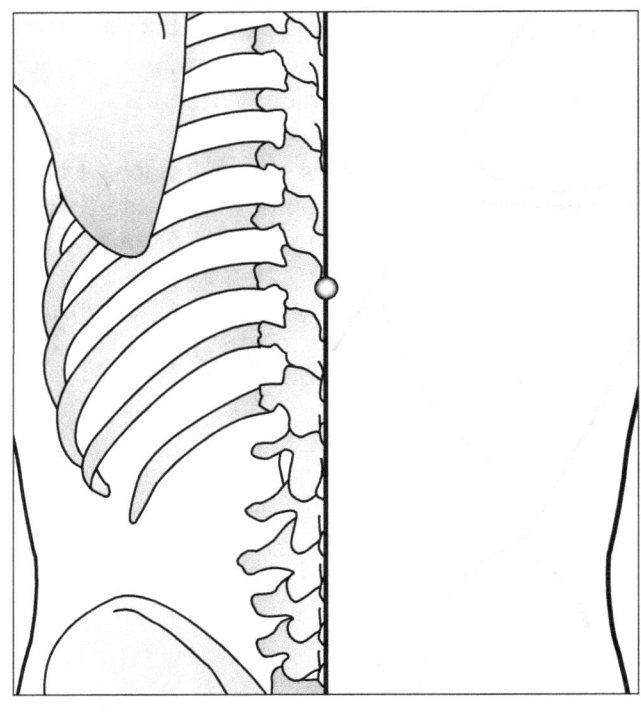

Location: On the back and on the posterior midline, in the depression below the spinous process of the 9th thoracic vertebra.

Functions: Manages the Stomach and Liver Qi, nourishes Kidneys, supports Spleen and back, extinguishes wind-damp, relieves pain and spasm, calms shen.

Indications: Pleurisy, intercostal neuralgia, hepatitis, cholecystitis, hysteria, epilepsy, seizures, pain of the Heart, gastric pain, suppressed anger.

Notes
_____
_____
_____
_____
_____
_____
_____
_____

Point Combinations
_____
_____
_____
_____
_____
_____

DU 9
ZHIYANG

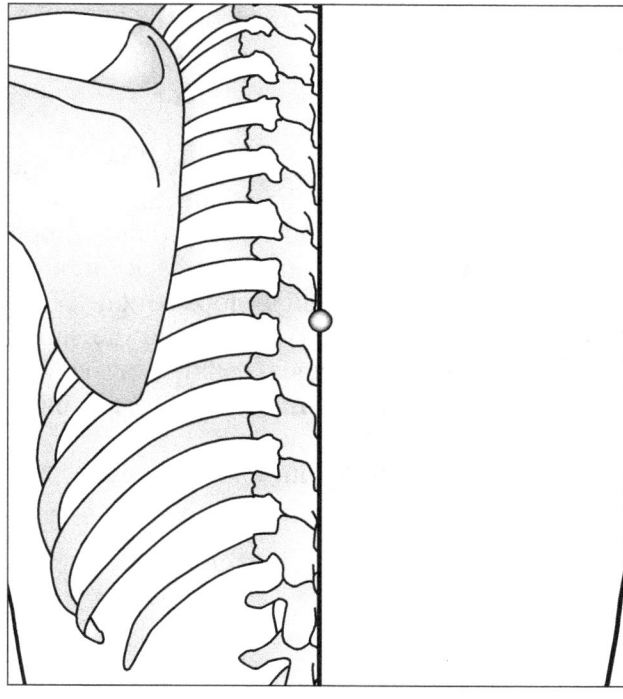

Location: On the back and on the posterior midline, in the depression below the spinous process of the 7th thoracic vertebra.

Functions: Removes blockages from the channel and stimulates the connecting vessels, nourishes Yang, manages the function of Qi, Liver and Gall Bladder and middle jiao, supports the Spleen, resolves damp-heat, opens chest and lungs, suppress cough.

Indications: Dysphasia, dyspnea, fullness of the chest, cough, hiccup, asthma, panting, pleurisy, chest, back, and stomach pain, intercostal neuralgia, cholecystitis, hepatitis, jaundice, malaria, round worm in bile duct, borborygmus, sighing.

Attributes: *Main point for cholecystitis and hepatitis.

Notes

Point Combinations

DU 10
LINGTAI

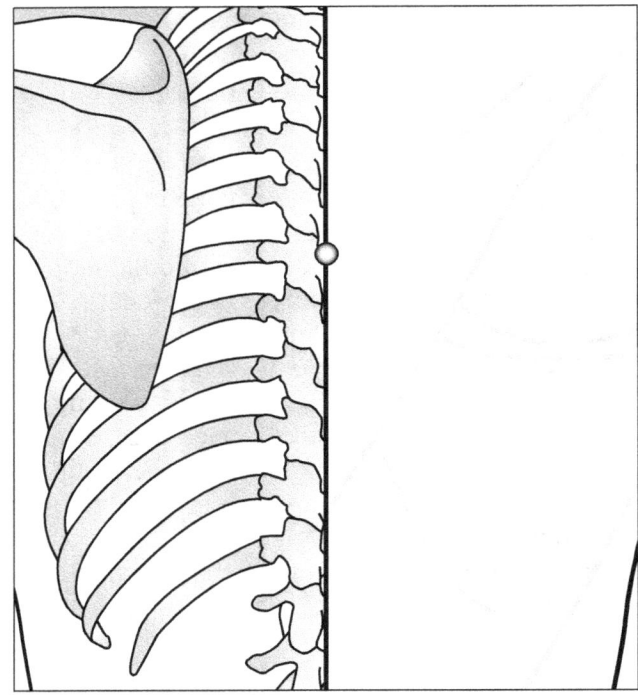

Location: On the back and on the posterior midline, in the depression below the spinous process of the 6th thoracic vertebra.

Functions: Removes blockages from the channel and stimulates the connecting vessels, clears heat, expels blood toxicity, cools blood heat, supports Heart, Lungs and back, unbinds and sooths chest and lungs, stops cough.

Indications: Stiff neck, pain along the spine, carbuncles, boils, dyspnea, asthma, bronchitis, cough, common cold, malaria, stomach pain, round worm in the bile duct.

Attributes: * Good point for boils on the neck and back.

Notes

Point Combinations

DU 11
SHENDAO

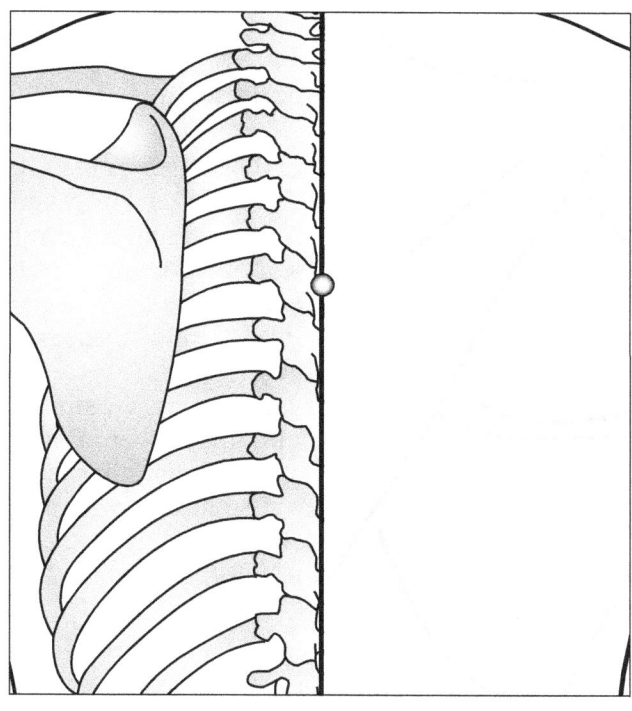

Location: On the back and on the posterior midline, in the depression below the spinous process of the 5th thoracic vertebra.

Functions: Manages yang and Heart Qi, nourishes Heart and Lung, cools Heart fire, pacify Heart, calms shen. relieves pain, unbinds and sooths chest, extinguishes wind and alleviate fright.

Indications: Dizziness, poor memory, shortness of breath, cough, anxiety, Heart disease, palpitations, pain and stiffness of the back, intercostal neuralgia, fever, malaria, seizures, sadness.

Notes

Point Combinations

DU 12
SHENZHU

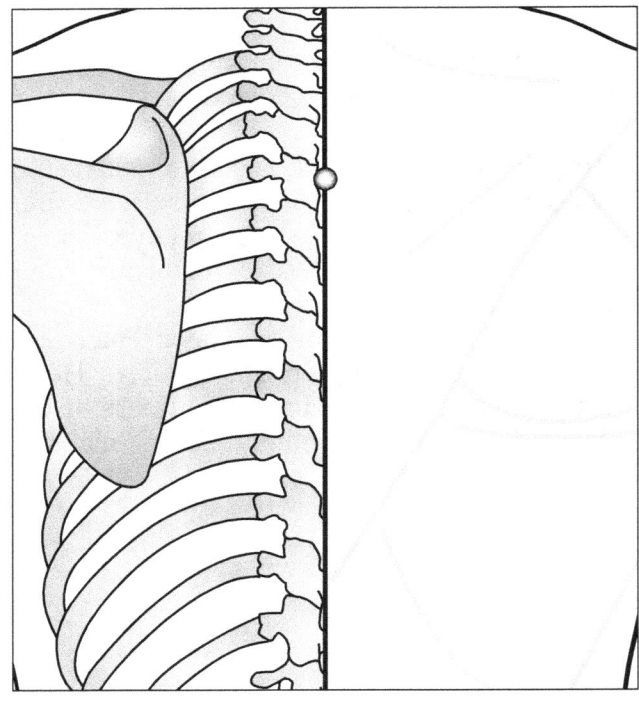

Location: On the back and on the posterior midline, in the depression below the spinous process of the 3rd thoracic vertebra.

Functions: Manages and distributes Lung Qi, nourish Lung Qi, clears heat from the Heart and Lungs, eliminates pathogens and sedates fever and spasms, pacifies Heart and calms shen, extinguishes wind and wind-heat, removes obstructions, unbinds and sooths chest, courses Qi counter flow and relieves cough.

Indications: Aphasia, cough, asthma, wheezing, pneumonia, pulmonary tuberculosis, bronchitis, chest and back pain, rage, hysteria, mental disease, epilepsy, seizures, pain and stiffness of the lower back.

Attributes: *Good point for mental and/or emotional disease.

Notes _____

_____

_____

_____

_____

_____

_____

_____

Point Combinations _____

_____

_____

_____

_____

_____

_____

DU 13
TAODAO

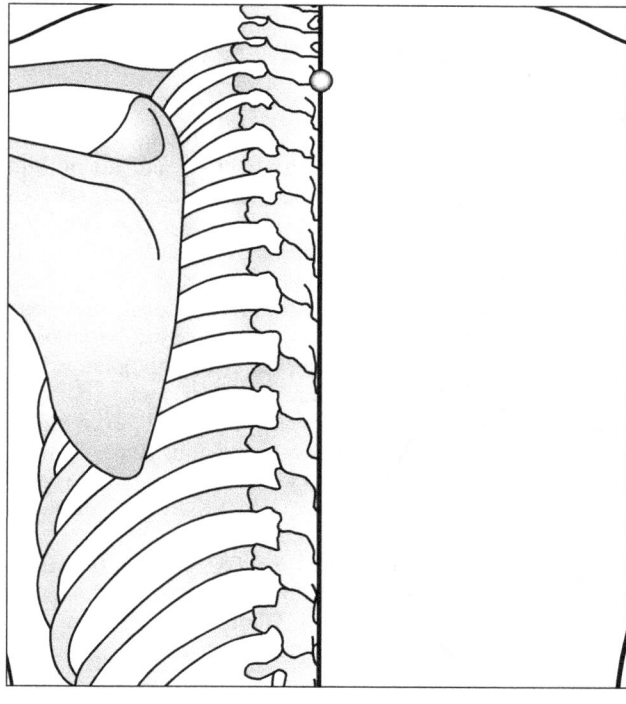

Location: On the back and on the posterior midline, in the depression below the spinous process of the 1st thoracic vertebra.

Functions: Rectifies Shaoyang, eliminates exterior pathogens and sedates fever, releases exterior, extinguishes wind and wind heat, clears fire and Lung heat, distributes Lung Qi, soothes collaterals, tonifies deficiency and Wei Qi, calms shen.

Indications: Fever, alternating chills and fever, anhidrosis, headache, dizziness, muscle spasm of head and neck, cough, pulmonary or infantile tuberculosis, low back pain, stiffness of the back, psychosis, seizures, malaria.

Attributes: Meeting point of DU and Urinary Bladder channels.

*Main point for malaria.

Notes

Point Combinations

DU 14
DAZHUI

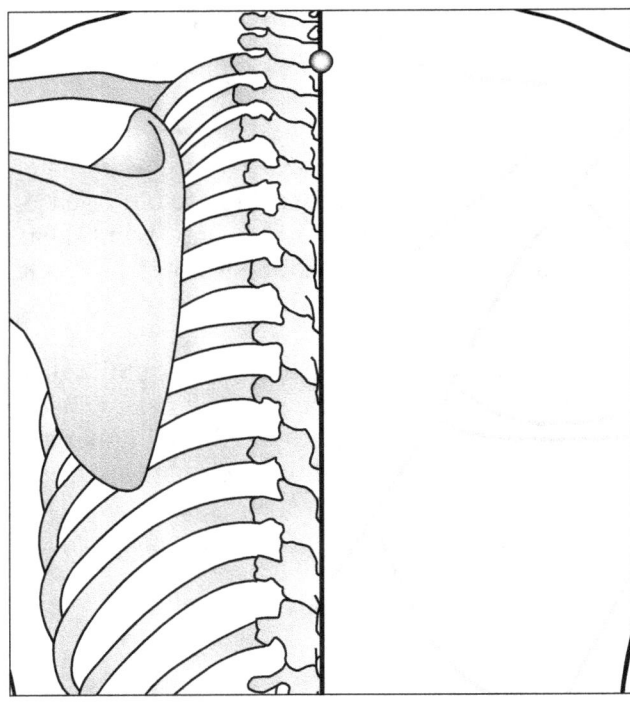

Location: On the back and on the posterior midline, in the depression below the spinous process of the 7th cervical vertebra.

Functions: Relieves exterior condition, eliminates exterior pathogens from yang channels and disinhibits yang Qi, extinguishes wind-heat, and lung heat, sedates fever, manages nutritive and defensive Qi, tonifies yang and defensive Qi, harmonizes Qi and rectifies yin collapse, soothes collaterals and calms shen.

Indications: Congestion of throat and chest, shortness of breath, asthma, bronchitis, pulmonary tuberculosis, cough, emphysema, common cold, cold pathogens, upper respiratory infection, asthma, shoulder and neck pain and stiffness, fever, tidal fever, chills and fever, night sweating, heat in the bones, hypertension, vomiting with or without blood, aversion to wind, yangming stage heat, taiyang disorder, heat stroke, hepatitis, blood diseases malaria, seizures, epilepsy, psychosis

Attributes: Meeting point of DU, Large Intestine, Stomach, Small Intestine, Urinary Bladder, San Jiao, and Gall Bladder channels. Sea of Qi point.
*Main point for malaria or high fever.

Notes

_____

_____

_____

_____

_____

_____

_____

Point Combinations

_____

_____

_____

_____

_____

_____

DU 15
YAMEN

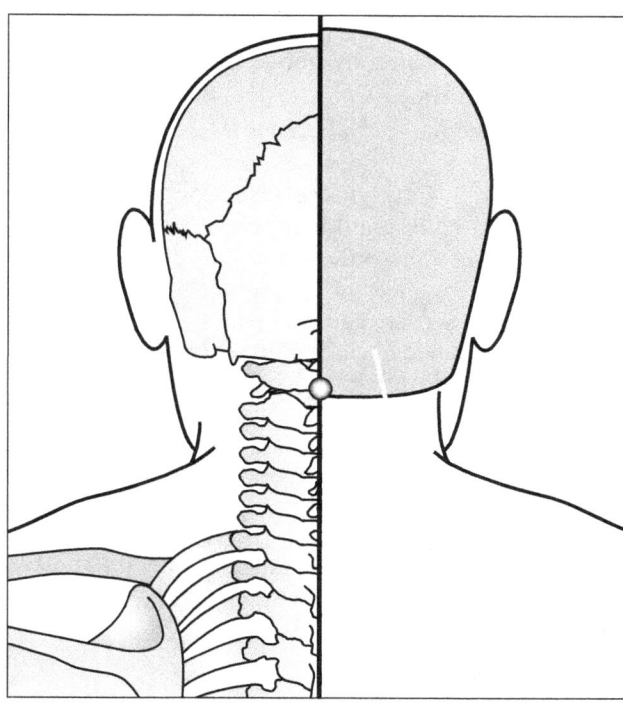

Location: On the neck and on the posterior midline, 0.5 cun directly above the midpoint of the posterior hairline. (in the depression below the spinous process of the 1st cervical vertebra)

Functions: Disinhibits the mind and liberates the senses, removes blockages in the channel and stimulates the connecting vessel, courses Qi, expels wind, encourages the quiet behavior of joints, assists the tongue, neck, and spine, lubricates the throat, encourages speech.

Indications: Loss of consciousness, occipital headache, nosebleed, deafness or muteness, post stroke apoplexy, flaccidity or stiffness of the tongue, sudden horse voice, aphasia, neck stiffness, chills and fever, anhidrosis, mental disorders, cerebral palsy, convulsions, epilepsy, mania, hysteria, depression.

Attributes: Meeting point of DU and Yang Wei channels, Window of the Sky point and Sea of Marrow point.

Notes

_____
_____
_____
_____
_____
_____
_____
_____
_____

Point Combinations

_____
_____
_____
_____
_____
_____
_____

DU 16
FENGFU

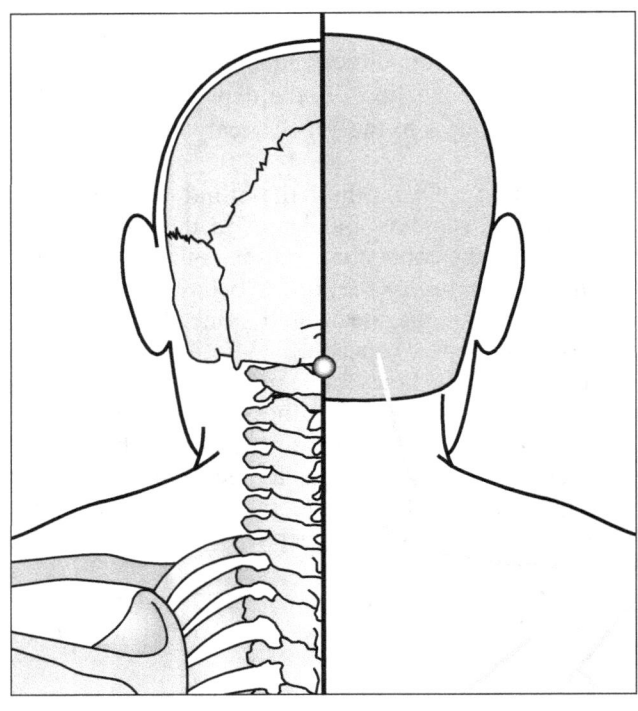

Location: On the neck and on the posterior midline, 1 cun directly above the midpoint of the posterior hairline. (in the depression below the external occipital protuberance).

Functions: Extinguishes interior and exterior wind, wind-cold, wind-heat, clears Heart heat and fire, nourishes the-Sea of marrow, encourages the quiet behavior of joints, disinhibits the mind and liberates the senses, calms shen.

Indications: Headache, blurred vision, dizziness, nose bleed, sore throat, sudden horse voice, aphasia, post stroke apoplexy, flaccidity of the tongue, stiff neck, hemiplegia, numbness of the limbs, common cold, aversion to cold, shivering with perspiration, stroke, mental illness, fear, sadness.

Attributes: Meeting point of DU, Yang Wei and Urinary Bladder channels. Ghost point, Window of the Sky point, and Sea of Marrow point.

Notes

Point Combinations

DU 17
NAOHU

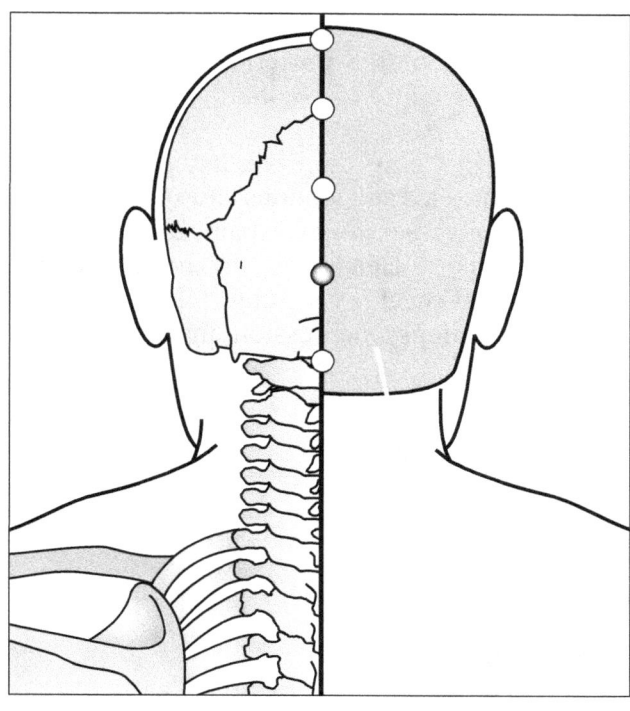

Location: On the head, 2.5 cun directly above the midpoint of the posterior hairline, and 1.5 cun above DU-16 Fengfu, in the depression on the upper border of the external occipital protuberance.

Functions: Extinguishes wind and clears heat, disinhibits the mind and liberates the senses, dissipates swelling, relieves pain, assists the eyes, stops spasm and tetany, calms shen.

Indications: Headache, dizziness, issues of the eye and vision, pain, stiffness, and swelling of the head, face and neck, lockjaw, goiter, laryngitis, dysphonia, aversion to wind, chills and fever, jaundice, mental issues, mania, seizure, epilepsy.

Attributes: Meeting point for DU and Urinary Bladder channels, Sea of Marrow point.

Notes

Point Combinations

DU 18
QIANGJIAN

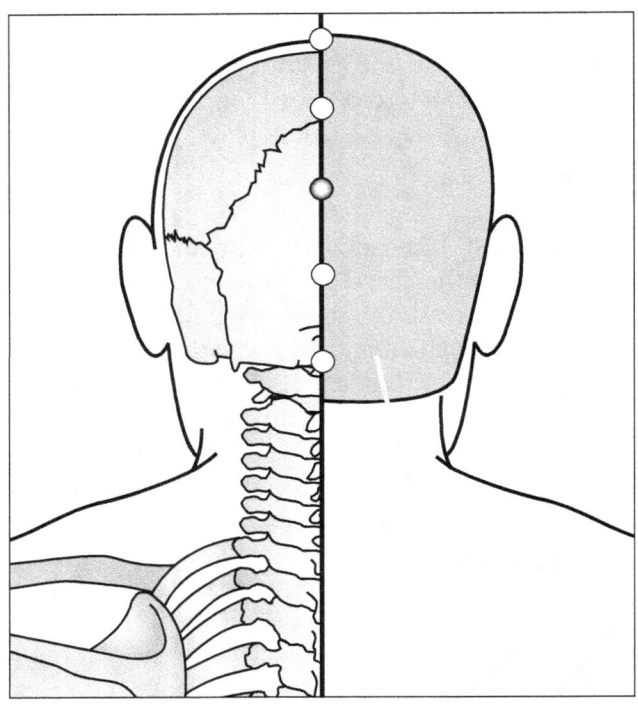

Location: On the head, 4 cun directly above the midpoint of the posterior hairline, 3 cun directly above DU-17 Naohu.

Functions: Calms the Liver and expels wind, soothes muscles and tendons and stimulates the connecting vessel, relieves pain, calms shen.

Indications: Headache, dizziness, blurred vision, stiff neck, vomiting bile, insomnia, seizures, epilepsy, depression, mania.

Notes

Point Combinations

DU 19
HOUDING

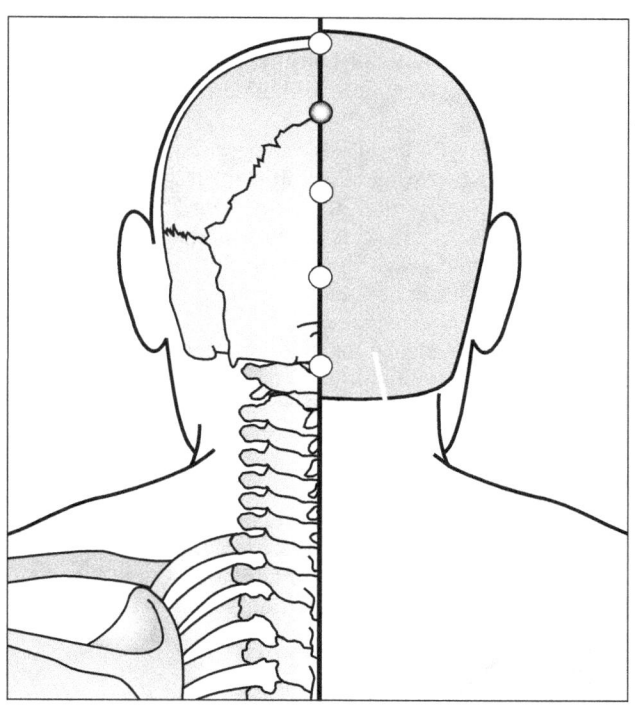

Location: On the head, 5.5 cun directly above the midpoint of the posterior hairline, 1.5 cun directly above DU-17 Naohu.

Functions: Supports the Heart, head and yang, calms the Liver, Heart and shen, suppress yang, extinguishes wind, and relieves pain.

Indications: Headache, migraine, dizziness, vertigo, insomnia, pain and stiffness of the head and neck, aversion to wind and cold, common cold, mania, severe anxiety, convulsions, seizures, epilepsy.

Notes

Point Combinations

DU 20
BAHUI

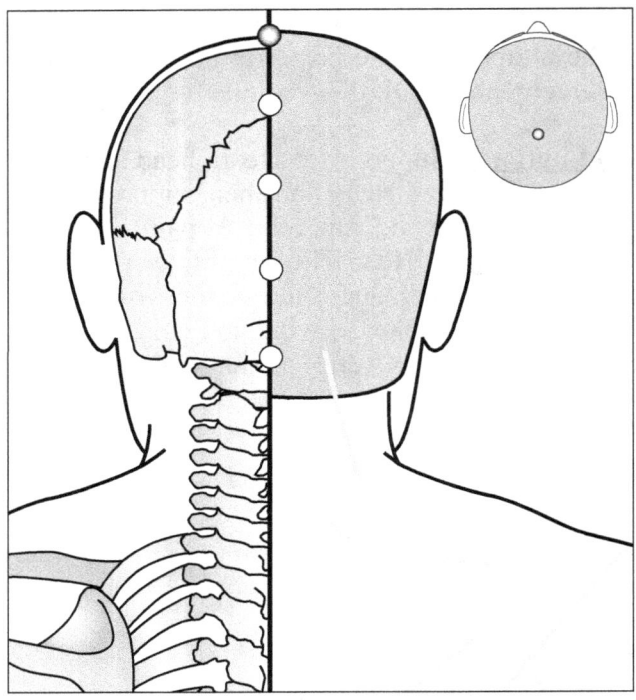

Location: On the head, 5 cun directly above the midpoint of the anterior hairline, at the midpoint of the line connecting the apexes of both ears.

Functions: Extinguishes interior and Liver wind, suppresses Liver yang, disinhibits the mind and liberates the senses, supports the head nourishes the mind, rectifies yang rising, clears heat, subdues extreme heat in yang channels, distributes Liver Qi, uplifts prolapse, facilitates resuscitation, calms shen.

Indications: Headache, dizziness, vertigo, frontal and vertex headache or pain at the vertex, eye or vision disorders, tinnitus, deafness, sinus and nasal obstruction or congestion, nosebleed, lockjaw, chest oppression, palpitations, hemorrhoids, diarrhea, rectal prolapse, prolapsed uterus, vaginal bleeding hyper/hypotension, loss of consciousness, shock, stroke, post stroke apoplexy, hemiplegia, tetany, seizures, epilepsy, emotional imbalances, malaria.

Attributes: Meeting point of DU, Ren, Large Intestine, Stomach, Small Intestine, Urinary Bladder, San Jiao, Gall Bladder and Liver channels, Sea of Marrow point.
*Main point for dizziness and hemorrhoids.

Notes _____
_____
_____
_____
_____
_____
_____
_____

Point Combinations _____
_____
_____
_____
_____
_____

DU 21
QIANDING

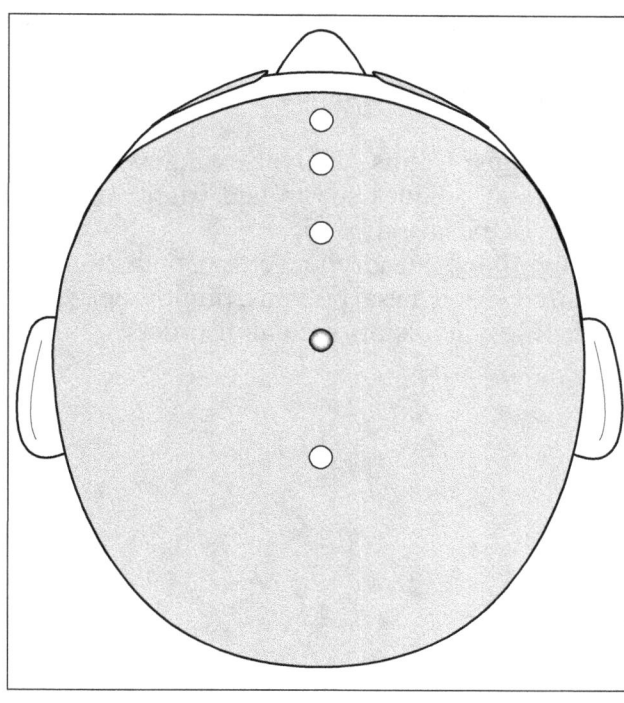

Location: On the head, 3.5 cun directly above the midpoint of the anterior hairline, 1.5 cun directly anterior to DU-20 Baihui.

Functions: Calms the Liver and cultivates yang, extinguishes wind-damp, extinguishes wind and suppresses tetany, invigorates the collaterals and dispels swelling, disinhibits and supports the mind, liberates the senses, and assists vision, calms shen and steady the mind.

Indications: Headache, vertical headache, dizziness, vertigo, blurred vision, nasal polypus, rhinorrhea, rhinitis and epilepsy.

Notes

Point Combinations

DU 22
XINHUI

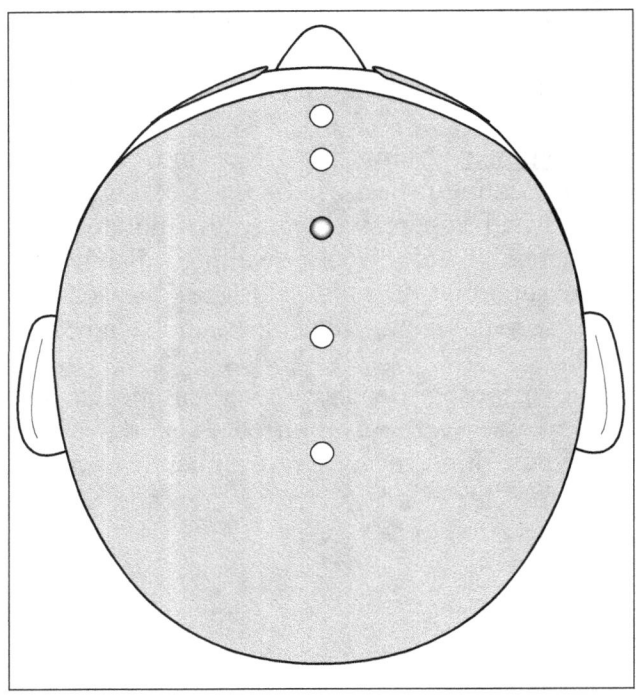

Location: On the head, 2 cun directly above the midpoint of the anterior hairline, 3 cun directly anterior to DU-20 Baihui.

Functions: Calms the Liver, extinguishes Liver wind and subdues spasm and fright, supports the eyes, nose and mind.

Indications: Headache, vertigo, opthalmalgia, blurred vision, nasal polypus, rhinitis, epistaxis, infantile convulsion, mental disorders.

Notes
_____
_____
_____
_____
_____
_____
_____
_____

Point Combinations
_____
_____
_____
_____
_____
_____
_____

DU 23
Shangxing

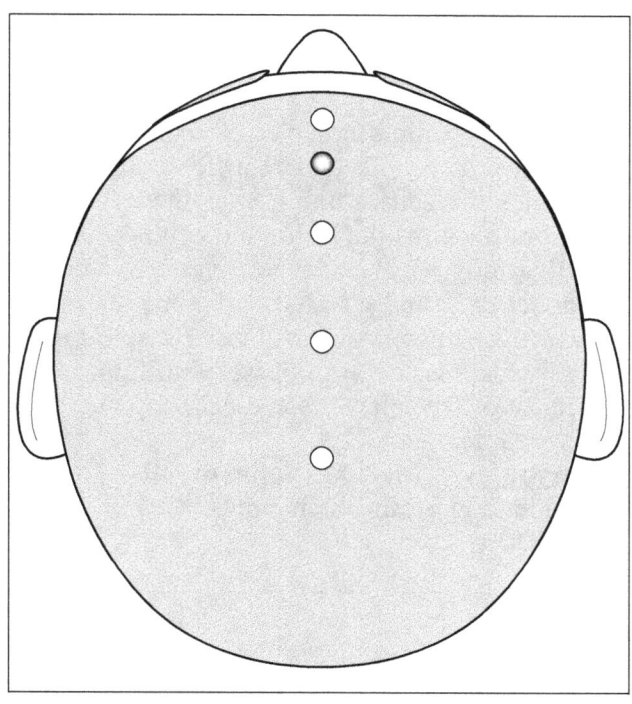

Location: On the head, 1 cun directly above the midpoint of the anterior hairline.

Functions: Extinguishes wind-heat, clears Liver heat and pathogens, manages local Qi, liberates the senses and assists the nasal passageways, eyes and vision, halt bleeding.

Indications: Headache, dizziness, opthalmalgia, facial edema, keratitis, myopia, any nasal or sinus problems, febrile disease, seizures, mental disorders.

Attributes: Ghost point.

*Good point for inflammation of the eye.

Notes

_____

_____

_____

_____

_____

_____

_____

_____

Point Combinations

_____

_____

_____

_____

_____

_____

_____

DU 24
SHENTING

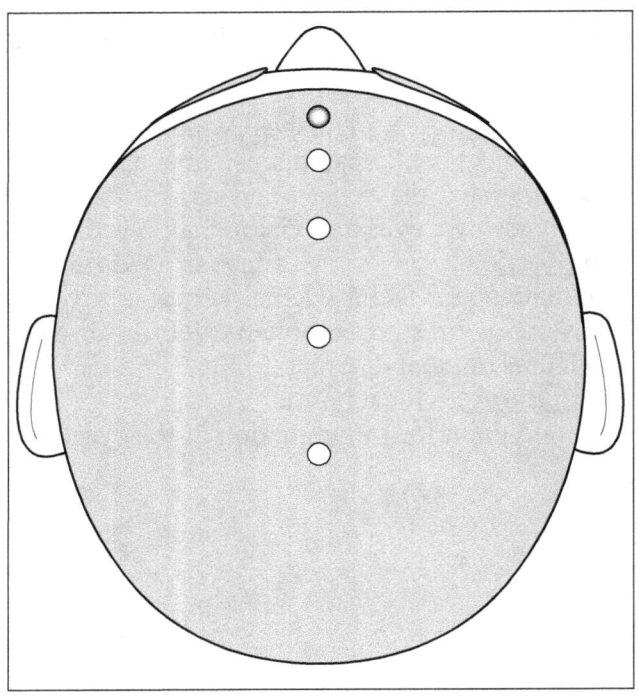

Location: On the head, 0.5 cun directly above the midpoint of the anterior hairline.

Functions: Calms the Liver, extinguishes wind-heat, restores yang and rectifies counterflow, liberates the senses and assists the eyes, nose and brain, calms the Heart and calms shen.

Indications: Headache, vertigo, frontal headaches (and sinus), dizziness, chills and fever insomnia, loss of consciousness, manic depression, epilepsy, vomiting, nasal congestion, dyspnea, nose bleed, copious clear dyspnea, fear, anxiety.

Attributes: Meeting point of DU, Urinary Bladder and Stomach channels.

Notes

_____
_____
_____
_____
_____
_____
_____
_____
_____

Point Combinations

_____
_____
_____
_____
_____
_____
_____

DU 25
SULIAO

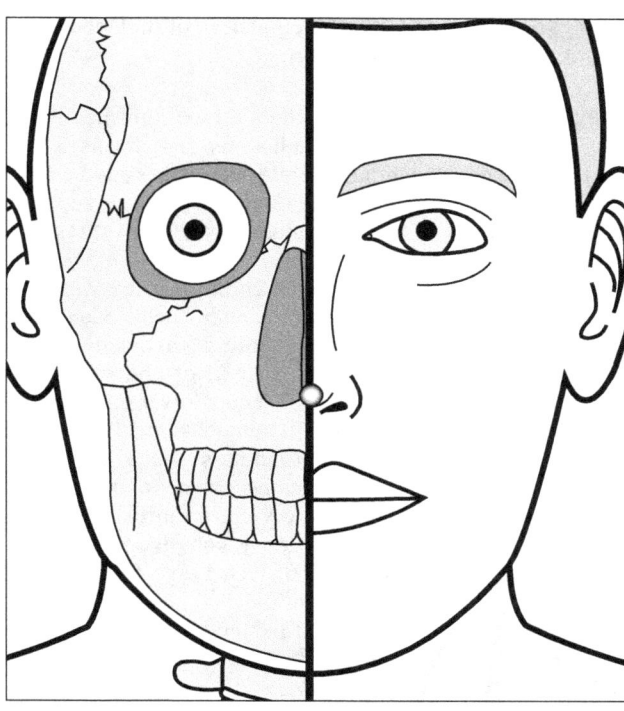

Location: On the face, on the tip of the nose.

Functions: Liberates the senses and assists the nose, unbinds the lungs and clears heat, nourishes yang and Qi and transforms stagnation.

Indications: Loss of consciousness, copious nasal discharge, epistaxis, rhinitis, extra tissue in the nose, nasal obstruction, polyps or sores, rosacea, drinkers nose, dyspnea, bradycardia, hyposmia, hypotension, infantile convulsions, shock.

Notes
_____
_____
_____
_____
_____
_____
_____
_____
_____

Point Combinations
_____
_____
_____
_____
_____
_____
_____

DU 26
RENZHONG

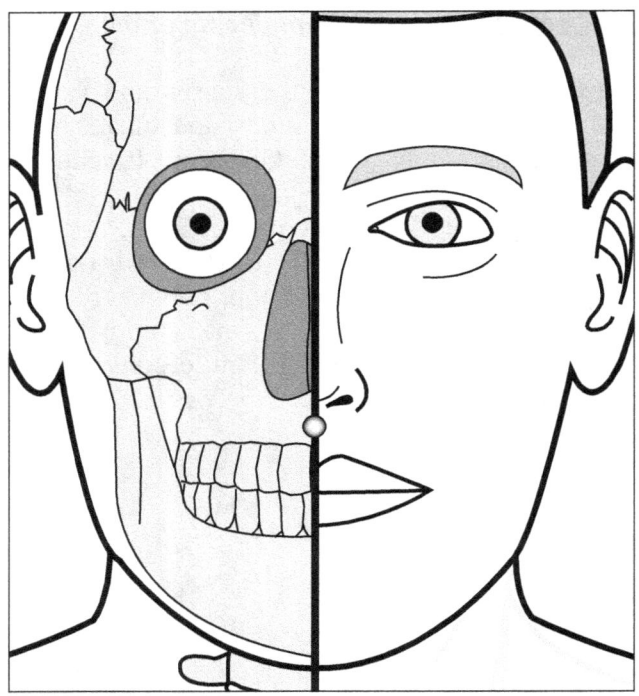

Location: On the face, at the junction of the upper third and middle third of the philtrum.

Functions: Manages DU channel, extinguishes wind, wind-phlegm and wind pathogens transforms Heart phlegm, clears the mind, liberates the senses and benefits the nose and face, clears interior heat in the nose, supports the lumbar spine, relieves pain, relaxes sinews, restores consciousness and calms shen.

Indications: Headache with chills and fever, spasm or malfunction of the eyes or mouth, facial edema, lip tremor, post stroke lockjaw, halitosis, hyposmia, nasal discharge or bleeding, pain in Heart or abdomen, pain and stiffness of the lower back, acute lower back sprain, edema, wasting disorder, unquenchable thirst, heat exhaustion, jaundice, motion sickness, shock, drowning, heat exhaustions, coma, unconsciousness, unexpected or inappropriate laughter or crying, insanity, psychosis, hysteria, mania, seizures, epilepsy, convulsions.

Attributes: Meeting point of DU, Large Intestine and Stomach channels. Ghost point.
*Good point for psychosis or hysteria.
**Main point for acute low back sprain.
***Main resuscitation point.

Notes

_____

_____

_____

_____

_____

_____

_____

_____

Point Combinations

_____

_____

_____

_____

_____

_____

_____

DU 27
DUIDAN

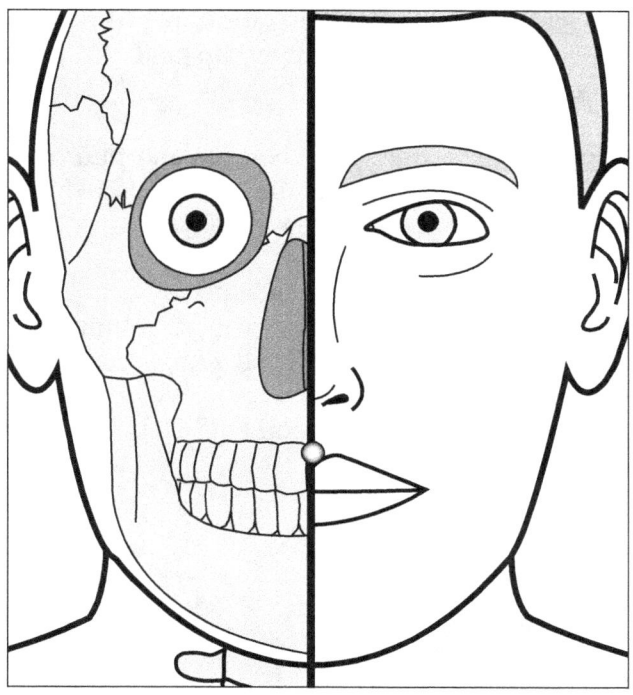

Location: On the face, at the upper boarder of the upper lip, where the skin of the phitrum and the upper lip meet.

Functions: Clears heat, Stomach and Heart heat, promote yin, engender fluid and benefits the mouth, calms shen.

Indications: Nasal obstruction, polyps or congestion, epistaxis, swelling, twitching, or stiffness of the lips, ulceration of the mouth, lockjaw, halitosis, pain or swelling of the gums, dry tongue, stomatitis, vomiting, wasting disorder, unquenchable thirst, dark urine, mental disorders, mania-depression, seizures, epilepsy.

Notes

Point Combinations

DU 28
YINJIAO

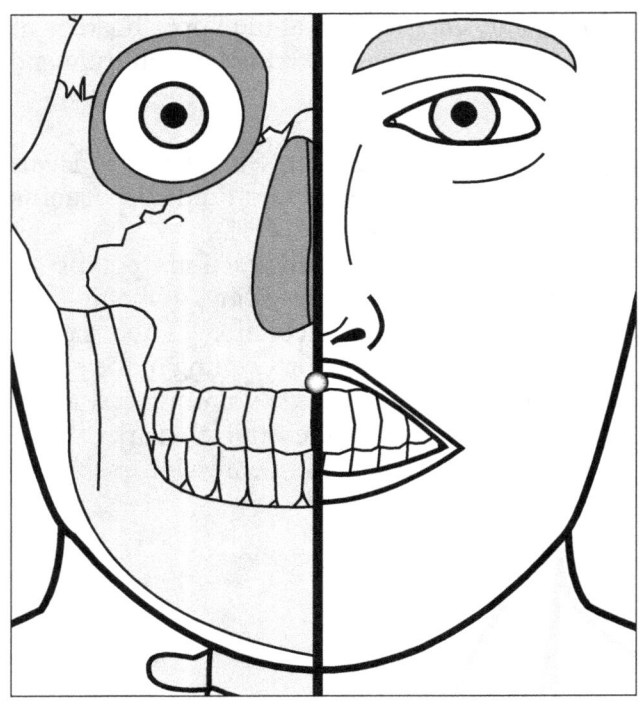

Location: On the inside of the upper lip, where the frenulum of the upper lip and the gum meet.

Functions: Illuminate the eyes and improves vision, clears heat and fire and stops itching, unbinds lungs and nasal passageways and liberates the senses, calms shen.

Indications: Rhinorrhea, neck pain and stiffness, nasal polypus, pain, swelling and bleeding around the teeth and gums, acute wrist sprain, mental disorders.

Attributes: Meeting point of DU, Ren and Stomach channels.

Notes _____

_____

_____

_____

_____

_____

_____

_____

_____

Point Combinations _____

_____

_____

_____

_____

_____

_____

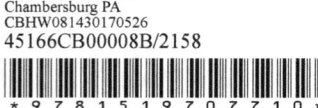